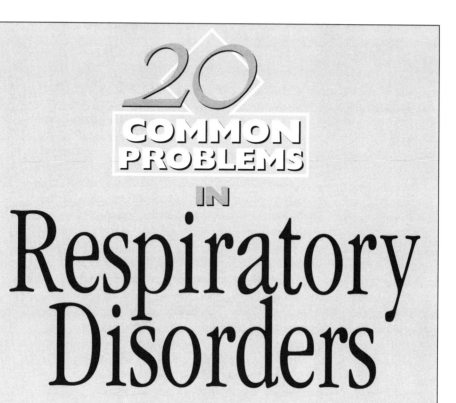

20 COMMON PROBLEMS IN Respiratory Disorders

Notice

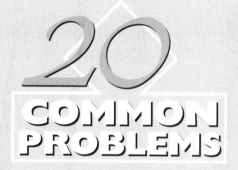

Respiratory Disorders

EDITOR

WILLIAM J. HUESTON, M.D.

Department of Family Medicine
Medical University of South Carolina
Charleston, South Carolina

SERIES EDITOR

BARRY D. WEISS, M.D.

Professor of Clinical Family and Community Medicine
University of Arizona College of Medicine
Tucson, Arizona

McGraw-Hill

Medical Publishing Division

New York   Chicago   San Francisco   Lisbon   London   Madrid   Mexico City
Milan   New Delhi   San Juan   Seoul   Singapore   Sydney   Toronto

McGraw-Hill

A Division of The McGraw·Hill Companies

20 COMMON PROBLEMS IN RESPIRATORY DISEASES

Copyright © 2002 by The McGraw-Hill Companies, Inc. All rights reserved. Printed in the United States of America. Except as permitted under the United States Copyright Act of 1976, no part of this publication may be reproduced or distributed in any form or by any means, or stored in a data base or retrieval system, without the prior written permission of the publisher.

1234567890 DOCDOC 098765432

ISBN 0-07-137526-0

This book was set in Garamond Light by Better Graphics, Inc.
The editors were Andrea Seils, Susan R. Noujaim,
and Muza Navrozov.
The production supervisor was Catherine H. Saggese.
The index was prepared by Alexandra Nickerson.

R.R. Donnelley & Sons was printer and binder.

The book is printed on acid-free paper.

Library of Congress Cataloging-in-Publication Data

20 common problems in respiratory disorders / editor, William J. Hueston.
        p. ; cm.
    Includes bibliographical references and index.
    ISBN 0-07-137526-0
    1. Respiratory organs--Diseases. 2. Primary care (Medicine) I. Title: Twenty common problems in respiratory disorders. II. Hueston, William J.
    [DNLM: 1. Respiratory Tract Diseases--diagnosis. 2. Respiratory Tract Diseases--therapy. WF 141 Z999 2003]
    RC731 .A15 2003
    616.2--dc21
                                                                    2001056220

INTERNATIONAL EDITION ISBN 0-07-121274-4
Copyright © 2002. Exclusive rights by The McGraw-Hill Companies, Inc., for manufacture and export. This book cannot be re-exported from the country to which it is consigned by McGraw-Hill. The International Edition is not available in North America.

Contents

Contributors

ALLERGIC RHINITIS: MECHANISMS, EVALUATION, AND TREATMENT
(CHAPTER 15)
Peter J. Carek, M.D.
Department of Family Medicine
Medical University of South Carolina
Charleston, South Carolina

Lori M. Dickerson, PharmD.
Department of Family Medicine
Medical University of South Carolina
Charleston, South Carolina

ASTHMA
(CHAPTER 16)
Barbara P. Yawn, M.D.
Olmsted Medical Center Research and Education
Rochester, Minnesota

COMMON COLD
(CHAPTER 4)
William J. Hueston, M.D.
Department of Family Medicine
Medical University of South Carolina
Charleston, South Carolina

Arch Mainous III, PhD.
Department of Family Medicine
Medical University of South Carolina
Charleston, South Carolina

COMMON OCCUPATIONAL RESPIRATORY DISEASES
(CHAPTER 18)
William M. Simpson, Jr., M.D.
Department of Family Medicine
Medical University of South Carolina
Charleston, South Carolina

COPD: MANAGEMENT OF ACUTE EXACERBATIONS AND CHRONIC STABLE DISEASE
(CHAPTER 17)
Melissa H. Hunter, M.D.
Department of Family Medicine
Medical University of South Carolina
Charleston, South Carolina

Dana E. King, M.D.
Department of Family Medicine
Medical University of South Carolina
Charleston, South Carolina

COUGH
(CHAPTER 1)
John Smucny, M.D.
Department of Family Medicine
SUNY-Upstate Medical Center
Syracuse, New York

CROUP, EPIGLOTTITIS, BRONCHIOLITIS, AND PERTUSSIS
(CHAPTER 10)
Mark A. Knox, M.D.
University of Pittsburgh Medical Center
School of Nursing Building
Pittsburgh, Pennsylvania

DYSPNEA AND SHORTNESS OF BREATH
(CHAPTER 2)
William J. Hueston, M.D.
Department of Family Medicine
Medical University of South Carolina
Charleston, South Carolina

EVALUATION AND MANAGEMENT OF ACUTE BRONCHITIS
(CHAPTER 9)
David L. Hahn, M.D.
Arcand Park Clinic
Madison, Wisconsin

IMMUNIZATION FOR RESPIRATORY DISEASES
(CHAPTER 19)
Richard K. Zimmerman, M.D.
Department of Family Medicine and Epidemiology
University of Pittsburgh
Pittsburgh, Pennsylvania

Inis Jane Bardella, M.D.
Department of Family Medicine and Epidemiology
University of Pittsburgh
Pittsburgh, Pennsylvania

LUNG CANCER
(CHAPTER 14)
Kevin C. Oeffinger, M.D.
Department of Family Practice
University of Texas-Southwestern Medical Center
Dallas, Texas

OTITIS MEDIA AND OTITIS EXTERNA
(CHAPTER 7)
Terrence E. Steyer, M.D.
Department of Family Medicine
Medical University of South Carolina
Charleston, South Carolina

William J. Hueston, M.D.
Department of Family Medicine
Medical University of South Carolina
Charleston, South Carolina

PHARYNGITIS
(CHAPTER 5)
Jonathan L. Temte, M.D.
Department of Family Medicine
University of Wisconsin
Madison, Wisconsin

PNEUMONIA
(CHAPTER 11)
William J. Hueston, M.D.
Department of Family Medicine
Medical University of South Carolina
Charleston, South Carolina

PREVENTION AND TREATMENT OF INFLUENZA
(CHAPTER 8)
Lori M. Dickerson, PharmD.
Department of Family Medicine
Medical University of South Carolina
Charleston, South Carolina

Peter J. Carek, M.D.
Department of Family Medicine
Medical University of South Carolina
Charleston, South Carolina

PULMONARY EMBOLISM
(CHAPTER 13)
Kesh Hebbar, M.D.
Department of Family Medicine
Medical University of South Carolina
Charleston, South Carolina

PULMONARY FUNCTION TESTING
(CHAPTER 3)
Harold A. Williamson, Jr., M.D.
Department of Family and Community Medicine
University of Missouri-Columbia School of Medicine
Columbia, Missouri

RESPIRATORY INFECTIONS IN THE IMMUNOCOMPROMISED PATIENT
(CHAPTER 12)
Robert Mallin, M.D.
Department of Family Medicine
Medical University of South Carolina
Charleston, South Carolina

Edwin A. Brown, M.D.
Department of Internal Medicine
Medical University of South Carolina
Charleston, South Carolina

SINUSITIS
(CHAPTER 6)

Morten Lindbaek, M.D.
Department of General Practice
University of Oslo
Oslo, Norway

John M. Hickner, M.D.
Department of Family Practice
Michigan State University
B100 Clinical Center
East Lansing, Michigan

SMOKING CESSATION
(CHAPTER 20)

Robert Mallin, M.D.
Department of Family Medicine
Medical University of South Carolina
Charleston, South Carolina

Preface

"The earth is suffocating. . . ."
Final words of Fredric Chopin, dying from tuberculosis

As long as people have breathed, they have had respiratory problems. Some of the common respiratory maladies that people face today were the same problems the people struggled with centuries ago. For example, influenza has been described as many as 400 years ago. Evidence of tuberculosis infection has been discovered in remains uncovered from ancient Egypt and probably dates back as far as neolithic time.

With the dawn of the Industrial Revolution, when large numbers of people began to populate the emerging industrial cities of Europe, the spread of respiratory infections became rampant. By the 1600s and 1700s, a quarter of all deaths in Europe were caused by "consumption." Until early in the last century, epidemics of respiratory infections caused periodic waves of death that could devastate entire populations. In the early 1700s, an epidemic of diphtheria killed one-third of all children and 2.5% of the entire population residing in New England. The influenza pandemic of 1918–1919 purportedly resulted in the deaths of 21 million people worldwide including over half a million in the United States. These respiratory epidemics were more than a periodic nuisance. People were not so much concerned that the flu would cause them to miss work. They feared that it would kill them.

Respiratory problems preyed most heavily on the vulnerable members of society. The youngest and oldest were at highest risk for being overwhelmed by pneumonia, "the old man's friend." Epidemics would wipe out entire generations of older individuals and most of the children in a community. Antibiotics and better living conditions have made pneumonia less lethal in modern times, but some populations remain at high risk from respiratory infections. Over three-quarters of deaths from pneumonia occur in the elderly[1] and the World Health Organization estimates that 2.6 million children under the age of 5 years continue to die of respiratory infections each year.[2]

While we have tamed many of the respiratory problems from the past, people continue to breathe. And so they continue to suffer from respiratory problems. And as we continue to breathe, we encounter new ways in which our environment is capable of injuring our respiratory system.

The Changing Scope of Respiratory Problems

As we have developed better ways to combat respiratory infections, other breathing problems are rising up to take their place. Instead of infectious agents, environmental problems appear to be fueling new respiratory diseases. Chronic obstructive pulmonary disease (COPD), highly associated with cigarette use, is now the fourth most common killer of Americans according to the 1998 national vital statistics data. The percentage of all individuals dying from COPD (4.8% of total) has surpassed that of pneumonia and influenza (3.9%).[3]

The popularity of smoking in the early part of this century not only spawned the COPD epidemic, but has made lung cancer the leading cause of cancer deaths in men and women. Tobacco is harmful enough when it is the only toxic substance inhaled into the lung. When combined with other environmental toxins such as radon and asbestos, the effects of smoking are magnified. In medical practice today, the most cost-effective preventive measure that physicians can employ is to counsel patients about smoking cessation.

The frequency of other respiratory diseases related to environmental exposures is also on the rise. In particular, the prevalence of asthma is increasing, especially in urban areas and in poorer populations where exposure to infections, environmental toxins, and allergens are more common. In addition to more children having asthma, the death reate from this disease is climbing as well.

Occupational exposures to pulmonary toxins have become a serious problem. Over the past decades, serious lung diseases in workers exposed to asbestos and harmful dusts while working in coal mines have resulted in severe morbidity and disability for many individuals. While health policy makers and industry have realized that respiratory diseases in the workplace must be addressed through better safety equipment and by limiting exposure, a significant number of workers continue to be exposed to dangerous materials as part of their employment.

The emerging environmental threats to our lungs have made respiratory problems chronic conditions rather than acute infections and changed the way we think about people with lung diseases.

Respiratory Problems in Primary Care

This is a textbook of common problems and there is no group of problems that is more common in primary care practice than respiratory diseases. In the National Ambulatory Medical Care Survey (NAMCS), the top three complaints encountered by primary care physicians were cough, sore throat, and earache—all respiratory problems.[4] When studies have looked at diagnoses rather than presenting complaints, respiratory diseases continue to make the top of the lists of reasons why people are seen by primary care clinicians.

This book will focus on the common respiratory problems seen in primary care practices. The book is separated into five sections: symptoms and evaluation of respiratory problems; upper respiratory infections; lower respiratory infections; noninfectious acute and chronic respiratory diseases; and prevention of respiratory problems.

The section on symptoms focuses on the kinds of problems for which patients see their clinicians. The chapters attempt to offer a guide to how to evaluate these common complaints and what to do when the initial evaluation does not reveal the underlying cause.

The sections on infectious causes of respiratory problems hone in on the major diagnoses encountered by primary care clinicians. These include problems generally seen in the ambulatory setting such as common colds, ear infections, acute bronchitis, and pharyngitis as well as more severe infections such as pneumonia. In addition, a chapter has been included on children since many infections are unique to this special population. Finally, special mention must be made of individuals who are immunosuppressed. The diagnosis of respiratory problems in this population is sometimes more difficult and treatment is sometimes more difficult.

The next section of the book looks at common respiratory problems that are not caused by infections. Acute conditions such as pulmonary embolism are covered along with chronic respiratory conditions (COPD, asthma) and lung cancer. Also included is a chapter on occupational respiratory illnesses since many workers have pulmonary problems that are caused or exacerbated by exposures on the job.

Finally, no book on primary care would be complete unless we considered how to prevent illness. Chapter 19 focuses on immunizations that are available to prevent respiratory infections in children and adults. Additionally, the last chapter of the book provides information about behavioral and pharmacologic advances in smoking cessation.

ters for the book. I am grateful for the time, commitment, and effort they have expended to make this book possible. I also would like to express my gratitude to Barry Weiss, MD, who coordinates the *20 Common Problems* series for McGraw-Hill, for proposing this topic and recommending me to be editor of this edition.

William J. Hueston, M.D.

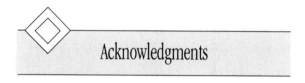

Acknowledgments

I am indebted to the many authors who have shared their expertise with me by writing chap-

References

1. Centers for Disease Control. Pneumonia and influenza mortality—United States, 1988–1989 season. *MMWR* 1989;38:97.
2. Pneumococcal vaccines. *Weekly Epidemiology Record* 1999;74:177–184.
3. Murphy SL: Deaths: final data for 1998. *National Vital Statistics Report* 2000;48(11):1–106.

Respiratory Symptoms and Their Evaluation

John Smucny

Cough

Cough is a very common symptom, with a prevalence of approximately 15 percent in children and 20 percent in adults.[1,2] One out of every ten people visits a clinician's office annually with a primary complaint of cough, and cough accounts for 3 percent of all office visits.[3]

Cough can lead to discomfort, sleeping difficulties, interference with one's routine activities, and a lower quality of life. Cough can also lead to a variety of complications, such as pneumothorax, pneumomediastinum, headache, syncope, herniated disk, inguinal hernia, rib fracture, subconjunctival hemorrhage, and urinary incontinence. Patients seek help for these troublesome symptoms and complications, as well as out of concern that the cough represents a potentially serious underlying condition.[4]

Many people manage their own or their children's symptoms at home without seeking medical advice. This is reflected in the observation that the annual cost of over-the-counter treatments for acute cough in the United States is in the billions of dollars per year.[5]

Cough Physiology

A cough is a protective mechanism that clears the tracheobronchial tree of secretions and foreign material. Detailed descriptions of the mechanics and physiology of cough can be found elsewhere,[5–7] and so they will only very briefly be considered here. A cough typically begins with a deep inspiration. Next, the glottis transiently closes and the expiratory muscles contract, which leads to high intrathoracic pressures. The glottis then opens and a forceful exhalation occurs that expels secretions or other material. The large airways are initially compressed during this exhalation, but as the lung volume decreases, smaller airways are compressed and larger airways open. With successive coughs, secretions and other materials are

mobilized from the smaller to the larger airways and then expelled.

The complex reflex arc that controls cough includes afferent receptors, a central pathway, and efferent motor outputs. Afferent receptors have been histologically shown to exist only in the pharynx, larynx, and lower respiratory tract, but are also believed to be located in the external auditory canals, eardrums, sinuses, diaphragm, pleura, pericardium, and stomach. These receptors respond to a variety of stimuli, such as chemical irritants, mechanical insults, and inflammatory mediators. The afferent receptors are innervated by branches of the vagus nerve and relay impulses to the central cough center. This central cough center is diffusely located in the medulla and involves opioid receptors at synapses. Efferent motor outputs from the cough center travel to the chest wall muscles, bronchial tree, and larynx through the vagus, phrenic, and other spinal motor nerves. People with abnormalities in the cough pathway have reduced effectiveness of cough and are more prone to developing aspiration syndromes and pneumonia.

Differential Diagnosis

There are more than 100 conditions that can cause cough. These include anything that causes inflammation of the respiratory tract (such as infections or exposure to toxic substances), mechanical insults (such as aspiration of secretions or foreign bodies, or pressure on structures of the tracheobronchial tree), chemical irritants (such as irritating gases or liquids), and thermal stimuli (such as cold air). From a practical standpoint, however, most coughs are caused by a relatively smaller and more manageable number of problems.

An adequate history and physical examination are usually sufficient to develop an empiric therapeutic plan, particularly for patients with acute cough. Red flags for potentially life-threatening conditions that can present as cough are also detected from the initial evaluation (see Table 1-1). Patients with these red-flag symptoms and signs might require a more urgent management.

It is useful to determine the duration of a patient's cough because this significantly narrows the differential diagnosis. Acute cough is defined as a cough of less than three weeks' duration, and chronic cough as a cough lasting three or more weeks.[6] Some authors also include a subacute category to cover durations of three to eight weeks.[8] Of course, all subacute or chronic coughs begin acutely at some point, but nonetheless the duration of cough at the time of presentation helps determine the most probable causes.

Acute Cough

There are no reported studies regarding the frequency of various conditions that cause acute cough. Consensus opinion holds that the most common cause is a viral upper respiratory tract infection (i.e., the common cold). Over 80 percent of people with colds have a cough during the first two days of their illness, and 25 percent are still coughing after two weeks.[8] Other common causes of acute cough include acute bacterial sinusitis, rhinitis due to allergies or environmental irritants (e.g., tobacco smoke), acute bronchitis, pneumonia, and exacerbations of chronic bronchitis and asthma (see Table 1-2); acute bronchiolitis and laryngotracheobronchitis (croup) are additional common causes in infants and children. Less common causes of acute

Table 1-1

Red-Flag Symptoms and Signs for Potentially Life-Threatening Conditions in Patients with Cough

RED FLAG	POSSIBLE CONDITION
Symptoms	
Dyspnea	Asthma, chronic bronchitis, pneumonia, pulmonary embolus, cancer, tuberculosis, congestive heart failure
Chest pain	Pulmonary embolus, pneumonia, cancer, tuberculosis
Hemoptysis	Cancer, pneumonia, tuberculosis
Weight loss	Cancer, tuberculosis
Signs	
Fever	Pneumonia, tuberculosis
Tachypnea	Asthma, chronic bronchitis, pneumonia, pulmonary embolus, cancer, tuberculosis, congestive heart failure
Tachycardia	Asthma, chronic bronchitis, pneumonia, pulmonary embolus, cancer, congestive heart failure
Wheezes, rhonchi	Asthma, chronic bronchitis, congestive heart failure
Rales	Pneumonia (especially if unilateral), congestive heart failure (especially if bilateral)
Dullness to percussion	Pneumonia, pleural effusion
Egophony, pectoriloquy	Pneumonia
Absent breath sounds	Pleural effusion, pneumothorax
Cyanosis	Asthma, chronic bronchitis, cancer, pneumonia

Table 1-2

Common Causes of Acute Cough

INFECTIOUS	NONINFECTIOUS
Viral upper respiratory infection	Allergic rhinitis
	Nonallergic rhinitis
Acute bacterial sinusitis	Acute exacerbation of
Acute laryngotracheitis (croup)*	chronic bronchitis†
	Asthma exacerbation†
Acute bronchitis	Pulmonary embolus
Pertussis	Pneumothorax
Influenza	Pleural effusion‡
Pneumonia	Congestive heart
Acute bronchiolitis*	failure

*Croup and bronchiolitis are only in children.
†Acute exacerbations of chronic bronchitis and asthma can be provoked by acute respiratory infections.
‡Pleural effusions can accompany pneumonia as well as noninfectious conditions.

cough include aspiration (of secretions, food, or foreign bodies), pulmonary embolus, pleural effusion, pneumothorax, and congestive heart failure.

INFECTIOUS CAUSES OF ACUTE COUGH

Infectious causes of acute cough can arise from either the upper or the lower respiratory tract. In addition to the common cold and bacterial sinusitis, acute cough can accompany pharyngitis (particularly if viral), laryngitis, and otitis media.

Cough can arise from both upper and lower respiratory tract infections. Typical symptoms of upper respiratory tract infections include nasal drainage and/or congestion, tearing, ear pain and/or fullness, postnasal drip, throat irritation, hoarseness, facial pain, and headache; those of lower respiratory tract infections include dyspnea and wheezing. Whether a cough is productive or causes chest pain is not helpful in differentiating upper and lower tract infections. Sputum can arise either from postnasal drip or

from the lower tracheobronchial tree; chest pain may be due to chest wall discomfort from the cough itself or may indicate a pleuropulmonary problem. Other symptoms that can be seen in both upper and lower tract infections include fever, chills, myalgia, nausea, and fatigue. Some pathogens, such as influenza and *Mycoplasma pneumoniae*, commonly cause both upper and lower respiratory tract symptoms.

UPPER RESPIRATORY TRACT INFECTIONS Regarding upper respiratory tract infections, it is difficult to clinically differentiate the common cold (viral rhinosinusitis) from acute bacterial sinusitis (bacterial rhinosinusitis). Since bacterial sinusitis is a complication in less than 2 percent of colds, the vast majority of patients with this syndrome have viral infections.[9] Cough is frequently seen with both viral and bacterial rhinosinusitis, and its presence does not help differentiate the two. Findings that are believed to be more likely in patients with bacterial sinusitis include purulent nasal discharge, maxillary toothache, unilateral facial pain or sinus tenderness, and worsening of symptoms after initial improvement. The greater the number of these indicators that are present, the more likely is a bacterial infection. The presence of purulent nasal discharge alone, however, is not very useful because the majority of patients with viral upper respiratory tract infections will develop yellow nasal discharge during their illness and still have spontaneous resolution of their symptoms.[10] Patients and physicians commonly, and erroneously, associate yellow discharge with infections that require antibiotic therapy.[11,12]

Sinus radiography is not routinely recommended because it may be abnormal in up to 40 percent of patients with the common cold. If radiographs are obtained, the findings of complete opacification or air-fluid levels are helpful (80 to 85 percent specific), but mucosal thickening is not (50 percent specific). The absence of all three findings effectively rules out bacterial sinusitis.

LOWER RESPIRATORY TRACT INFECTIONS Regarding lower respiratory tract infections, it is important to identify patients who have pneumonia because antibiotic treatment is initially indicated for these patients.[13] Fortunately, the physical examination is very sensitive at detecting pneumonia in most patients. For immunocompetent, community-dwelling adults, pneumonia is unlikely if all vital signs and the chest examination are normal.[14] In elderly and immunosuppressed patients, the physical examination is less sensitive, so obtaining a chest radiograph is appropriate even if the examination is normal. If pneumonia is suspected clinically, guidelines recommend obtaining a chest radiograph for confirmation because the physical findings are not specific.[13] In addition to appropriate antibiotic therapy, management of pneumonia includes possible admission for observation and/or supportive care. Prognostic indicators are useful in determining which patients require more aggressive care.[13]

Patients with lower respiratory tract infections who do not have pneumonia are commonly diagnosed with "acute bronchitis." The usefulness of this term has recently been questioned because physicians use varying definitions and do not consistently differentiate it clinically from upper respiratory tract infections.[15,16] For example, a survey of family physicians reported that 58 percent stated that the cough in acute bronchitis should be productive and 28 percent that wheezing or rhonchi should be present on examination, while the remainder did not think a productive cough was needed for the diagnosis.

Other lower respiratory tract infections for which adequate antimicrobial therapy exists include pertussis and influenza, so it is important to determine whether or not a patient may have these infections. In some series, more than 20 percent of adults with cough of more than 1 to 2 weeks' duration had pertussis.[17] Pertussis should be suspected in patients who have been in close contact with a known case, or if the cough is paroxysmal or induces vomiting. However, many immunized people have a mild illness that is indistinguishable from other acute or subacute causes of cough.[17,18] Antibiotic treatment of pertussis is clearly effective at reducing the severity and decreasing the infectivity of the illness only if it is begun within the early catarrhal phase of the illness. Household contacts of patients in the cough phase should receive prophylactic antibiotics, however.[17]

Influenza should be considered whenever the influenza virus is circulating in a community. The definition of an influenza-like illness includes feverishness plus two of the following symptoms: cough, headache, myalgia, or sore throat. Approximately 80 percent of patients with an influenza-like illness who have both cough and fever within 48 h of symptom onset during the influenza season have culture-proven influenza.[19] Treatment with antiviral agents within this time period can reduce the duration of illness and may prevent some complications.[20] Rapid serologic tests can confirm a clinical suspicion of influenza; most currently available tests are 90 percent specific, although somewhat less sensitive.[21]

NONINFECTIOUS CAUSES OF ACUTE COUGH

Clues to noninfectious causes of acute cough can be gathered from additional history taking, including exacerbating factors and past medical history, and from the physical examination. For example, a springtime cough in a patient with known seasonal allergies is commonly due to postnasal drip from allergic rhinitis. In patients who do not have a prior history of respiratory problems and whose symptoms do not appear to be due to infection, a comprehensive examination may be necessary to uncover the diagnosis. In addition to the respiratory system, this should include a thorough evaluation of the ears (e.g., cerumen), nose (e.g., polyps), throat (e.g., postnasal drip), heart (e.g., third heart sound), and extremities (e.g., unilateral edema). When the diagnosis is still in question, chest radiographs and other tests may be indicated.

ACUTE COUGH IN CHILDREN

Causes of acute cough in children include infections such as the common cold, sinusitis, croup, bronchiolitis, and pneumonia; and noninfectious causes such as foreign body aspiration and acute exacerbations of asthma.

Colds and sinusitis in children are usually due to viral infections. Young children with bacterial sinusitis may not have the typical symptoms seen in adults; those with persistent nasal discharge and daytime cough that is not improving after 10 to 14 days meet the criteria for bacterial sinusitis.[22] As in adults, sinus radiographs are not routinely recommended to diagnosis sinusitis.[22]

Croup (acute laryngotracheobronchitis) is a viral infection in children aged 6 months to 3 years that presents as a barking cough with or without stridor or hoarseness. On occasion, croup can lead to severe respiratory distress. Anteroposterior plain films of the neck may demonstrate narrowing of the subglottic area.

Bronchiolitis is a viral infection in infants that presents as acute obstructive respiratory disease that occurs within a few days of the onset of rhinorrhea and cough. It is the most common form of lower respiratory tract infection in infants, and can lead to severe respiratory compromise and death. Chest films may show hyperinflation with or without atelectasis or consolidation.

Influenza in children may not cause all the typical symptoms seen in adults. Common presentations in children include only fever and cough with or without rhinorrhea, and croup. The availability of rapid tests for influenza has been shown to decrease the use of antibiotics for suspected bacterial infections in children.[23]

Pneumonia can be clinically excluded in infants and young children if the respiratory rate and lung auscultatory findings are normal and if the child does not demonstrate increased work of breathing. As with adults, positive findings are not specific and therefore do not rule in pneumonia.[24]

Foreign body aspiration should always be considered in children with acute cough who do not have an obvious infection. A history of a choking episode is 86 to 96 percent sensitive and 76 to 82 percent specific for identifying aspiration of a foreign body.[25,26]

Chest radiographs are only 60 to 70 percent sensitive, so a negative film does not rule out foreign body aspiration. Bronchoscopy is both diagnostic and therapeutic.

Chronic Cough

The most common causes of chronic cough in adults have been delineated in multiple prospective studies (see Table 1-3). The differential diagnosis hinges on whether patients smoke. In nonsmokers, the most common causes of chronic cough are postnasal drip, asthma, eosinophilic bronchitis, and gastroesophageal reflux disease (GERD). In smokers, chronic bronchitis and lung cancer are additional concerns. Less common causes of chronic cough in both smokers and nonsmokers include angiotensin-converting enzyme–inhibitor therapy, bronchiectasis, chronic interstitial lung disease, and tuberculosis. Patients may have a prolonged postinfectious cough following an acute respiratory infection that spontaneously resolves over the course of a few months or longer. Postinfectious cough may be due to either postnasal drip or airway inflammation. Finally, psychogenic cough can present as chronic cough, although this is rare in adults. Chronic cough may be due to more than one cause in 18 to 62 percent of patients.[6]

POSTNASAL DRIP

Postnasal drip is the most common cause of chronic cough in most series, ranging from 8 to 87 percent of patients with a chronic cough.[6] It can be caused by a variety of conditions, including allergic rhinitis, nonallergic rhinitis, chronic bacterial or fungal sinusitis, and rhinitis medicamentosa (from nasal decongestants or cocaine). Postnasal drip also can persist for a prolonged

Table 1-3

Causes of Chronic Cough

ADULTS	CHILDREN
COMMON	
Postnasal drip	Postnasal drip
Asthma	Asthma
Postinfectious cough	Postinfectious cough
Gastroesophageal reflux disease	Gastroesophageal reflux disease
Eosinophilic bronchitis	Psychogenic (habit) cough
Chronic bronchitis	Congenital anomalies (in infants)
Angiotensin-converting enzyme inhibitor therapy	Environmental exposures (e.g., tobacco smoke)
LESS COMMON	
Lung cancer	Mediastinal and lung masses
Bronchiectasis	Cystic fibrosis
Chronic interstitial pulmonary disease	Congenital heart disease
Tuberculosis	Chronic aspiration

period after a viral upper respiratory infection. In addition to cough, patients with postnasal drip typically complain of nasal congestion and/or discharge, and a sensation of something (such as a tickle) in the throat. The timing and quality of the cough itself do not differentiate postnasal drip from other causes of chronic cough.[27] The physical examination may reveal nasal drainage and/or abnormal mucosa, pharyngeal drainage, and cobblestoning.

Once it has been determined that the cough is due to postnasal drip, the precise cause of postnasal drip can be determined through additional tests, such as sinus imaging studies and allergy testing. Sinus radiography is over 95 percent sensitive but only 75 percent specific at diagnosing chronic sinusitis as a cause of chronic postnasal drip with cough.[6] Therefore, negative radiographs rule out chronic sinusitis as an etiology, but positive ones do not necessarily rule it in. Some patients without typical symptoms and signs of postnasal drip do respond to antihistamine-decongestant therapy and are believed to have "silent" postnasal drip.[6]

ASTHMA

Asthma is another common cause of chronic cough. Many patients with asthma may have a chronic cough in addition to other typical asthma symptoms such as chest tightness, dyspnea, and wheezing. Others, however, may complain of cough only, and therefore have what is termed cough-variant asthma. The actual prevalence of cough-variant asthma is unclear; it ranges from 6 to 57 percent of asthmatics in different studies.[6] Some experts believe that it is now overdiagnosed, especially in children.[5]

Clues to asthma as a cause of a patient's cough include the presence of the above symptoms and coughing triggered by allergens, irritants, cold air, and exercise. The physical examination at the time of the visit may be normal, particularly for patients with cough-variant asthma. Wheezing, if present, is highly specific for obstructive airway disease.[28] Pulmonary function tests, along with methacholine or histamine challenge tests for airway hyperresponsiveness, may be helpful in diagnosing asthma. The sensitivity and specificity of a methacholine challenge test in diagnosing asthma as a cause of chronic cough are 100 percent and 70 percent, respectively.[6] Therefore, a normal challenge test essentially rules out asthma, but a positive one does not rule it in. Patients with abnormal challenge tests who have symptom resolution within 1 week of beta-agonist asthma therapy meet the criteria for cough-variant asthma.[29] If such tests are not available, the diagnosis may be attempted by observing the response to therapy with beta-agonists or inhaled corticosteroids. If the cough improves after corticosteroids, however, this does not definitively prove that asthma is the underlying diagnosis, because other inflammatory lung diseases may also respond to corticosteroids.

EOSINOPHILIC BRONCHITIS

Eosinophilic bronchitis is a recently recognized cause of chronic cough that may be responsible for 10 to 15 percent of cases.[2] Patients with this syndrome have a chronic cough with sputum eosinophilia (3 percent eosinophils), but none of the other abnormalities seen with asthma. Specifically, these patients have no symptoms suggestive of variable airflow obstruction, normal pulmonary function tests, and normal responses to methacholine challenge tests. Inhaled and systemic corticosteroids seem to be effective treatment.[2,6]

GASTROESOPHAGEAL REFLUX DISEASE

GERD is responsible for chronic cough in 8 to 40 percent of cases.[30] It may cause cough through a variety of mechanisms, including irritation of the larynx, aspiration into the bronchial tree, and stimulation of an esophageal-bronchial cough reflex. Reflux of gastric contents also may be a consequence of cough, and this can lead to a perpetual cough-reflux-cough cycle. Up to 75 percent of patients with GERD-induced cough may not have coexisting reflux symptoms of heartburn or acid regurgitation. Also, most GERD-related cough occurs while people are upright during the day and not when they are lying down at night.

The diagnosis of GERD as a cause of a patient's cough is most certain when the cough resolves with appropriate therapy. This includes lifestyle modifications and proton-pump inhibitors, histamine-2 receptor antagonists, and/or metoclopramide.[30] Since it may take up to 3 months to notice a significant improvement, an alternative diagnostic strategy is 24-h esophageal pH monitoring. This test is highly sensitive (100 percent negative predictive value) and reasonably specific (89 percent positive predictive value) in diagnosing GERD-induced cough.[30] Surgical interventions, such as fundoplication, may help patients who do not respond to medical therapy.

CHRONIC BRONCHITIS

Chronic bronchitis, one form of chronic obstructive pulmonary disease, is defined as cough with phlegm production on most days over a period of at least 3 months for 2 consecutive years in a patient in whom other causes of chronic cough have been excluded. Although it is a common cause of cough in community surveys, it accounts for only 5 percent of patients who present to a physician with chronic cough.[6] Chronic bronchitis is rare in nonsmokers, unless they have long-term exposure to dust or fumes. Patients with chronic bronchitis are most likely to cough upon awakening. Patients with advanced disease have signs of right-sided heart failure, such as peripheral edema and central cyanosis. Although chronic bronchitis is a clinical definition, patients may have abnormalities on chest radiographs and/or pulmonary function testing because of concomitant emphysema.

LUNG CANCER

Lung cancer accounts for only 2 percent of patients that present with chronic cough.[6] Patients who smoke are at greatest risk. Smoking cessation decreases a person's risk, although the risk remains elevated indefinitely compared to that of people who have never smoked.[31] Other known risk factors are exposures to carcinogens, such as asbestos, radon, uranium, and second-hand smoke. In addition to cough, which occurs in over 70 percent of patients with lung cancer, patients may also have hemoptysis, wheezing, dyspnea, and weight loss (particularly in advanced disease). Diagnostic tests include chest radiographs and computed tomography (CT) scans, sputum cytology, and bronchoscopy. Because nonsmokers have a low probability of lung cancer, normal chest radiographs rule out cancer as a cause of their cough. However, because smokers are more likely to have cancer, normal chest films do not rule out the disease in these cases. Therefore, CT scans and sputum cytology are appropriate for patients whose cough persists after they quit smoking. Both tests have been shown to detect cancers at early and treatable stages in patients with normal plain chest radiographs.[6,32,33] If these tests are negative, bronchoscopy can be considered, although it has a low yield in patients with negative imaging studies.[6]

ANGIOTENSIN-CONVERTING ENZYME INHIBITOR-INDUCED COUGH

Chronic cough is a potential adverse effect of angiotensin-converting enzyme inhibitor (ACEI) therapy. The prevalence of cough in people who take ACEIs is approximately 10 percent.[6] ACEIs are believed to increase the sensitivity of the cough reflex by increasing the concentration of cough mediators such as bradykinin, substance P, and prostaglandins. The onset of the cough ranges from 1 week to 1 year after beginning ACEIs.

The cough associated with ACEIs is usually described as an irritating, tickling, or scratching sensation in the throat, but some patients may cough hard enough to induce vomiting. Since cough has been reported with all ACEIs and is not usually dose-dependent, replacing the ACEI with another ACEI or decreasing the dose may not be effective. Cough due to ACEIs should improve within days and resolve completely within 2 weeks of discontinuing the ACEI.[34] For patients who must continue to take ACEIs, possibly effective treatments for the cough include nifedipine, sulindac, baclofen, theophylline, and cromolyn.[34] The incidence of cough from angiotensin receptor blockers is less than that from ACEIs and similar to that from placebo.[35]

BRONCHIECTASIS

Bronchiectasis is an uncommon cause of chronic cough, but it has been reported in about 4 percent of cases.[6] The incidence is decreasing because fewer people have poorly treated recurrent or chronic respiratory infections (e.g., pneumonia or tuberculosis). In addition to cough, most patients with bronchiectasis produce sputum, often in substantial amounts. Other chronic or intermittent symptoms may include wheezing, hemoptysis, fatigue, and weight loss. The diagnosis is suggested clinically and with chest radiographs, and can be confirmed with high-resolution CT scanning.

CHRONIC INTERSTITIAL PULMONARY DISEASE

Chronic interstitial pulmonary disease includes a variety of specific conditions that are characterized by diffuse infiltration of the lung tissue with inflammatory cells or collagen. Among these conditions are collagen vascular diseases, sarcoidosis, and idiopathic pulmonary fibrosis.[36] Patients with chronic interstitial disease can have chronic cough, but they are more likely to present with dyspnea. The diagnosis is suggested clinically, radiographically, and with pulmonary function tests, but transbronchial or open lung biopsy may be needed for confirmation. Depending on the specific condition, serologic tests may also be useful. The optimal treatment depends on which specific disease a patient has.

TUBERCULOSIS

Although tuberculosis (TB) is an uncommon cause of chronic cough in studies, it should be considered in patients at risk. Patients at risk include recent immigrants from countries in which TB is endemic, contacts of patients with TB, the homeless, and those who are immunocompromised. Most patients with pulmonary TB have a chronic cough with an insidious onset.[37] Other common symptoms include weight loss, fatigue, fever, and night sweats. Less common symptoms include anorexia, chest pain, dyspnea, and hemoptysis.

Chest radiographs in patients with TB are usually abnormal and may show infiltrates, adenopathy, solitary masses, and effusions. Sputum smears are 40 to 60 percent sensitive and 99 percent specific. Sputum cultures take weeks to grow, but are much more sensitive (80 percent) and equally specific. Skin tests may be falsely negative in patients with acute TB because of anergy, or falsely positive in patients with prior TB infection who have another cause of their current symptoms.

CHRONIC COUGH IN CHILDREN

The prevalence of various causes of chronic cough has not been studied as thoroughly in children as it has in adults. A single retrospective study showed that the most common causes were asthma, postnasal drip, GERD, congenital anomalies, and psychogenic cough.[6] Congenital anomalies include vascular rings (e.g., aberrant innominate artery, double aortic arch, pulmonary artery sling), tracheomalacia, tracheoesophageal fistulas, and bronchogenic cysts. Congenital heart disease can also cause cough, as well as other respiratory symptoms. Psychogenic cough (or habit cough) is the final diagnosis in up to 10 percent of children with chronic cough and is more common in girls. It often follows an acute respiratory tract infection, occurs only during the day, and has a barking or honking quality. Other causes of chronic cough in children include bronchiectasis (in cystic fibrosis, immotile cilia syndrome, and immunodeficiency), chronic aspiration (especially in children with abnormal swallowing), and exposure to environmental irritants such as tobacco smoke.[1]

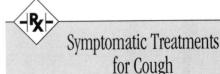

Symptomatic Treatments for Cough

Treatments for cough can either be directed specifically at the cause of the cough or be used simply for the control of symptoms. Specific treatments are discussed in great detail in later chapters of this book, and so the discussion in this section will be mostly devoted to nonspecific symptomatic therapies.

Symptomatic treatments for cough are divided into two categories: antitussives and protussives. Antitussives are meant to decrease the frequency and/or severity of cough; protussives are meant to improve the clearance of secretions. Symptomatic treatments with other actions that may improve cough symptoms include antihistamine-decongestant combinations, bronchodilators, and anti-inflammatory drugs. A summary of effective treatments for cough is presented in Table 1-4.

Antitussives

Antitussives are indicated when the cough serves no useful function, causes distress, and is unresponsive to specific therapies. Few placebo-controlled trials of antitussives for patients with cough have been reported. Most studies have been conducted in animal models or have involved experimentally induced cough in humans and may not be directly applicable to patient care.

Antitussives that are available in the United States and that have been shown to be effective

Table 1-4

Cough Treatments with Demonstrated Effectiveness in Controlled Trials

MEDICATION	INDICATIONS
Codeine	Cancer or other chronic conditions for which specific therapy is not available
Dextromethorphan	Cancer or other chronic conditions for which specific therapy is not available; possibly for common cold
Guaifenesin	Acute upper respiratory tract infections in adults
Combination first-generation antihistamine-decongestant	Postnasal drip from various etiologies
N-acetylcysteine/carbocysteine	Chronic bronchitis, bronchiectasis
Beta-agonists	Asthma, chronic bronchitis; possibly acute bronchitis
Ipratropium	Chronic bronchitis, postinfectious cough, nonallergic rhinitis
Corticosteroids	Asthma, eosinophilic bronchitis, chronic interstitial lung diseases, acute croup; possibly chronic bronchitis
Cromolyn/nedocromil	Asthma
Proton-pump inhibitors	Gastroesophageal reflux disease
Antibiotics	Pneumonia, bacterial sinusitis, exacerbations of chronic bronchitis, bronchiectasis, tuberculosis, pertussis (if used early)

in one or more placebo-controlled trials in people with pathologic cough are codeine, dextromethorphan, and diphenhydramine. Benzonatate and carbetapentane are two other agents that are available, but for which controlled trials that demonstrate effectiveness are lacking. Antitussives that are available in other countries that may be effective in controlling cough include levodropropizine, glaucine, guaimesal, caramiphen, viminol, and moguisteine.[6]

CODEINE

Codeine suppresses cough by binding to opioid receptors in the central cough center. In doses of 30 to 60 mg four times daily it is an effective antitussive for pathologic chronic cough in such conditions as cancer and pulmonary fibrosis.[6] However, it is no more effective than placebo for coughing associated with acute upper respiratory tract infections in children and adults.[38]

The use of codeine clearly has drawbacks. Therapeutic doses can lead to significant adverse effects, such as sedation, dizziness, nausea, vomiting, and constipation. Toxic doses can lead to respiratory arrest. It also is addicting. For these reasons, the American Academy of Pediatrics Committee on Drugs does not recommend its routine use in children with cough.[39]

Prescription cough medications containing narcotics other than codeine are available, but their effectiveness has not been reported in published trials. Presumably their efficacy and adverse effect profile would be comparable to those of codeine at equipotent doses.

DEXTROMETHORPHAN

Dextromethorphan is derived from opiates and has a similar mechanism of action. Dextromethorphan is more effective than placebo and of similar effectiveness to codeine for patients with chronic cough. The effectiveness of dextromethorphan for cough associated with upper respiratory infections is not clear because placebo-controlled trials have shown conflicting results.[38] One series of three successive single-dose trials demonstrated decreased coughing in patients given dextromethorphan, but a similar smaller trial did not detect any difference between dextromethorphan and placebo.[38] Repeated-dose trials have not shown dextromethorphan to be more effective than placebo in children or adults.

Dextromethorphan is less sedating, constipating, and addicting than codeine, but it can cause confusion, excitation, nervousness, and irritability in usual doses.[40] High doses can lead to dysphoria and respiratory depression, and occasional cases of abuse have been reported.[39] Because dextromethorphan is metabolized by the cytochrome P-450 enzyme 2D6, caution is needed in using it in patients taking drugs that inhibit this enzyme (e.g., fluoxetine, paroxetene). The American Academy of Pediatrics does not recommend the routine use of dextromethorphan for children with cough.[39]

Carbetapentane (or pentoxyverine) is an antitussive related to dextromethorphan that is found in some over-the-counter preparations. Published controlled trials demonstrating its effectiveness are lacking.

BENZONATATE

Benzonatate is chemically related to topical anesthetics and is believed to anesthetize the stretch receptors in the respiratory tree and thereby reduce the cough reflex. Oral formulations are FDA-approved for the symptomatic relief of cough. Controlled trials have not been published, however, so it is difficult to evaluate the effectiveness of this drug. A recent small, uncontrolled study showed that it decreased cough in cancer patients whose cough was not responding to opioids.[41] The approved dose for adults is 10 mg three times daily.

Adverse effects of benzonatate include hypersensitivity reactions, local anesthetic effects on the oral mucosa (if the medication is chewed or allowed to dissolve in the mouth), and various gastrointestinal and central nervous system side effects. It can cause seizures and cardiac arrest in toxic amounts,[42] and its safety in children has not been established.

Protussives

There are two classes of protussives: expectorants and mucolytics. Expectorants increase the production of respiratory fluid, which may decrease the viscosity of mucus so that it more easily undergoes mucociliary transport and is expectorated. Mucolytics decrease viscosity more directly by breaking mucopolysaccharide fibers or mucoproteins.

EXPECTORANTS

Guaifenesin, the only FDA-approved expectorant, is a very commonly used over-the-counter and prescribed cough medication. Very few controlled studies evaluating its effectiveness for patients with cough have been published. Two placebo-controlled studies in adults with acute viral upper respiratory tract infections have shown some benefit.[38] In one, 75 percent of patients who were given guaifenesin noted improvements in cough frequency and intensity, as compared with 31 percent in the placebo group. A second study showed no difference in cough frequency or severity between groups, but the guaifenesin group did note a decrease in sputum thickness and quantity. In patients with asthma or chronic bronchitis guaifenesin is not more effective than placebo at decreasing sputum viscosity.[6]

Guaifenesin is generally safe. In high doses, however, it can cause headache, drowsiness, dizziness, nausea, vomiting, diarrhea, abdominal pain, and rash.[39]

MUCOLYTICS

There are a variety of mucolytics, but few have demonstrated any effectiveness for the treatment of cough. For chronic bronchitis, oral *N*-acetylcysteine decreases the incidence of acute exacerbations and improves symptoms,[43] but oral iodide has not been shown to be useful, and iodinated glycerol was removed from the U.S. market because of concerns over toxicity and lack of proven benefit.[44] Aerosolized amiloride and rhDNase may be helpful in patients with cystic fibrosis.[6,45]

Antihistamine-Decongestant Therapy

Combination antihistamine-decongestant therapy has been studied in both children and adults with acute cough due to the common cold.[38] One study in adults showed that the combination of dexbrompheniramine and pseudo-ephedrine was more effective than placebo in reducing cough severity, and a second showed that the combination of loratadine and pseudoephedrine was not better than placebo. The efficacy of the former combination has been attributed to the anticholinergic properties of first-generation antihistamines, which may decrease postnasal drip in nonallergic conditions. On the other hand, neither of the two trials comparing first-generation antihistamine-decongestant combinations with placebo for acute cough in children has demonstrated any benefit.[38] Combination first-generation antihistamines and decongestants have decreased chronic cough due to postnasal drip from nonallergic and postviral rhinitis in uncontrolled studies in adults.[6]

One small trial showed that diphenhydramine alone decreased cough more than placebo in patients with chronic bronchitis or sarcoidosis.[6] This may be due to effects on the central cough center.[40] Two trials of terfenadine (a second-generation antihistamine that is no longer available) did not find it to be more effective than placebo for adults with acute cough.[38] Two trials of first-generation antihistamincs (clemastine and chlorpheniramine) alone in children with acute cough did not find them to be more effective than placebo.[38]

Bronchodilators

Beta-agonists are standard bronchodilating therapy for patients with asthma. They also decrease cough in cough-variant asthma.[29] Their effectiveness in cough due to acute respiratory tract infections in patients without underlying lung disease is not clear.[45] Two controlled trials have shown that patients given albuterol were less likely to still be coughing after 1 week than patients given placebo or erythromycin, but two other studies have not shown beta-agonists to be clearly better than placebo. One trial showed a benefit only for a subgroup of patients who were wheezing on presentation. Trials in children with acute cough or recurrent, persistent cough have not found beta-agonists to be more effective than placebo.[45,46] Adverse effects of beta-agonists include tremor, palpitations, and nervousness.

Inhaled ipratropium is beneficial in decreasing the frequency and severity of cough in patients with chronic bronchitis and in postinfectious cough.[6] On the other hand, neither ipratropium nor oxitropium is more effective than placebo in decreasing cough in patients with acute respiratory tract infections who do not have underlying lung disease.[47,48] Adverse effects of inhaled anticholinergic drugs are similar to those of beta-agonists, although anticholinergics are more likely to cause dry mouth and a paradoxical increase in cough, and less likely to cause nervousness.

There is no evidence that theophylline is effective for patients with acute cough or with chronic cough due to underlying pulmonary problems.[6]

Anti-inflammatory Drugs

Anti-inflammatory medications are the mainstay of treatment for patients with asthma. Inhaled nedocromil and corticosteroids have both been shown to improve cough in these patients.[6] Of the two, corticosteroids are believed to be more effective than nedocromil for both typical and cough-variant asthma. In adults, the maximal benefit from inhaled steroids in cough-variant asthma may take 8 weeks to achieve, and rare patients with this condition seem to improve only with high-dose oral corticosteroids. There is experimental evidence that leukotriene antagonists, which are effective for other asthma symptoms, may not decrease cough sensitivity in asthmatics.[49]

Inhaled corticosteroids also decrease cough in eosinophilic bronchitis,[2] but not in patients with idiopathic chronic cough who do not have sputum eosinophilia.[50] Oral corticosteroids are effective for many of the conditions that cause chronic interstitial lung disease[36] and for acute exacerbations of chronic bronchitis.[51] Inhaled corticosteroids as chronic therapy for chronic bronchitis may decrease symptoms in patients with more severe disease.[44] Regarding acute cough in patients without underlying lung disease, one trial showed that inhaled steroids are no more effective than placebo when added to diphenhydramine and tetracycline.[52] Finally, uncontrolled studies have shown a 2-week course of oral corticosteroids to be beneficial in postinfectious cough.[6]

The nonsteroidal anti-inflammatory drug naproxen has been shown to decrease cough and other cold symptoms in a single placebo-controlled trial of experimentally induced rhinoviral infections in adults when given within 6 h of exposure to the virus.[53]

Combination Therapies

There are numerous over-the-counter and prescribed medications that combine two or more of these ingredients. There are limited data showing that combinations are effective in adults, but no evidence of effectiveness in children.[38] A combination of dextromethorphan and albuterol was more effective than either placebo or dextromethorphan alone in decreasing the severity of night cough in patients with acute upper respiratory tract infections, but had no

effect on daytime symptoms. Another study showed that a combination of dextromethorphan, ephedrine, doxylamine, and acetaminophen led to better overall symptom control than placebo in patients with the common cold. Combination therapies in which an antitussive is combined with an expectorant for patients with acute respiratory infections have not been shown to be more effective than placebo in children,[54] nor than guaifenesin alone in adults.[55]

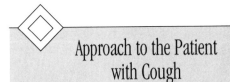

Approach to the Patient with Cough

Establishing the duration of the cough is the most useful first step in approaching the patient with a cough. Once the duration of coughing is established, the remainder of the history and physical examination can then determine likely diagnoses, whether there is a need for additional diagnostic tests, and which, if any, empiric therapy would be beneficial. Algorithms describing useful approaches to acute and chronic cough in immunocompetent adults are presented in Figs. 1-1 and 1-2. These algorithms may oversimplify the medical decision-making process because clinicians commonly entertain multiple diagnoses concurrently. Nonetheless, the algorithms do point to common conditions that should be considered.

Approach to the Patient with Acute Cough

Determining whether an acute cough is due to an infection is a useful first step. If it appears to be due to an infection, the next step is to see whether pneumonia can be ruled out. In immunocompetent, community-dwelling adults, this can be done if all vital signs and the chest examination are normal. If the vital signs are abnormal or the chest examination suggests consolidation (rales and/or decreased breath sounds), then a chest radiograph should be obtained to confirm pneumonia.

If pneumonia is excluded in patients with an acute infection causing cough, influenza should be considered if the signs and symptoms are suggestive and if influenza is present in the com-

Figure 1-1

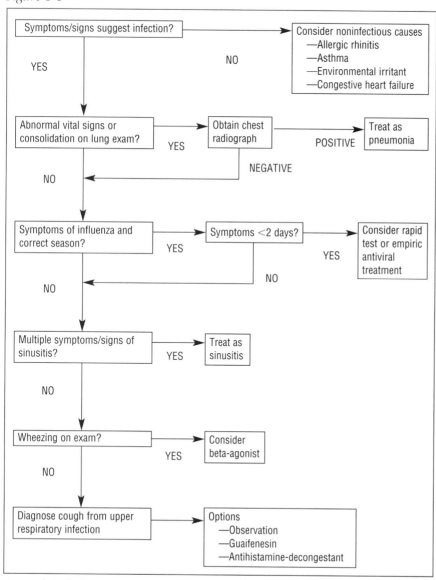

Approach to the immunocompetent adult patient with acute cough.

Figure 1-2

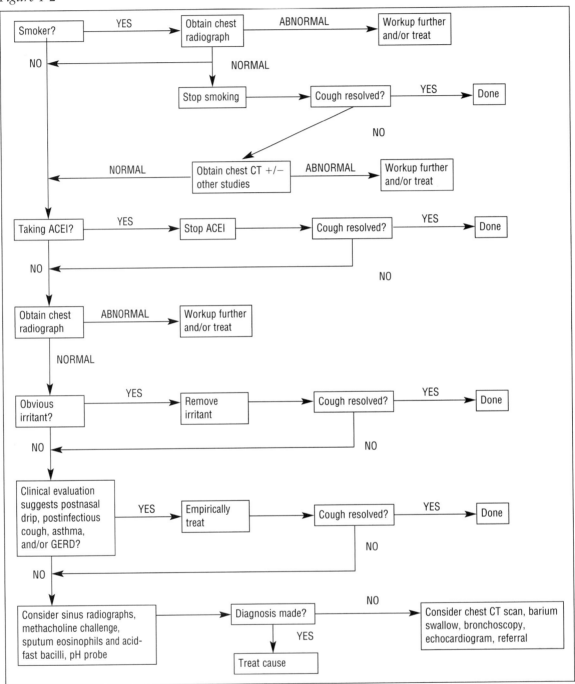

Approach to the immunocompetent adult patient with chronic cough.
Abbreviations: CT, computed tomography; ACEI, angiotensin-converting enzyme inhibitor;
GERD, gastroesophageal reflux disease.

munity. For patients with influenza-like illnesses of less than 2 days' duration, empiric treatment with anti-influenza drugs or rapid serologic testing can be considered. Patients without pneumonia or influenza who have multiple symptoms and signs of acute bacterial sinusitis might benefit from empiric antibiotic therapy, particularly if they are not improving after 7 days of illness. Adjunctive treatment with decongestants with or without antihistamines may be offered as well.

Patients with acute infectious cough who do not have pneumonia or influenza and do not have symptoms of acute bacterial sinusitis are not likely to derive any benefit from any particular therapy. In particular, antibiotics are unlikely to be beneficial. Strategies to decrease the unnecessary use of antibiotics without sacrificing patient satisfaction include explanation and delayed antibiotic prescribing.[56,57] Reassurance is the best option for many patients with uncomplicated acute cough, but symptomatic treatments may help some feel better. Analgesics and antipyretics benefit patients with pain and fever. Although trials regarding the effectiveness of beta-agonists are inconsistent, these agents might decrease the duration of cough for some patients, particularly those with wheezing on initial evaluation. Other symptomatic treatments that may be offered to patients with acute cough include guaifenesin and combination first-generation antihistamine-decongestants. Patients should be informed, however, that the evidence regarding the effectiveness of symptomatic treatments for acute cough is limited, and that adverse effects are possible.

For patients with acute cough who do not seem to have an infectious etiology, one should consider allergic or nonallergic rhinitis if symptoms are primarily in the upper respiratory tract. Symptoms that are seasonal or are associated with obvious allergens make allergic rhinitis more likely, and empiric treatment with intranasal corticosteroids or antihistamines and/or allergy testing are options. Patients with allergic rhinitis may have concomitant asthma and may need to be treated for both conditions.

Patients with acute cough and no evidence of rhinitis should be questioned about environmental exposures that might lead to cough. Patients with underlying heart disease should be carefully evaluated for congestive heart failure. Other less common causes of acute cough that may be suggested by the history and examination and that require additional testing to confirm include pneumothorax, pleural effusion, and pulmonary embolus.

Approach to the Patient with Chronic Cough

Protocols for the evaluation of adults with chronic cough have been shown to accurately diagnose and effectively treat approximately 90 percent of patients with chronic cough.[6,58-60] These protocols are characterized by a combination of diagnostic tests and empiric therapies. It is important to note that the characteristics and timing of the cough are not very helpful in establishing a diagnosis and that up to 60 percent of patients may have more than one etiology of their chronic cough.[6] An approach that incorporates items from a number of studies is outlined in Fig. 1-2.

Smokers who present with a chronic cough should have an initial chest radiograph and be counseled about smoking cessation. If the chest film is suggestive of cancer, then further evaluation is necessary. If the film is negative, then effective smoking cessation strategies should be provided and the patient should be reevaluated after a few weeks. If the cough has resolved, then no further evaluation is necessary. If the cough persists, however, then further evaluation with a chest CT scan, sputum cytology, and/or bronchoscopy is indicated. Former smokers who develop a chronic cough should also have further diagnostic testing if their initial chest film is negative.

Nearly all nonsmokers with chronic cough should also have an initial chest radiograph. The sensitivity of a chest film in diagnosing the cause of chronic cough in nonsmokers is very good, with a specificity ranging from 54 to 76 percent. The only patients who do not require an initial chest film are those who take an ACEI. In these patients, discontinuation of the ACEI should lead to cessation of cough within 2 weeks if that is the cause of the cough. If the chest film clearly suggests a specific diagnosis, then further evaluation and/or treatment is undertaken as appropriate. For nonsmokers whose chest film is negative, careful inquiry into possible environmental irritants should be made. If these can be identified, then avoidance should be undertaken if possible. If this is successful, then no further studies or treatment are needed.

Of nonsmokers with chronic cough who do not take ACEIs and have negative chest films, nearly all have either postnasal drip, asthma, or GERD.[6] If the history and physical examination clearly suggest one of these conditions, then empiric therapy for that condition should be implemented. If the cough resolves, then continued treatment is provided as needed. If the cough fails to completely resolve with empiric treatment, further tests and treatment are needed. If the cough partially improves, then the partially successful treatment should be continued while further study is undertaken.

If a patient does not clearly have postnasal drip, asthma, or GERD, then diagnostic tests for these three conditions as well as for eosinophilic bronchitis and TB should be sequentially obtained. These tests include sinus radiography, allergy testing, pulmonary function testing with a methacholine challenge test, sputum for eosinophils and acid-fast bacilli, and 24-h esophageal pH monitoring. If any of these tests suggests a diagnosis, appropriate treatment is provided. Resolution of cough confirms the diagnosis; if the cough persists, additional studies are needed. These could include a chest CT scan, barium swallow, bronchoscopy, and echocardiogram. Alternatively, referral to a pulmonologist is appropriate when the diagnosis is not made with the initial sequence of tests and empiric therapies.

References

1. Chang AB, Powell CVE: Non-specific cough in children: diagnosis and treatment. *Hosp Med* 59:681–684, 1998.
2. Brightling CE, Pavord ID: Eosinophilic bronchitis: an important cause of prolonged cough. *Ann Med* 32:446–451, 2000.
3. Schappert SM: Ambulatory care visits to physician offices, hospital outpatient departments, and emergency departments: United States, 1997. *Vital Health Stat* [13] 143:1–39, 1999.
4. Bergh KD: The patient's differential diagnosis: unpredictable concerns in visits for acute cough. *J Fam Pract* 46:153–158, 1998.
5. Chang AB: Cough, cough receptors, and asthma in children. *Pediatr Pulmonol* 28:59–70, 1999.
6. Irwin RS, Boulet L-P, Cloutier MM, et al: Managing cough as a defense mechanism and as a symptom. A consensus panel report of the American College of Chest Physicians. *Chest* 114:133S–181S, 1998.
7. Widdicombe JG: Advances in understanding and treatment of cough. *Arch Monaldi* 54:275–279, 1999.
8. Irwin RS, Madison JM: Primary care: the diagnosis and treatment of cough. *N Engl J Med* 343:1715–1721, 2000.
9. Hickner JM, Bartlett JG, Besser RE, et al: Principles of appropriate antibiotic use for acute rhinosinusitis in adults: background. *Ann Intern Med* 134:498–505, 2001.
10. Puhakka T, Makela MJ, Alanen A, et al: Sinusitis in the common cold. *J Allergy Clin Immunol* 102:403–408, 1998.
11. Mainous AG III, Zoorob RJ, Oler MJ, et al: Patient knowledge of upper respiratory infections: implications for antibiotic expectations and unnecessary utilization. *J Fam Pract* 45:75–83, 1997.
12. Dosh SA, Hickner JM, Mainous AG III, et al: Predictors of antibiotic prescribing for nonspecific upper respiratory infections, acute bronchitis, and acute sinusitis. An UPRNet study. *J Fam Pract* 49:407–414, 2000.
13. Bartlett JG, Breiman RF, Mandell LA, et al: Community-acquired pneumonia in adults: guidelines for management. *Clin Infect Dis* 26:811–838, 1998.
14. Metlay JP, Kapoor WN, Fine MJ: Does this patient have community-acquired pneumonia? Diagnos-

ing pneumonia by history and physical examination. *JAMA* 278:1440–1445, 1997.

15. Hueston WJ, Mainous AG III, Dacus EN, et al: Does acute bronchitis really exist? A reconceptualization of acute viral respiratory infections. *J Fam Pract* 49:401–406, 2000.

16. Oeffinger KC, Snell LM, Foster BM, et al: Diagnosis of acute bronchitis in adults: a national survey of family physicians. *J Fam Pract* 45:402–409, 1997.

17. Wright SW: Pertussis infection in adults. *South Med J* 91:702–708, 1998.

18. Yaari E, Yafe-Zimmerman Y, Schwartz SB, et al: Clinical manifestations of *Bordetella pertussis* infection in immunized children and young adults. *Chest* 115:1254–1258, 1999.

19. Monto AS, Gravenstein S, Elliott M, et al: Clinical signs and symptoms predicting influenza infection. *Arch Intern Med* 160:3243–3247, 2000.

20. Couch RB: Drug therapy: prevention and treatment of influenza. *N Engl J Med* 343:1778–1787, 2000.

21. Luber SR: Influenza year 2001 update: epidemiology, diagnosis, and outcome-effective guidelines for neuraminidase inhibitor therapy. *Primary Care Consensus Reports* 1–16, Feb. 1, 2001.

22. O'Brien KL, Dowell SF, Schwartz B, et al: Acute sinusitis—principles of judicious use of antimicrobial agents. *Pediatrics* 101:174–177, 1998.

23. Noyola DE, Demmler GJ: Effect of rapid diagnosis on management of influenza A infections. *Pediatr Infect Dis J* 19:303–307, 2000.

24. Margolis P, Gadomski A: Does this infant have pneumonia? *JAMA* 279:308–313, 1998.

25. Metrangolo S, Monetti C, Meneghini L, et al: Eight years' experience with foreign-body aspiration in children: What is really important for a timely diagnosis? *J Pediatr Surg* 34:1229–1231, 1999.

26. Zerella JT, Dimler M, McGill LC, et al: Foreign body aspiration in children: value of radiography and complications of bronchoscopy. *J Pediatr Surg* 33:1651–1654, 1998.

27. Mello CJ, Irwin RS, Curley FJ: Predictive value of the character, timing, and complications of chronic cough in diagnosing its cause. *Arch Intern Med* 156:997–1003, 1996.

28. Holleman DR, Simel DL: Does the clinical examination predict airflow limitation? *JAMA* 273:313–319, 1995.

29. Irwin RS, French CT, Smyrnios NA, et al: Interpretation of positive results of a methacholine inhalation challenge and 1 week of inhaled bronchodilator use in diagnosing and treating cough-variant asthma. *Arch Intern Med* 157:1981–1987, 1997.

30. Irwin RS, Richter JE: Gastroesophageal reflux and chronic cough. *Am J Gastroenterol* 95:S9–S14, 2000.

31. Burns DM: Primary prevention, smoking, and smoking cessation. *Cancer* 89:2506–2509, 2000.

32. Henschke CI, McCauley DI, Yankelevitz DF, et al: Early Lung Cancer Action Project: overall design and findings from baseline screening. *Lancet* 354:99–105, 1999.

33. Petty TL: The early identification of lung carcinoma by sputum cytology. *Cancer* 89:2461–2464, 2000.

34. Luque CA, Vazquez Ortiz M: Treatment of ACE inhibitor-induced cough. *Pharmacotherapy* 19:804–810, 1999.

35. Pylypchuk GB: ACE inhibitor- versus angiotensin II blocker-induced cough and angioedema. *Ann Pharmacother* 32:1060–1066, 1998.

36. Reynolds HY: Diagnostic and management strategies for diffuse interstitial lung disease. *Chest* 113:192–202, 1998.

37. Long R, Cowie R: Tuberculosis: 4. Pulmonary disease. *Can Med Assoc J* 160:1344–1348, 1999.

38. Schroeder K, Fahey T: Over-the-counter medications for acute cough in children and adults in ambulatory settings (Cochrane Review), in *The Cochrane Library*, Issue 3. Oxford, Update Software, 2001.

39. Berlin CM Jr, McCarver-May DG, Notterman DA, et al: Use of codeine- and dextromethorphan-containing cough remedies in children. *Pediatrics* 99:918–920, 1997.

40. Over-the-counter (OTC) cough remedies. *Med Lett Drugs Ther* 43:23–25, 2001.

41. Doona M, Walsh D: Benzonatate for opioid-resistant cough in advanced cancer. *Palliative Med* 12:55–58, 1998.

42. Crouch BI, Knick KA, Crouch DJ, et al: Benzonatate overdose associated with seizures and arrhythmias. *J Clin Toxicol* 36:713–718, 1998.

43. Stey C, Steurer J, Bachmann S: The effect of oral *N*-acetylcysteine in chronic bronchitis: a quantitative systematic review. *Eur Respir J* 16:253–262, 2000.

44. Ferguson GT: Update on pharmacologic therapy for chronic obstructive pulmonary disease. *Clin Chest Med* 21:723–738, 2000.

45. Smucny J, Flynn C, Becker L, et al: Beta-2 agonists for acute bronchitis (Cochrane Review), in *The Cochrane Library, Issue 3. Oxford*, Update Software, 2001.

46. Chang AB, Phelan PD, Carlin JB, et al: A randomised, placebo controlled trial of inhaled salbutamol and beclomethasone for recurrent cough. *Arch Dis Child* 79:6–11, 1998.

47. Lowry R, Wood A, Higenbottam T: The effect of anticholinergic bronchodilator therapy on cough during upper respiratory tract infections. *Br J Clin Pharmacol* 37:187–191, 1994.

48. Salzman GA, Chen M, Willsie-Ediger SK: The effect of inhaled ipratropium bromide on the acute transient cough during viral respiratory illness. *Chest* 98:129S, 1990.

49. Dicpinigaitis PV, Dobkin JB: Effect of zafirlukast on cough reflex sensitivity in asthmatics. *J Asthma* 36:265–270, 1999.

50. Pizzichini MM, Pizzichini E, Parameswaran K, et al: Nonasthmatic chronic cough: no effect of treatment with an inhaled corticosteroid in patients without sputum eosinophilia. *Can Respir J* 6:323–330, 1999.

51. Sherk PA, Grossman RF: The chronic obstructive pulmonary disease exacerbation. *Clin Chest Med* 21:705–721, 2000.

52. Frank A, Dash CH: Inhaled beclomethasone dipropionate in acute infections of the respiratory tract. *Respiration* 48:122–126, 1985.

53. Sperber SJ, Hendley JO, Hayden FG, et al: Effects of naproxen on experimental rhinovirus colds. A randomized, double-blind, controlled trial. *Ann Intern Med* 117:37–41, 1992.

54. Taylor JA, Novack AH, Almquist JR, et al: Efficacy of cough suppressants in children. *J Pediatr* 122:799–802, 1993.

55. Croughan-Minihane MS, Petitti DB, Rodnick JE, et al: Clinical trial examining effectiveness of three cough syrups. *J Am Board Fam Pract* 6:109–115, 1993.

56. Hamm RM, Hicks RJ, Bemben DA: Antibiotics and respiratory infections: are patients more satisfied when expectations are met? *J Fam Pract* 43:56–62, 1996.

57. Dowell J, Pitkethly M, Bain J, et al: A randomised controlled trial of delayed antibiotic prescribing as a strategy for managing uncomplicated respiratory tract infection in primary care. *Br J Gen Pract* 51:200–205, 2001.

58. McGarvey LPA, Heaney LG, Lawson JT, et al: Evaluation and outcome of patients with chronic non-productive cough using a comprehensive diagnostic protocol. *Thorax* 53:738–743, 1998.

59. Marchesani F, Cecarini L, Pela R, et al: Causes of chronic persistent cough in adult patients: the results of a systematic management protocol. *Arch Monaldi* 53:510–514, 1998.

60. Pratter MR, Bartter T, Lotano R: The role of sinus imaging in the treatment of chronic cough in adults. *Chest* 116:1287–1291, 1999.

William J. Hueston

Dyspnea and Shortness of Breath

Dyspnea refers to the sensation that it is difficult to catch one's breath. Inherent in the definition is that this is an uncomfortable sensation. In contrast to the normal respiratory effort, which is minimal and unconscious, individuals with dyspnea are aware that their act of breathing is noticeable and that the effort required is more than usual.

Dyspnea typically occurs when oxygen supply cannot meet oxygen demand, but it can occur even when oxygen levels match requirements. For example, patients with lung dysfunctions such as emphysema will note the additional effort required to move air into and out of their lungs and will complain of dyspnea. The sensation of dyspnea in the face of normal oxygen supply also occurs in older patients in whom the ability to sense a respiratory load increases. This heightened appreciation of respiratory elastic loads in older individuals can lead to a greater sensation of difficulty breathing at the same level of respiratory effort.[1] Thus, as patients age, chronic obstructive changes in their lung function may cause worsening dyspnea despite fairly stable pulmonary function.

Shortness of breath is usually not painful, but it does cause anxiety. Often the anxiety that accompanies dyspnea can create diagnostic confusion, since anxiety can also cause a feeling of breathlessness. It can be difficult to ascertain which came first: the dyspnea or the anxiety.

Assessing Severity

Dyspnea can be graded on the basis of the level of activity required to produce shortness of breath. For individuals with good gas exchange, moderately intense exercise is required before the demand for oxygen exceeds the ability of the lungs and vascular system to supply it. Individuals with mild lung disease may be comfortable at rest but experience dyspnea with high levels of exertion. As the lung disease worsens, less activity is required to cause shortness of breath. In severe cases, the patient may be dyspneic even at rest. However, the degree of exertion needed to produce dyspnea is dependent on the level of

conditioning previously attained by a particular individual. For example, a very fit runner with a pulmonary embolism may be able to continue to exercise at what would seem to be very high levels of functioning for someone who was not so well conditioned. Therefore, any change in an individual's ability to perform at his or her previous level of exertion without shortness of breath should prompt further evaluation.

The severity of respiratory problems can be assessed quickly by using a scoring scale developed and tested by Gulsvik and Refvem.[2] The scale takes about 6 min to complete and includes four subscales that determine a wheezing score, a cough score, an attacks of breathlessness score, and a dyspnea score. Each subscale includes four statements of varying degrees of severity (e.g., "I never have wheezing in the chest" to "I have wheezing in the chest all day/night") that are presented along a visual analog scale. Investigators evaluating this tool found that the cough score was useful in distinguishing between smokers and nonsmokers and could predict the amount of smoking. In addition, each point increase in the dyspnea and cough scores predicted a drop in the peak flow rate of 7 to 12 percent.

Epidemiology

The prevalence of dyspnea increases with advancing age. This is probably related to greater sensation of respiratory loads,[3] plus additional exposure over time to toxic agents, such as cigarette smoke, that result in progressive lung damage.

The biggest risk factor for developing dyspnea over time is the use of cigarettes. Conversely, smoking cessation has a positive effect on symptoms of shortness of breath. In one multisite study, patients who discontinued smoking experienced a 50 percent drop in their shortness of breath and other respiratory symptoms over

13 years of observation compared to others in the cohort who had continued to smoke.[4]

The risk of having dyspnea also appears to be related to occupation. A French study found that the percentage of older individuals who complained of chronic shortness of breath was associated with their type of occupation and the work they performed during their lifetime.[5] For example, while 37 percent of farm workers over age 65 complained of chronic shortness of breath, only 18 percent of seniors who had been schoolteachers had this problem. The highest adjusted risk for dypsnea was seen in older individuals who had been employed as farm workers, farm managers, domestic service employees, and other blue-collar workers. The lowest risk was seen in a class titled "intellectual occupation," which included most indoor work in a professional setting. In a younger population, a study in New Zealand found higher risks of shortness of breath in hairdressers and bakers, while nurses had the lowest levels of dyspnea.[6] The study also found that working in occupations involving exposure to vapors, gases, dust, or fumes was associated with future development of respiratory diseases that cause shortness of breath.

Dyspnea also is common in patients with end-stage cancer. Between one-fifth and four-fifths of patients with advanced cancer will have dyspnea near the end of their lives.[7] Dyspnea usually worsens in severity and frequency as patients get closer to death. In these circumstances, attention to palliative efforts to relieve dyspnea (see "Managing Chronic Dyspnea" later in this chapter) is more appropriate than attempting to correct gas exchange abnormalities.

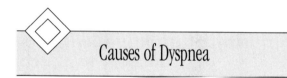

Causes of Dyspnea

Dyspnea can result from a variety of causes, but these can be categorized into four general groupings: (1) decreased oxygen supply from lung dysfunction, (2) decreased oxygen delivery from cardiovascular problems, (3) decreased oxygen-carrying capacity in the circulation, or (4) increased oxygen demand.

Decreased Oxygen Supply from Lung Dysfunction

Oxygen-carrying capacity is dependent on adequate air exchange in the lung and the ability to transport oxygen on hemoglobin. For adequate gas exchange to occur, the chest wall must function appropriately to provide adequate inspiratory and expiratory forces, alveolar spaces need to be healthy to permit adequate gas exchange, vascular flow to the lung must be unobstructed, and the oxygen-carrying capacity of the blood must be adequate. A disruption in any of these four systems will result in mismatches of oxygen delivery and demand, resulting in shortness of breath.

NEUROMUSCULAR PROBLEMS RESULTING IN HYPOVENTILATION

Inspiratory effort is dependent upon appropriate neurologic input to the respiratory muscles, suitable muscle strength to respond to the stimulation, and chest wall integrity. Problems in any of these areas can lead to shortness of breath (Table 2-1).

Disruption in the integrity of the thorax or its ability to generate appropriate negative and positive pressures during inspiration and expiration will result in progressive hypoventilation and dyspnea. This occurs with malformations of the thorax, such as kyphosis or scoliosis. The loss of chest wall integrity seen with multiple rib fractures or open chest wounds also will impair the ability to create a negative pressure. An open wound, such as a pneumothorax, may result in sucking of air into the pleural space with inspiration rather than into the lung.

Disorders in the nervous system that drives muscular coordination or effectiveness also will result in hypoventilation and shortness of breath.

Table 2-1

Neuromuscular Diseases Causing Shortness of Breath

Chest mechanical abnormalities
  Fractured ribs
  Severe kyphosis or scoliosis
  Ankylosing spondylitis
  Tension pneumothorax
Neurologic diseases that impair respiration
  Amyotrophic lateral sclerosis
  Guillain-Barré syndrome
  Multiple sclerosis
Muscular diseases that impair chest wall
  motion
  Poliomyelitis
  Myasthenia gravis
  Muscular dystrophy

These include central nervous system abnormalities such as multiple sclerosis, spinal cord disorders such as amyotrophic lateral sclerosis, and peripheral neuropathies such as Guillain-Barré syndrome.

Finally, syndromes that result in progressive muscle weakness can lead to inability to get an appropriate breath. These include primary muscle diseases as well as muscular atrophy from malnutrition or cachexia associated with end-stage cancer.

ALVEOLAR OBSTRUCTION LEADING TO DECREASED GAS EXCHANGE

The alveolar space provides a large surface area for gas exchange between inspired air and pulmonary capillaries. The alveolar-arterial gradient allows oxygen to flow from more highly oxygenated air into the bloodstream, with a corresponding outflow of carbon dioxide from the blood to the alveolar space. For gas exchange to occur efficiently, the alveolar surface area needs to be unobstructed and the interstitium of the alveolus needs to be thin to allow gas transport. Problems such as obstruction of the alveolus or

its proximal bronchial tree, collection of material in the alveolar space that blocks gas transport, or thickening of the interstitial space all will result in reduced gas exchange.

BRONCHIAL AIRWAY OBSTRUCTION A number of problems can cause obstruction of the airways and result in hypoventilation (Table 2-2). In several of these cases, specific signs and symptoms can be elicited that will indicate the area of obstruction. For example, with inflammation of the epiglottis and larynx, stridor is usually present. However, the site of airway obstruction is not always obvious. Further evaluation may be necessary to identify the area of obstruction.

Table 2-2

Causes of Airway Obstruction Leading to Dyspnea

Epiglottic/laryngeal obstruction
  Viral infection (croup)
  Epiglottitis (*Haemophilus influenzae*)
  Laryngeal cancer
Tracheal obstruction
Bronchial inflammation or obstruction
  Chronic bronchitis
  Neoplasms
    Lung cancers, especially squamous cell
      and adenocarcinoma
  Asthma
  Gastroesophageal reflux with chronic
    aspiration
Alveolar obstruction
  Pneumonia
  Cystic fibrosis
  Pulmonary edema
    Congestive heart failure/cardiac shock
    Ischemic lung injury (adult respiratory
      distress syndrome)
    Toxin-mediated pulmonary edema
      (e.g., smoke inhalation)
  Drowning
  Pulmonary alveolar proteinosis
  Pulmonary hemorrhage

ALVEOLAR SPACE DISEASES Any problems that allow the accumulation of fluid or other material in the alveolar space will reduce the surface area available for gas exchange. The material in the alveolar space can be pus, extrusion of capillary fluid into the alveolar space, external fluid that is inspired, or other materials produced by the lung (Table 2-2).

INTERSTITIAL AIRWAY DISEASES Interstitial diseases reduce the ability of gas to flow between the pulmonary capillaries and the alveoli. In addition to progressive dyspnea, patients with interstitial lung diseases have restrictive changes on pulmonary function testing and diffuse infiltrates on chest x-ray (Table 2-3). A variety of conditions can result in obstruction of gas exchange in the interstitium. These include interstitial pneumonitis from infections (usually viral), toxic expo-

sures, materials that produce hypersensitivity reactions, or drugs. Problems also develop as a result of infiltration of new tissue into the interstitial spaces by deposition of either new connective tissue (such as in the collagen vascular diseases) or other cellular material (such as granulomata in sarcoidosis or Wegener's granulomatosis). An increased interstitial gradient to gas exchange also can occur as a result of additional lymph fluid secondary to obstruction of lymphatic outflow. This usually occurs as a result of lymphatic spread of cancer from adjoining regions such as the breast, lung, and stomach. Finally, alveolar mucosal disease can result in a barrier to gas exchange and mimic findings of interstitial diseases.

Decreased Oxygen Delivery from Cardiovascular Problems

Three major cardiovascular problems can produce shortness of breath: embolism of the pulmonary artery; reductions in systolic blood flow from chronic heart failure, acute ischemia, or infarction; and pulmonary hypertension (see Table 2-4).

EMBOLIC DISEASES

Pulmonary embolic disease usually results from embolism of a clot from a deep venous thrombosis of the lower extremity or pelvis to the pulmonary vasculature. The diagnosis and management of this condition is presented in more detail in Chapter 13. In addition to clots, dyspnea can occur from emboli of other materials, such as fat, amniotic fluid, and air.

Fat embolism occurs in the presence of a fracture of a long bone or, more rarely, after orthopedic surgery. Embolism usually occurs 24 h to 3 days following the trauma and results in the rapid onset of dyspnea, tachypnea, confusion, and petechiae. The treatment of fat embolism is supportive, although there is some suggestion that the syndrome can be prevented with admin-

Table 2-3

Interstitial Lung Diseases

Primary pulmonary fibrosis
Interstitial pneumonitis
   Infection (e.g., CMV pneumonitis)
   Chronic toxic exposures (e.g., asbestosis,
     radiation pneumonitis, pneumoconiosis)
   Hypersensitivity pneumonitis (e.g., farmer's
     lung, bird fancier's lung)
   Drugs (e.g., amiodarone, bromocriptine,
     cyclophosphamide, nitrofurantoin,
     penicillamine)
Collagen vascular diseases
   Scleroderma
   Rheumatoid arthritis
   Systemic lupus erythematosis
   Polymyositis-dermatomysositis
Lymphatic obstruction (usually from metastatic
   disease)
Sarcoidosis
Wegener's granulomatosis
Langerhans cell granulomatosis (histiocytosis X)

ABBREVIATIONS: CMV, cytomegalovirus.

Table 2-4

Cardiovascular Causes of Shortness of Breath

Pulmonary embolism
 Thromboembolic disease
 Fat embolism
 Amniotic fluid embolism
 Air embolism
Myocardial ischemia
Valvular heart disease
Cardiomyopathies
 Diabetic cardiomyopathy
 Late hypertensive cardiomyopathy
 Postpartum cardiomyopathy
 Postmyositis cardiomyopathy
 Idiopathic cardiomyopathy
Pulmonary hypertension
 Secondary to other disorders
 External compression
 Primary pulmonary hypertension
  Secondary to drugs (e.g., L-tryptophan,
   anorectic agents)
  Idiopathic primary pulmonary hypertension
Pericarditis and cardiac tamponade

istration of prophylactic corticosteroids (methyl-prednisolone at a dose of 2.5 mg/kg every 6 h for 4 days) after extensive lower extremity trauma. Administration of steroids after the development of symptoms is not beneficial.[8]

Amniotic fluid embolism is a dramatic, usually fatal condition that occurs during labor. Symptoms include acute onset of dyspnea with rapid progression to respiratory distress, circulatory collapse, and often death. The mechanism of injury is entry of amniotic fluid into the venous circulation, with rapid activation of the thrombotic system. Deposition of amniotic fluid in the lungs results in fibrin deposition in the pulmonary vasculature, occlusion of blood flow, pulmonary hypotension, and complete circulatory obstruction. Similar events occur in other end-organ tissues. While this event is rare, it is usually devastating. No risk factors are associated with the occurrence of amniotic fluid

embolism, and no treatment beyond supportive measures such as oxygen supplementation and mechanical ventilation has been shown to reduce mortality.

Air embolism can result in acute obstruction of pulmonary artery blood flow, circulatory collapse, and death. Small amounts of air embolism can cause severe dyspnea and hypotension. Patients at risk for air embolism include anyone with a central venous catheter line. Since inspiration produces a significant negative intrathoracic pressure, a leak in such a line can result in significant amounts of air being pulled into the vascular system during inspiration.

PULMONARY HYPERTENSION

Pulmonary hypertension usually results from either left heart failure or chronic hypoxia associated with chronic obstructive pulmonary disease (Chapter 17), cystic fibrosis, neuromuscular disorders that result in hypoventilation, and interstitial lung diseases. Usually, pulmonary hypertension does not develop in interstitial lung disease until the diffusing capacity of the lung is less than 50 percent of normal. Additionally, pulmonary vascular obstruction can occur with compression from extraarterial structures such as aneurysms, neoplasms, and granulomas. However, several other conditions can cause pulmonary hypertension from direct effects on the pulmonary vasculature. These include the use of a number of drugs, such as cocaine, L-tryptophan, rapeseed oil, and amphetamine-like anorexic agents; thromboembolic disease; sickle cell disease; pulmonary vasculitis; and primary pulmonary hypertension.

While pulmonary hypertension is a secondary manifestation of most of the disorders noted previously and is usually recognized as a complication of these disorders, primary pulmonary hypertension can be difficult to diagnose. Primary pulmonary hypertension usually begins early in life and is most common in individuals between the ages of 20 and 50. It is twice as common in women as in men, and there appears to be a higher genetic predisposition in children of affected individuals. This disorder should be suspected in younger patients with few risk factors who present with gradually increasing shortness of breath in the absence of other significant cardiopulmonary findings.

Symptoms of pulmonary hypertension are usually gradual in onset, with dyspnea as a prominent feature. Dyspnea usually starts out with exertion only and progresses in severity until patients have shortness of breath at rest. Other symptoms such as fatigue, chest pain, and syncope also occur more frequently as the severity of disease escalates. Symptoms of right heart failure, such as edema, jugular venous distention, and hepatic enlargement, are usually a late finding and indicate that significant pulmonary hypertension has been present for a substantial time period.

Decreased Oxygen-Carrying Capacity in the Circulation

The amount of oxygen dissolved in the blood, as opposed to that bound to hemoglobin, is very small. Increasing oxygen saturation in the patient who is unable to transport oxygen on hemoglobin has little overall benefit. Consequently, the concentration of hemoglobin in the bloodstream and its ability to bind and release oxygen are important factors in determining whether oxygen is available to tissues.

Problems with oxygen-carrying capacity can be broken down into two general categories: (1) lack of hemoglobin (i.e., anemia) and (2) ineffectual oxygen binding and release from hemoglobin (Table 2-5).

Just because an adequate supply of hemoglobin is available does not assure that oxygen-carrying capacity is normal. In heavy smokers or in individuals who work in poorly ventilated areas, carbon monoxide binding to hemoglobin may render a sizable percentage of the hemoglobin unable to transport oxygen. Heavy smokers may have carboxyhemoglobin levels of 8 to

Table 2-5

Oxygen Delivery Problems Causing Dyspnea

Acquired anemia
  Blood loss
  Hemolysis
  Underproduction
Congenital abnormalities in hemoglobin
  production and function
  Thalassemias
  Sickle cell disease
  Sickle cell–hemoglobin C disease
  Hereditary spherocytosis
Acquired dysfunction in hemoglobin function
  Carbon monoxide poisoning

10 percent of their total hemoglobin. Usually these individuals will respond over time with a secondary polycythemia to compensate for the ineffective hemoglobin.

Individuals exposed to high levels of carbon monoxide at work or through poorly ventilated exhaust systems in their home run the risk of acute carbon monoxide poisoning. This condition should be suspected in patients presenting with shortness of breath and headaches who are heating their homes. Less reliable mechanisms of home heating, such as an indoor gas heater or wood stove, are more commonly involved with carbon monoxide poisoning. However, even reliable commercial furnaces can develop exhaust leaks that can lead to the accumulation of carbon monoxide.

Increased Oxygen Demand

A number of conditions are associated with shortness of breath when oxygen supply and delivery are normal. These include situations in which oxygen need is increased as a result of hypermetabolic states such as hyperthyroidism or beriberi. Some drugs, such as amphetamines or cocaine, can result in hypermetabolic states that produce shortness of breath (see Table 2-6).

Table 2-6

Other Causes of Shortness of Breath

Hyperthyroidism
Drugs that produce a hypermetabolic state
Cocaine
Amphetamines
Fat embolism
Generalized anxiety disorder
Panic disorder

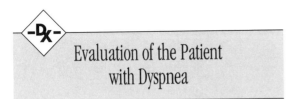

Evaluation of the Patient with Dyspnea

History

Several key points should be elicited in the history of the patient with dyspnea. An important point to determine is how rapidly the symptoms developed. Symptoms that develop over a matter of minutes or an hour usually indicate an acute event, such as pulmonary embolism, pulmonary edema, myocardial infarction, infection, or aspiration of a foreign body. Other conditions develop over a matter of days and point to a progressive failure in oxygenation, such as that caused by pneumonia or bronchial obstruction from asthma or infection, or a worsening ability to deliver oxygen, such as in acute blood loss or escalating heart failure. Symptoms that worsen gradually over a period of weeks suggest a slowly progressing disorder such as hyperthyroidism, slowly developing anemia, or a slowly developing obstruction from a neoplasm. Finally, chronic lung diseases such as pulmonary fibrosis, pulmonary hypertension, or chronic obstructive pulmonary disease initially cause symptoms over a period of months or years.

A thorough cardiopulmonary history and review of systems for cardiac or respiratory problems should be performed. The presence of respiratory symptoms such as a cough, wheezing, laryngitis, or hemoptysis increases the probability that the problem is in the airways. Chest pain, orthopnea, lower extremity edema, and a history of cardiac problems in the past can lead to more investigation of the heart. The presence of symptoms attributable to the respiratory or cardiac systems is specific, but not very sensitive. The failure to elicit any pulmonary or cardiac symptoms on history does not exclude the possibility that the heart or lungs are contributing to the shortness of breath. In the absence of clear indications of other problems, such as anemia or thyroid disease, further evaluation of the cardiopulmonary system may be necessary.

In addition to the current history, the past medical history can be useful in identifying sources of dypsnea. Individuals with prior cardiac problems may be more likely to experience congestive heart failure or ischemic heart disease. Patients who have had a prior history of a deep venous thrombosis, who are taking oral contraceptives, or who have a hypercoagulable state associated with cancer or pregnancy are at higher risk for a pulmonary embolus. Those who have had gastrointestinal bleeding in the past or who are on anticoagulants may be more prone to develop anemia. Therefore, careful attention to past medical problems and current medication use can be helpful in directing the physical examination and other studies.

Finally, other risk factors for pulmonary problems should be elicited. These include a history of smoking, a history of occupational exposures to respiratory toxins in the patient and family members, and a family history of respiratory or cardiac diseases.

Physical Examination

The vital signs and initial general appearance of the patient can be very helpful in giving an initial impression of the severity of shortness of breath. The respiratory rate and pulse are both elevated in most acute and severe problems causing dypsnea. Additionally, an initial assessment of the work involved in breathing can indicate the level of respiratory distress being experienced by the patient. The findings of tachypnea, tachycardia, and air hunger are hallmarks of acute hypoxia and have been described as the triad for pulmonary embolism, although they may be present in any instance of acute, severe decline in oxygenation. Altered mental status is a sign of severe hypoxia and an indication that immediate attention is needed to prevent further deterioration.

The presence of a fever may indicate an acute infection, although the absence of a fever does not necessarily exclude pneumonia. In older patients or those who are immunosuppressed, pneumonia may not cause a fever. In particular, geriatric patients may exhibit atypical symptoms such as falls or confusion in the presence of a pneumonia. Instead of a fever, tachypnea is the most reliable sign of pneumonia in this population.

The physical examination should be complete, but particular attention should be paid to the cardiopulmonary system. Examination of the lungs should include determination that aeration is present bilaterally and whether wheezing, rales, or rhonchi are present. Decreased breath sounds will be found with a pneumothorax, pleural effusion, or total obstruction of the lung by a mass or a foreign body. Percussion of the lung can help differentiate pneumothorax (hyperresonant chest) from a pleural effusion (dullness to percussion). Focal areas of decreased breath sounds can be found in cases of consolidation. Eliciting changes in fremitus and the presence of egophony can indicate that consolidation is present.

When abnormal lung sounds are found, attention to the location of the findings may be useful. For example, unilateral wheezing should raise suspicion for aspiration of a foreign body (in a younger patient or an individual with an impaired level of consciousness) or an obstructing mass (in an older patient). Bilateral wheezing may occur with asthma, acute bronchitis, or toxic exposures such as smoke or chemical inhalations. Similarly, focal areas of rales may be indicative of pneumonia. Bilateral rales, especially those starting at the lung bases and progressively moving upward, are more typical of pulmonary edema.

The cardiac examination should focus on specific signs of heart failure or ischemia. The heart rate and rhythm can reveal whether a dysrhythmia is present that can cause reduced cardiac output. The presence of an S_3 along with displacement of the point of maximal impulse denotes a dilated left ventricle. Checking for jugular venous distention and lower extremity edema may provide other signs of congestive heart failure.

In addition to the cardiopulmonary examination, other findings may help point to causes of shortness of breath. Individuals should be evaluated for signs of anemia, such as orthostatic hypotension or pale mucous membranes. An abdominal examination including evaluation of the stool for occult blood can indicate gastrointestinal sources of bleeding. A thyroid examination should be performed to evaluate for tenderness that can accompany Graves' disease or thyroiditis.

Laboratory and Imaging Studies

While the laboratory and imaging sequence should follow the clinical cues suggested by the history and physical examination, logical sequences for staging the patient with acute and chronic shortness of breath are shown in Figs. 2-1 and 2-2.

PULSE OXYMETRY

Probably the quickest and most useful assessment that can be performed in the patient with

Figure 2-1

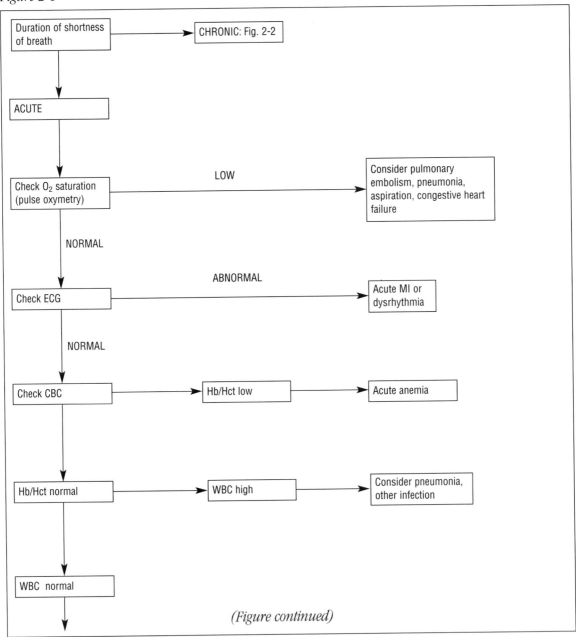

An approach to evaluating acute dyspnea.

ABBREVIATIONS: ECG, electrocardiogram; MI, myocardial infarction; CBC, complete blood count; Hb/Hct, hemoglobin/hematocrit; WBC, white blood count; COPD, chronic obstructive pulmonary disease.

Figure 2-1 (Continued)

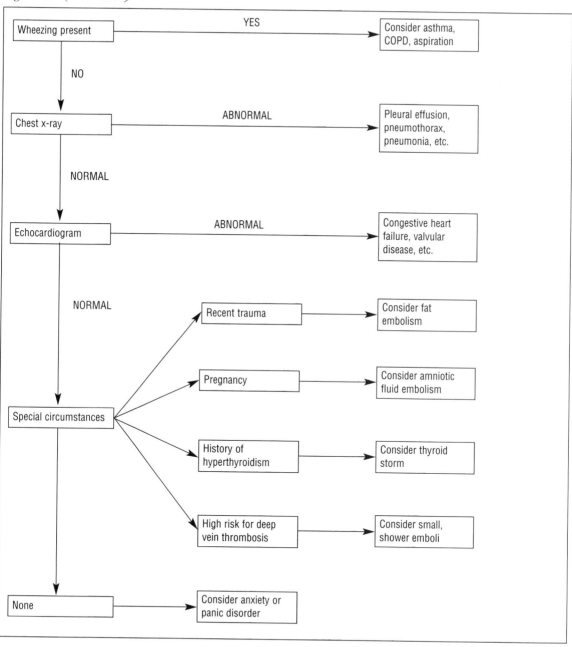

Figure 2-2

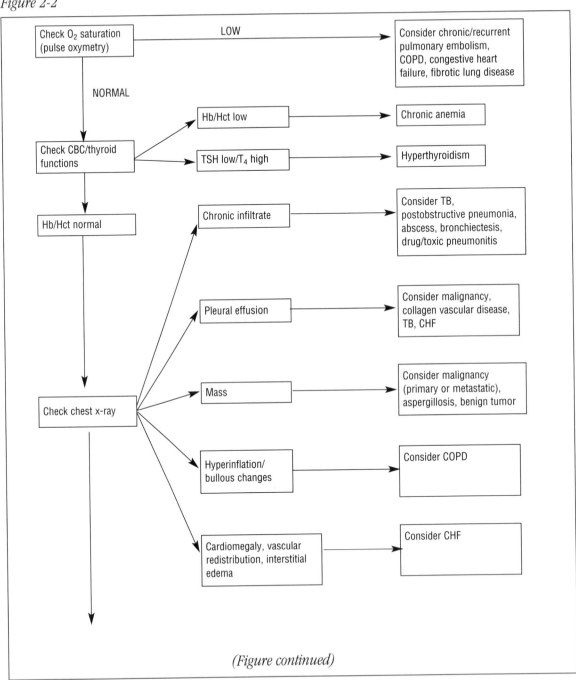

Suggested approach to chronic shortness of breath.
ABBREVIATIONS: COPD, chronic obstructive pulmonary disease; CBC, complete blood count; Hb/Hct, hemoglobin/hematocrit; TSH, thyroid stimulating hormone; TB, tuberculosis; CHF, congestive heart failure; DLCO, diffusion of the lung for carbon monoxide.

Figure 2-2 (Continued)

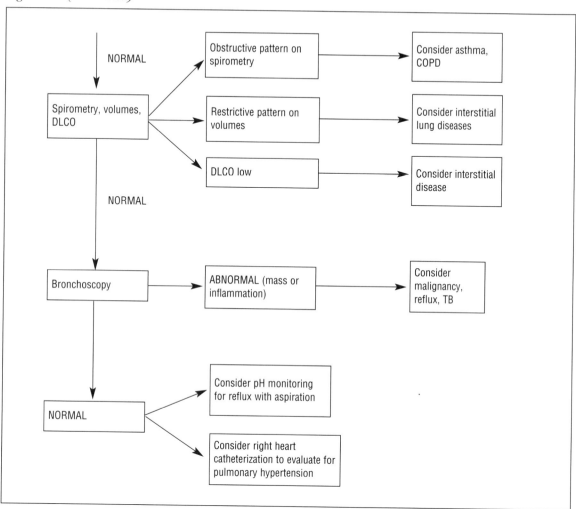

acute shortness of breath is measuring oxygen saturation with a pulse oxymeter. Pulse oxymetry is widely available, noninvasive, and reliable in providing oxygen saturation if used properly in a cooperative individual. Normal oxygen saturation levels in healthy individuals should be between 96 and 100 percent. Significant reductions in oxygen saturation indicate that oxygen transport to the bloodstream is the source of the problem. However, it should be noted that many patients with chronic obstructive pulmonary disease have decreased oxygen saturation levels on a chronic basis. If there is a question about the accuracy of a pulse oxymetry measurement, abnormal oxygen saturation can be confirmed with an arterial blood gas, which can determine ventilatory ability (from P_{CO_2}), acid-base status, and percentage of carboxyhemoglobin as well.

BLOOD TESTS

A complete blood count can be useful initially to test for anemia. In addition, if anemia is present, red cell indices can provide clues to the etiology of the anemia. The white cell count and platelets can be useful to determine whether other cell lines are depressed as well or whether the anemia is present because of leukemic suppression. Even when anemia is not present, a complete blood count is useful because the white cell count and differential can provide some indication of an infectious process.

CHEST X-RAY

In most patients with shortness of breath, a chest x-ray is the first imaging study that should be obtained. A plain x-ray can determine whether a pneumothorax is present, indicate the presence of a pleural effusion, show an infiltrate and the pattern of the infiltrate, provide information about interstitial disease, and detect the presence of cardiomegaly and pulmonary vascular congestion. Depending upon these findings, appropriate follow-up testing is indicated; this is discussed further in the chapters dedicated to specific pulmonary disorders.

ELECTROCARDIOGRAM AND ECHOCARDIOGRAM

In addition to a chest x-ray, patients who are at high risk for cardiac abnormalities should have a resting electrocardiogram (ECG). The ECG can provide greater precision in determining the heart rate and cardiac rhythm and provide additional data, including evidence for ventricular hypertrophy, acute ischemia, and past myocardial injury. In patients with possibly pathological murmurs on physical examination or evidence of chamber enlargement on the ECG, an echocardiogram can evaluate valvular function and estimate cardiac output.

PULMONARY FUNCTION TESTING

If the initial evaluation of the oxygen saturation, chest x-ray, complete blood count, and ECG are normal, pulmonary function testing may be useful. Included in this evaluation should be determination of forced expiratory volume in one second (FEV_1), forced expiratory volume

between 25 and 75 percent of the vital capacity (FEV_{25-75}), and total vital capacity (VC). For patients with suspected interstitial lung disease, a diffusion of the lung for carbon monoxide (DLCO) is useful. This test will be abnormal in conditions that alter the ability of gases to move across the arterial-alveolar barrier. More information about pulmonary function testing is provided in Chapter 3.

OTHER TESTS

If the pulmonary function tests are normal as well, further testing can include thyroid function testing, esophageal pH monitoring, and bronchoscopy. Bronchoscopy should be performed in any patient with hemoptysis or any other sign of pulmonary obstruction or inflammation, such as those with a chronic cough. If all of these tests are normal as well, alternative diagnoses such as generalized anxiety disorder or panic disorder should be considered.

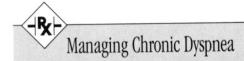

Managing Chronic Dyspnea

In nearly all cases, the approach to managing dyspnea is to identify the problem causing the shortness of breath and attempt to intervene. However, for many patients, such as those with severe chronic obstructive pulmonary disease, advanced pulmonary fibrosis, or dyspnea associated with cancer, treatment of the underlying problem is not an option. In these patients, management of dyspnea involves assisting patients with the anxiety and physical discomfort that accompanies shortness of breath.

A variety of modalities have been examined to determine if they can provide patients with chronic respiratory diseases with some relief from their sensation of feeling short of breath (Table 2-7). One useful measure is placing a fan so that air blows onto the patient's face.[9] It has been hypothesized that air moving over the face

Table 2-7

Approaches to Management of Chronic Dyspnea

> Nonpharmacologic interventions
>   Relaxation therapy
>   Supportive counseling
>   Music therapy
> Pharmacologic interventions
>   Morphine infusion
>   Chronic codeine therapy
>   Chronic promethazine therapy

stimulates trigeminal nerve cold receptors that somehow block the sensation of dyspnea.[10] Other nonpharmacologic approaches such as music therapy,[11] supportive and relaxation psychotherapy,[12] and progressive relaxation therapy[13] have been shown to be useful as well. Acupuncture also has been used to treat dyspnea,[14] but the evidence is conflicting as to whether there is any benefit to this modality or not.[15]

Pharmacological approaches to dyspnea are more limited. Physicians often prescribe benzodiazepines to treat the anxiety associated with shortness of breath, but there is little evidence that these drugs provide effective relief. For patients with end-stage disease, morphine has been shown to be effective at reducing both dyspnea symptoms and the anxiety that accompanies being short of breath.[16] Similar effects can be obtained by the use of chronic codeine or promethazine administration in ambulatory patients.[17]

References

1. Tack M, Altose MD, Cherniack NS: Effect of aging on respiratory sensations produced by elastic loads. *J Appl Physiol Respir Environ Exer Phys* 50:844–850, 1981.
2. Gulsvik A, Refvem OK: A scoring system on respiratory symptoms. *Eur Respir J* 1:428–432, 1988.
3. Rubin S, Tack M, Cherniack NS: Effect of aging on respiratory responses to CO_2 and inspiratory resistive loads. *J Gerontol* 37:306–312, 1982.
4. Krzyzanowski M, Robbins DR, Lebowitz MD: Smoking cessation and changes in respiratory symptoms in two populations followed for 13 years. *Int J Epidemiol* 22(4):666–673, 1993.
5. Nejjari C, Tessier JF, Dartigues JF, et al: The relationship between dyspnea and main lifetime occupation in the elderly. *Int J Epidemiol* 22:848–854, 1993.
6. Fishwick D, Bradshaw LM, D'Souza W, et al: Chronic bronchitis, shortness of breath, and airway obstruction by occupation in New Zealand. *Am J Respir Crit Care Med* 156:1440–1446, 1997.
7. Ripamonti C: Management of dyspnea in advanced cancer patients. *Supp Care Cancer* 7:233–243, 1999.
8. Schonfeld SA, Ployongsang Y, DiLisio R, et al: Fat embolism prophylaxis with corticosteroids: a prospective study in high-risk patients. *Ann Intern Med* 99:436–443, 1983.
9. LaGrand SB, Walsh D: Palliative management of dyspnea in advanced cancer. *Curr Opin Oncology* 11:25–34, 1999.
10. Burgess WR, Whitelaw WA: Effects of cold receptors on pattern of breathing. *J Appl Physiol* 64:371–376, 1988.
11. McBride S, Graydon J, Sidani S, Hall L: The therapeutic use of music for dyspnea and anxiety in patients with COPD who live at home. *J Holistic Nursing* 17:229–250, 1999.
12. Corner J, Plant H, A'Hern R, Bailey C: Non-pharmacological intervention for breathlessness in lung cancer. *Palliative Med* 10:299–305, 1996.
13. Renfroe KL: Effect of progressive relaxation on dyspnea and state anxiety in patients with chronic obstructive pulmonary disease. *Heart Lung* 17:408–413, 1988.
14. Filshie J, Penn K, Ashley S, Davis CL: Acupuncture for the relief of cancer-related breathlessness. *Palliative Med* 10:145–150, 1996.
15. Jobst KA: A critical analysis of acupuncture in pulmonary disease: efficacy and safety of the acupuncture needle. *J Alternat Complement Med* 1:57–85, 1995.
16. Cohen MH, Anderson AJ, Krasnow SH, et al: Continuous intravenous infusion of morphine for severe dyspnea. *South Med J* 84:229–234, 1991.
17. Ricc KL, Kronenberg RS, Hedemark LL, Niewoehner DE: Effects of chronic administration of codeine and promethazine on breathlessness and exercise tolerance in patients with chronic airflow obstruction. *Br J Dis Chest* 81:287–292, 1987.

Harold A. Williamson Jr.

Pulmonary Function Testing

Medical scientists since the time of Aristotle have attempted to quantify respiratory effort. Devices to measure both volume and flow rates have been constructed in order to better understand human anatomy, normal lung function, and disease states. John Hutchinson, a mid-nineteenth-century British physician, is generally regarded as the father of spirometry. By 1854, he had used a volumetric device to measure the lung capacities in 4000 subjects and had established the linear relationship between height and vital capacity.[1]

The basic mechanics of spirometric measurement changed little until technologic advances allowed the miniaturization of machines, and several decades of respiratory research enabled spirometry to help diagnose and manage diseases commonly encountered by family physicians.

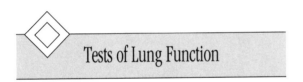

Tests of Lung Function

Although some measures of flow and volume are arcane and their interpretations subtle, the volumes and flow rates that are of most interest to physicians are quite straightforward.

Vital Capacity

Figure 3-1 shows some commonly used volumes and capacities. The most useful is the vital capacity, which is the total volume of exhaled air from deepest inspiration to total exhalation. This maneuver may be done in a leisurely manner but is usually done as part of a forced exhalation, which also allows measurement of expiratory flow rates.

Forced Expiratory Volume in 1 s (FEV₁)

Figure 3-2 shows the relationship between volume and time during a forced exhalation. The exhaled volume in 1 s (FEV_1) is the most useful measure for detecting obstruction.

Figure 3-3 shows the relationship between flow rates and volumes during a forced exhalation. This relationship creates a *flow-volume loop* of characteristic size and shape. Experienced pulmonologists can often arrive at a diagnosis from visualization of this curve. However, for clinicians less familiar with its use, numeric methods of organizing data are more useful.

Peak Expiratory Flow

Peak expiratory flow (PEF) is the maximum flow rate achieved during the forced exhalation

Figure 3-1

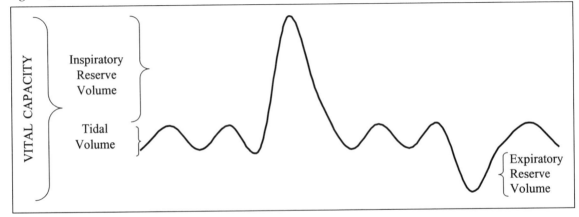

Lung capacity and volumes.

Figure 3-2

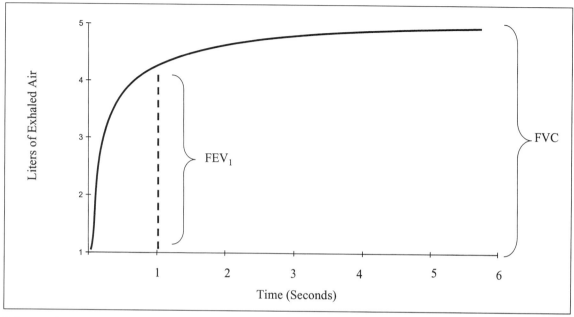

Volume and time.

(Fig. 3-3). PEF rates are reported as a part of standard spirometry but also can be measured using simple, inexpensive peak flow meters. Peak flow rates have been promoted as a way to help patients and clinicians monitor the course of asthma and in particular to detect early increases in obstruction. This is particularly helpful with asthmatic patients during the course of an acute viral respiratory illness or during allergy season. Much anecdotal evidence has fueled interest in the use of these meters. However, there is very little direct evidence that their routine use improves outcomes. Despite recommendations by prominent national consensus panels, primary care physicians have been slow to adopt routine spirometry PEF meters in practice.[2,3]

Some clinicians may be tempted to use peak expiratory rates in an office setting as a substitute for formal spirometry. Unfortunately, PEF is much more effort-dependent than FEV$_1$, and the range of normal is so broad as to minimize the utility of PEF for this purpose. On the other hand, reproducibility is very good for individual patients using one brand of peak flow meter over time. For these reasons, it is a practical monitoring device for patients with asthma, but not a good diagnostic tool.

Reversibility Testing with Bronchodilators

The addition of beta-agonist inhalation to standard spirometry allows an assessment of reversible obstruction. A baseline spirometric analysis is accomplished and followed by administration of an inhaled bronchodilator, either by a metered-dose inhaler or by a nebulizer. After 15 min, spirometry is repeated. An improvement in FEV$_1$ of 10 to 15 percent is considered a positive response, i.e., diagnostic of reversible airway disease. In the absence of an acute viral infection, this degree of improvement in FEV$_1$ is sufficient evidence for a diagnosis of asthma. Although a positive response suggests that bronchodilators will be clinically useful, a negative response does not rule out the use of a

Figure 3-3

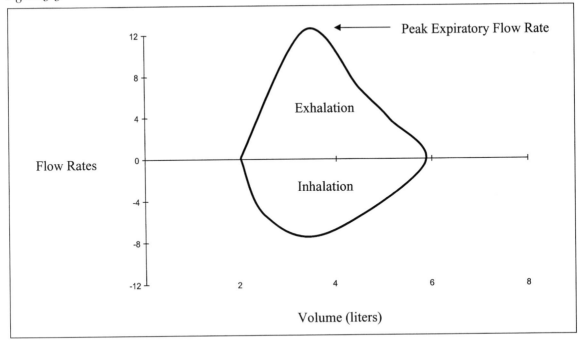

Flow-volume loop.

bronchodilator. Sometimes days or weeks of bronchodilator therapy is required before a benefit is confirmed.

Challenge Testing

Challenge testing allows the diagnosis of reversible airway obstruction in more subtle cases. A variety of potentially inciting stimuli (allergens, methacholine, histamine, exercise, cold air) can be used as a challenge test in an individual with undiagnosed dyspnea, cough, or wheeze. Normal individuals experience a decline in FEV_1 when exposed to these stimuli at high concentrations, but individuals with asthma respond to lower challenge doses. Such challenge testing should probably be limited to pulmonary function laboratories, where potential adverse effects

are more easily managed and where personnel are familiar with interpretation of the results.

Numerous other capacities, volumes, and flow rates are measurable and are occasionally of use in subtle or borderline conditions. They do not add much value in a primary care setting.

Instruments to Measure Lung Volumes and Flow

Advances in technology have reduced the size and cost of pulmonary function testing machines, making spirometry accessible to many office practices where the patient volume is adequate and trained office staff are available.

There are two main types of spirometers: volume sensing and flow sensing. Volume-sensing spirometers accumulate and measure exhaled air using a rubber bellows, a rolling seal, or a water seal. Traditionally, a tracing is recorded as exhaled air in the volume device moves a pen across a paper graph, from which volume and flows can be hand-calculated (e.g., Fig. 3-2). Most modern machines produce an automated analysis using an internal microprocessor or an attachment to a desktop computer.

Flow-sensing devices use one of several methods to measure the flow rates of exhaled air and integrate these data with the time of exhalation to provide an automated printout of preselected volumes and flow rates. This type of machine has gained favor for office use because of its smaller size, ease of use, lower cost, and disposable parts, which minimize cleaning and maintenance.

Regardless of the type of unit used, office spirometers, like those based in hospitals or pulmonary clinics, require maintenance and frequent calibration and should be operated by trained personnel.

A consensus statement from the National Lung Health Education Program calls for the development of spirometers that are designed specifically for office practices.[4] This projected new category of machines for use in the office will be distinguished from the sophisticated diagnostic-quality spirometers used in hospitals and other settings where formal testing usually takes place. Since most office practices do not need the level of sophistication present in these more expensive machines, office-based spirometers may make spirometry more accessible and affordable for patients in the ambulatory setting.

In addition to calling for the development of office-based spirometers, the National Lung Health Education Program also recommends replacing the currently used forced vital capacity (FVC) with FEV_6 (forced expiratory volume in 6 s). This change is recommended because measurement errors in FVC occur most often as a result of failed attempts at a full exhalation between

6 and 10 s. Establishing FEV_6 as the standard would eliminate this uncertainty. Instead of the FEV_1/FVC ratio being used for assessing pulmonary function, the new FEV_1/FEV_6 would become the standard for obstructive airway disease.

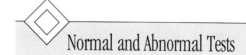

Normal and Abnormal Tests

Several factors other than disease influence lung function and affect test variability. In order of importance, these are gender, height, ethnicity, and age.[5] Most automated spirometers adjust for these variables when reporting the patient's performance versus a norm.

Rigorous standards for the performance and interpretation of spirometry have been proposed, revised, and updated by the American Thoracic Society (ATS).[6] Physicians who plan to include spirometry in their office practice should be familiar with these guidelines and should recognize that their attainment in an office practice is not easy.

Pulmonary function testing in infants and children is technically difficult, and interpretation of spirograms in these age groups requires experience.[7] Performance of such tests in a laboratory that is familiar with testing young children is preferable. Most adolescents, however, can be tested successfully in a well-equipped and experienced primary care office.

The traditional normal values for the FEV_1/FVC ratio were defined as 0.7 to 0.75. This is generally expressed as a percentage of FEV_1 to FVC of 70 to 75 percent. While most spirometry units will calculate a single predicted value for a given age and height, the actual normal range for other flows and volumes is defined as the predicted value plus or minus 20 percent of this value. For example, patients should be considered normal if their FEV_1 is 80 percent or more of the predicted value. Predicted values are based on either literal or electronic nomograms and are adjusted for height, gender, and race. Experts on pulmonary function testing acknowledge that establishing norms in such a way is arbitrary and does not allow a clinician to understand the patient's lung function in a comparative, quantitative fashion. Using predicted values also overestimates disease in tall and young individuals.[5] Therefore, experts are now calling for a change in the definition of norms such that percentiles of performance are reported instead of using the predicted value.

When discussing results with patients, the concept of "80 percent of predicted" is especially problematic. Therefore, some find it helpful to define respiratory obstruction for patients in qualitative terms, such as "mild obstruction" (60 to 70 percent of predicted), "moderate obstruction" (50 to 60 percent of predicted), and "severe obstruction" (less than 50 percent of predicted).

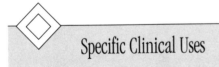

Specific Clinical Uses

Figure 3-4 shows a simplified algorithm for interpreting spirometry. Unfortunately, in clinical practice, the use of spirometry is not always so straightforward.

Keeping in mind the patient's clinical presentation, the first step in interpretation is usually evaluating whether obstruction is present. This is done by determining the FEV_1/FVC ratio. If this ratio is lower than 70 percent, obstruction is present. If the obstruction is reversible with a beta-agonist inhalation, asthma is the most likely diagnosis. Patients with chronic obstructive pulmonary disease (COPD) may have reversibility, but it is usually minor.

If the FEV_1/FVC ratio is greater than 70 percent but the FVC is low, a restrictive defect is indicated. As discussed later in this chapter, a restrictive pattern on spirometry can have a num-

ber of causes, and detection of this pattern should trigger careful evaluation using other diagnostic modalities.

Asthma

Spirometry may be needed to make the initial diagnosis and is sometimes helpful to follow the course of the disease—particularly response to medications.

Airway wall thickening and inflammation resulting in airway hyperactivity is the hallmark of asthma. Most symptomatic patients with asthma demonstrate obstruction on spirometry, with at least some degree of reversibility after bronchodilator. However, it is important to remember that airway hyperactivity is often transient in patients with asthma, and therefore spirometry may be normal within hours of a clear-cut "asthma attack." It is also true that patients with asthma may appear to have a fixed obstruction (i.e., they do not respond acutely to an inhaled bronchodilator), but marked improvement in obstruction may follow prolonged treatment with anti-inflammatories and bronchodilators.

Chronic Obstructive Pulmonary Disease

Normal nonsmokers show a gradual loss of FEV_1 over time of about 1 percent per year. Some cigarette smokers, those who are destined to develop COPD, experience a decline in lung function that is five times more rapid than normal. Many years before the development of dyspnea, most COPD patients exhibit an accelerated decline in FEV_1 that is detectable by serial spirometry. For this reason, many practitioners recommend periodic spirometric evaluation of smokers, even those without symptoms. The ratio FEV_1/FVC is the most appropriate indicator of developing COPD.

Aside from diagnosis, spirometry is helpful in following the course of emphysema and chronic bronchitis and measuring the response to med-

Figure 3-4

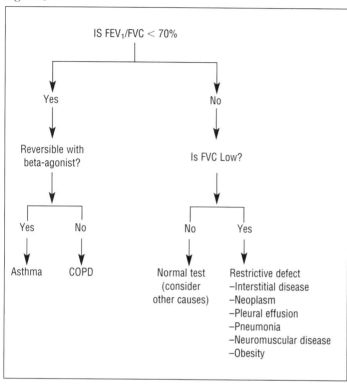

Patient with respiratory symptoms and a technically acceptable spirogram.
ABBREVIATIONS: FVC, forced vital capacity; COPD, chronic obstructive
pulmonary disease.

ication, and perhaps in counseling smokers about cessation efforts.

Patients with COPD may have some element of reversibility on spirometry and therefore may occasionally be difficult to distinguish from those with asthma. Patients with severe COPD may also exhibit an element of restrictive defect with a decline in FVC, probably as a result of lung scarring.

Restrictive Disorders

A low FVC with a normal FEV_1/FVC ratio should raise suspicion of disease causing a restrictive defect. Restrictive patterns should be interpreted with caution, however, particularly outside of an experienced laboratory.

Evaluation of a restrictive defect should include consideration of intrinsic lung diseases, such as pneumonia, sarcoid, and interstitial fibrosis. Chest wall disorders, obesity, pleural effusion, and severe kyphoscoliosis also may cause a restrictive defect. Neuromuscular diseases such as spinal cord injuries and myasthenia gravis may lead to volume changes on spirometry. Finally, congestive heart failure should be considered in a patient with a restrictive defect on spirometry.

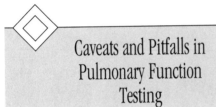

Caveats and Pitfalls in Pulmonary Function Testing

Despite general agreement that primary care physicians underutilize spirometric testing, a number of studies suggest caution in recommending widespread use of spirometry in office practices. Several studies indicate that spirometry in office settings lacks quality control and that ATS guidelines are infrequently met in clinical practice.[8,9] Furthermore, research has demonstrated a substantial discrepancy between primary care physicians' interpretations of spirometry and those of pulmonologists.[9,10]

Specific training for office staff and physicians is often recommended. One study found that training was successful at standardizing tests, but that the quality of the spirometry still did not generally satisfy ATS criteria for acceptability and reproducibility.[9] Consequently, primary care physicians are faced with a dilemma. Referral of patients to another facility such as a hospital for formal pulmonary function testing is inconvenient. Formal testing also increases the cost of pulmonary function testing. On the other hand, the quality of tests performed in the usual office setting does not seem to meet current standards, and interpretations of the test by primary care physicians may be lacking. Early detection of COPD, accurate diagnosis of asthma, and efficient evaluation of respiratory symptoms are all deemed important responsibilities of primary care physicians, but primary care physicians may have to carefully select patients for study in order to balance the cost and inconvenience of testing with the likely benefits.

As a response to this dilemma, a recent consensus statement from the National Lung Health Education Program has called for the development of office spirometry standards that differ from those in pulmonary laboratories.[4] Machines that coach patients and technicians through instructive displays (e.g., "insufficient duration of exhalation," "blow harder") may reduce testing variability and improve our ability to reliably assess respiratory symptoms.

As with other forms of medical testing, clinicians rarely make a diagnosis from spirometry alone. Spirometry is most useful when it is understood in the context of the patient's clinical presentation and the clinician's evaluation. Spirometry is a valuable adjunct in evaluating symptoms and following the course of respiratory disease but is rarely used as a stand-alone evaluation.

References

1. Spriggs EA: The history of spirometry. *Br J Dis Chest* 72:165–180, 1978.
2. Fried RA, Miller RS, Green LA, et al: The use of objective measures of asthma severity in primary care: a report from ASPN. *J Fam Pract* 41:139–143, 1995.
3. Picken HA, Greenfield S, Teres D, et al: Effect of local standards on the implementation of national guidelines for asthma. *J Gen Intern Med* 13:659–663, 1998.
4. Ferguson GT, Enright PL, Buist AS, et al: Special report: office spirometry for lung health in adults: a consensus statement from the National Lung Health Education Program. *Chest* 117:1146–1161, 2000.
5. Crapo RO: Pulmonary function testing, in Baum GL, Crapo JD, Celli BR, Karlinsky JB (eds): *Textbook of Pulmonary Diseases*, 6th ed. Philadelphia, Lippincott-Raven, 1998.
6. American Thoracic Society: Standardization of spirometry: 1994 update. *Am J Respir Crit Care Med* 152:1107–1136, 1995.
7. Pfaff JK, Morgan WJ: Pulmonary function in infants and children. *Pediatr Clin North Am* 41:401–423, 1994.
8. Dowson LJ, Yeung A, Allen MB: General practice spirometry in North Staffordshire. *Arch Monaldi* 54:186–188, 1999.

9. Eaton T, Withy S, Garrett J, et al: Spirometry in primary care practice: the importance of quality assurance and the impact of spirometry workshops. *Chest* 116:416–423, 1999.

10. Hnatiuk O, Moores L, Loughney T, Torrington K: Evaluation of internists' spirometric interpretations. *J Gen Intern Med* 11:204–208, 1996.

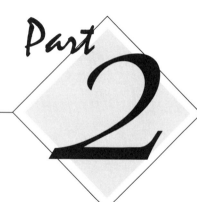

Part

2

Upper
Respiratory
Infections

William J. Hueston
Arch G. Mainous III

Chapter

4

Common Cold

Management of uncomplicated upper respiratory tract infections (URIs) has always been challenging. For years, there have been unsuccessful efforts to identify cures for these infections. Out of frustration at the unavailability of agents to fight these infections, clinicians have often resorted to prescribing antibiotics in an effort to please patients and in the belief that antibiotics might prevent potential complications. For some providers, antibiotics are expensive placebos for URIs. The recent increase in antibiotic-resistant bacteria has made this approach less desirable.[1] The use of antibiotics in circumstances in which they are ineffective (e.g., viral illnesses) creates an environment for the development of antibiotic-resistant bacteria, placing both populations and individual patients at risk. Thus, appropriate treatment of acute respiratory tract infections has become a challenge for both patients and health care providers.

Colds seem like a trivial clinical problem, but they have a big effect on both primary care practices and health care expenses. Although they are self-limited illnesses, URIs are among the most common reasons for visits to a clinician and account for significant absenteeism from work and school. The direct cost to the health care system for URIs only starts with the physician office visit. There may be additional costs for microbiologic and laboratory diagnostic tests that are of dubious clinical value.[2] The direct costs for colds also include treatment. The vast majority of prescribed antibiotics are given for the outpatient treatment of respiratory tract infections, and this contributes significantly to the huge cost of care associated with colds.[3] Not only are antibiotics prescribed frequently (and unnecessarily) for colds, but Americans spend another $1 to $2 billion annually on the more than 800 over-the-counter cough and cold preparations.[4,5]

Respiratory tract infections can exist throughout the respiratory tract, with inflammation and involvement of the mucosal surfaces of the individual's nose, sinuses, throat, ears, and chest. Many diagnoses used for respiratory tract infections have significant symptom overlap with others (e.g., acute sinusitis and common cold; common cold and acute bronchitis).[6] The inflammatory response to the pathogen produces swelling, discharge, and local pain. Different pathogens are more common at certain sites than others, thereby providing a guide for treatment.

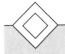

Epidemiology

URIs are a common infectious condition. Adults typically have two to four URIs each year, and children in day care have as many as six or seven.[7,8] Although URIs are mild, tend to get better on their own, and are of short duration, they are a leading cause of sickness and of industrial and school absenteeism. Each year, URIs account for 170 million days of restricted activity, 23 million days of school absence, and 18 million days of work absence.[9]

The transmission of pathogens associated with URIs commonly occurs through contact with inanimate objects[10] like playing cards as well as through direct hand-to-hand contact like that which occurs with a handshake.[11] URIs have a seasonal variation; in the United States, there is an increased prevalence between September and March. It is unclear why this variation exists, although it may be related to increased crowding of indoor populations in the colder months. Temperature is not the key to seasonal variation without the presence of a pathogen. Evidence from Antarctica shows that spacious, well-ventilated rooms reduce transmission of colds compared to crowded, poorly ventilated rooms, regardless of temperature.[12]

Pathophysiology/Etiology

A recent study established that the vast majority of colds are caused by viruses.[13] Rhinoviruses were the most common type of virus, found in 53 percent of the patients (Table 4-1). Coronaviruses were the second most common cause. Identified bacterial pathogens were *Chlamydia pneumoniae, Haemophilus influenzae, Streptococcus pneumoniae,* and *Mycoplasma pneumoniae.* In terms of bacterial pathogens, infections without evidence of a viral infection occurred in only 0.05 percent of the cases.

Viral respiratory infections are rarely severe enough to require hospitalization. However, this is not true for patients with severe underlying pulmonary problems, in whom respiratory viral infections can result in acute respiratory compromise that requires hospitalization.[14] Patients from lower-income populations with chronic underlying pulmonary illnesses are at greatest risk for severe compromise associated with a viral respiratory infection.

Finally, many patients tell their doctors that they are "susceptible" or "prone" to URIs. Greater susceptibility to respiratory viruses appears to be based on genetic factors related to processes that mediate host defenses against

Table 4-1

Causes of Colds in 200 Patients in Finland

Rhinovirus	53%
Coronavirus	9%
Influenza virus	6%
Other viruses	2%
No cause established	31%

From Makela MJ et al,[13] with permission.
Note: Total may exceed 100% because patients may have more than one virus.

viruses.[15] It is thought that these defenses are most vulnerable between the ages of 6 and 17 months of life, when URIs may be more common and may result in complications such as otitis media.

Diagnosis

URIs are often thought to be of short duration, but symptoms actually can last 12 to 14 days. In a study looking at the effectiveness of a saline nasal spray for URIs, Adam and colleagues found that the median time for recovery from an uncomplicated cold is 15.5 days.[16] Telling patients that colds last no longer than a week underestimates the actual natural history of an uncomplicated viral respiratory tract infection and leads patients to believe that symptoms persisting beyond a week are not normal.

Nasal Discharge

In general, early in the development of a URI, the nasal discharge is clear. As more inflammation develops, the discharge may take on some coloration. Yellow-, green-, or brown-tinted nasal discharge is an indicator of inflammation, not of secondary bacterial infection. Discolored nasal discharge does raise the likelihood of a sinusitis being present, but the presence of discolored nasal discharge alone in the absence of other signs of sinusitis is a weak predictor of bacterial infection. In their study of predictors of sinusitis, Williams and Simel found that patients with only one predictor (such as discolored nasal discharge) were three times less likely to have sinusitis than not to have it.[17] In the presence of other signs of sinusitis, though, discolored discharge may be a useful sign. A number of studies have shown that patients with discolored discharge do not appear to respond to antibiotics any better than they respond to placebos.[18,19]

Despite the evidence that the presence of discolored discharge does not indicate a more serious infection, patients place a great deal of emphasis on the color of their discharge. While healthy people in the community do not think that they should go to the doctor for a URI, Mainous and colleagues observed that many individuals report that when the nasal discharge becomes colored, they feel that they should seek care from a clinician.[20] More educated individuals recognized the symptoms of a URI when the scenario had clear discharge, but when it was changed to include discolored discharge, they believed that they should consult a doctor. So it appears that patients understand that they do not need to consult their doctor when they have a simple cold, but they are not aware that a discolored discharge is a common finding with a cold.

Follow-up studies have indicated that primary care physicians would prescribe antibiotics for individuals with symptoms consistent with a URI who had discolored nasal discharge.[21] So, it seems that not only are patients not certain of the symptoms of a cold, but they are not receiving appropriate advice from their health care providers.

Differential Diagnosis

The differential diagnosis of colds includes complications of the cold such as sinusitis or otitis media, acute bronchitis, and noninfectious rhinitis (Table 4-2).

SINUSITIS

Differentiating sinusitis from URIs can be difficult and is made more complex by the observation that computed tomography (CT) scans of patients with uncomplicated colds show that

Table 4-2

Differential Diagnosis for Congestion and Rhinorrhea

Common cold
Sinusitis
Viral
Allergic
Bacterial
Fungal
Seasonal allergic rhinitis
Vasomotor rhinitis
Rhinitis secondary to alpha-agonist withdrawal
Drug-induced rhinitis (e.g., cocaine)
Nasal foreign body

about half (47 percent) have evidence of sinus mucosal thickening consistent with sinus inflammation.[22] However, most of these patients do not develop signs and symptoms of bacterial sinusitis, and their colds resolve just like those of patients without sinus inflammation. Therefore, sinus tenderness or a "fullness" in the sinuses can be a common complaint of patients with colds, but is not indicative of acute bacterial sinusitis.

Williams and Simel studied a variety of patient symptoms and physical examination findings and determined which of these were associated with sinusitis as diagnosed by sinus x-ray.[17] In their study, four factors in combination increased the diagnosis of sinusitis (listed in order of strength of the association): maxillary toothache (positive likelihood ratio of 2.5); purulent secretions visualized (positive likelihood ratio of 2.1); poor response to decongestants (positive likelihood ratio of 2.1); abnormal transillumination (positive likelihood ratio of 1.6); and history of colored nasal discharge (positive likelihood ratio of 1.5). Combining the factors was most useful in predicting sinusitis, as shown in Table 4-3. As shown in Table 4-3, having two of these factors does not alter the likelihood of patients' having sinusitis. Having just one or none of them reduces the chance that the patient has sinusitis. It is only when three or four are present that the

Table 4-3

Likelihood Ratio for Sinusitis Based on the Number of Signs and Symptoms Present

NUMBER OF SIGNS AND SYMPTOMS PRESENT	LIKELIHOOD RATIO OF HAVING SINUSITIS
4	6.4
3	2.6
2	1.1
1	0.5
0	0.1

Adapted from Williams JW, Simel DL,[17] with permission.

history and physical examination findings are useful in raising the likelihood that a person has sinusitis.

Other studies have examined additional potential predictors for sinusitis. In a study of patients with sinusitis confirmed by CT scanning, it was found that so-called double sickening—that is, patients with colds experiencing mild symptoms for a few days followed by a period where they get sicker—also predicted sinusitis.[23] These investigators also found that purulent rhinorrhea or the presence of purulent material in the nose was helpful, as was an elevated sedimentation rate.

It should be emphasized, though, that not all sinusitis is bacterial. Indeed, most cases of sinusitis are probably viral in origin. Many patients with acute sinusitis associated with a cold have viral inflammation of the sinuses and will get better with no antibiotic therapy. While the absolute percentage of patients with viral sinusitis is difficult to know, estimates from the placebo arms of studies show that between about 60 and 75 percent of adults[24,25] and 43 percent of children[26] get better within 10 days. In most studies, antibiotics have achieved higher success rates, presumably indicating that some patients do have bacterial infections that are responsive to antibiotics. Yet even in the antibiotic arms of these trials, response rates have only been in the 70 to 80 percent range for adults and the 60 to 65 percent range for children.

Differentiating viral from bacterial sinusitis is difficult. One group of investigators examined signs and symptoms of sinusitis as confirmed by the presence of purulent material obtained on aspiration of the maxillary sinus. In this study, none of the symptoms or signs that are associated with radiologic evidence of sinusitis predicted a positive aspirate. Only an elevated sedimentation rate and raised C-reactive protein levels predicted purulent material on aspiration.[27]

While the symptoms and physical findings associated with sinusitis are limited in that they do not necessarily predict bacterial sinusitis, studies have shown that clinicians still rely on these symptoms and signs when diagnosing sinusitis. Most evidence shows that clinicians rely on sinus tenderness, sinus pressure, discolored discharge, and a prior history of sinusitis in making their diagnosis, even though none of these factors indicate the presence of sinusitis.[28,29]

ACUTE BRONCHITIS

Acute bronchitis refers to an infection in the lower respiratory tract, but it has symptoms that often overlap with those of a URI. In a survey of family physicians, Oeffinger and colleagues found little consensus about what symptoms define acute bronchitis.[30] For example, 58 percent of physicians required a productive cough, while 39 percent stated that whether or not the cough was productive did not matter. Variation also existed based on the experience of the clinician and whether he or she practiced in a community or academic setting. In contrast to Oeffinger's findings, a similar survey of physicians in the Netherlands suggested that clinicians did not rely on any specific sign or symptom, but rather relied on the total number of symptoms to differentiate acute bronchitis from a cold.[31]

The lack of a true definition of what constitutes acute bronchitis probably contributes to a great deal of overdiagnosis of this problem and the prescribing of antibiotics for common colds.

The amount of overlap between acute bronchitis and colds has even led some investigators to suggest that the two are not separate entities but represent different ends of a spectrum of virally mediated respiratory infections.[6] The only possible value in differentiating acute bronchitis from a cough associated with a URI is that albuterol has been shown to reduce the duration of a cough associated with acute bronchitis,[32,33] whereas it does not appear to be useful in nonspecific coughs associated with URIs.[34]

NONINFECTIOUS RHINITIS

In addition to these other respiratory infections, noninfectious problems also can cause significant rhinorrhea similar to that caused by a URI. These include allergic reactions, rhinitis secondary to withdrawal of topical nasal vasoconstrictors, and foreign bodies in the nasal cavity.

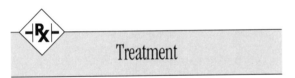

Treatment

Before discussing treatment strategies for patients with colds, it should be pointed out that most patients with URIs do not come to the doctor. In one Canadian community-based study, only 1 percent of people reported seeking care from a physician for a recent cold.[35] The people who were most likely to seek care for a cold were those who had multiple symptoms or who felt that the symptoms were lasting longer than expected.

Antibiotic Therapy

Despite the viral cause of URIs, several studies have shown that the majority of cases of URIs that are seen by doctors are treated with antibiotics.[36,37] Randomized controlled trials of antibiotic treatment of URIs have consistently demonstrated no benefit from taking antibi-

otics.[18,38–41] In a meta-analysis of the use of antibiotics for colds, no benefit was found to support the use of antibiotics, and an increase in side effects was found with their use.[42]

The concern about the use of antibiotics for URIs comes amidst evidence that in both the United States and Great Britain, antibiotic use has risen considerably in the last two decades.[3,43] This has occurred despite the fact that clinicians recognize that not all antibiotic prescriptions are essential. In one British study, general practitioners admitted that one-third of 1089 patients for whom antibiotics had been prescribed probably did not need them.[44] This is in addition to another 20 percent for whom the physicians confessed that antibiotics clearly were not needed!

A study of patients' attitudes toward colds showed that most patients recognized that a visit to the doctor was not necessary if they had a cold and that most people with colds do not come to see a clinician.[45] When they do come to see a clinician, however, they may have expectations regarding the treatment they would like to receive. For example, when researchers have surveyed patients who come to the doctor for upper respiratory symptoms, between 30 and 60 percent of parents of children or adult patients with colds said that they expect antibiotics.[46,47] Adults who think that antibiotics will be helpful tend to believe that they have a severe cold that has lasted too long or have received antibiotics for cold before.[46] Others also have found that one of the key factors influencing patients' belief that antibiotics are necessary is having received antibiotics for similar viral problems in the past.[48] Therefore, one of the best ways to discourage patients from coming to the doctor for antibiotics for their cold is to not get them into the habit of doing so in the first place. Also reassuring, though, is evidence that if the doctor spends some time explaining that the illness is caused by a virus and that antibiotics will not work, patients are satisfied.[47] Even patients who come to the doctor expecting an antibiotic are satisfied; in fact, they are just as satisfied with their care as those who came to the doctor not expecting an antibiotic.

A final strategy to reduce antibiotic use for colds has been to provide patients with a "backup" prescription for them to fill only if they feel that they are not getting better. Researchers who have tested the use of a backup prescription have found that only about 50 percent of patients report that they get the prescription filled during their illness episode.[49] The researchers' interpretation of these data is that providing backup prescriptions reduces antibiotic use because the remaining half of the patients who received a backup prescription did not receive an antibiotic. However, it should be remembered that *none* of these people actually needed an antibiotic. Those that filled the backup prescription represent a population that should not have received antibiotics in the first place. Because of the harm done by injudicious antibiotic use for patients with viral illnesses, providing patients with an antibiotic prescription, even if the prescription is not filled right away, does not appear to be a responsible solution.

In addition to promoting antibiotic resistance, antibiotic use constitutes a fairly substantial percentage of the cost of care for an episode of illness. When the billing claims for patients covered by Medicaid were examined, it was found that antibiotics alone were responsible for 23 percent of the total cost of the episode for patients diagnosed with a cold.[50] Based on one observation of antibiotic use in patients with URIs, it is believed that over $37 million a year is spent on antibiotics for Medicaid patients diagnosed with the common cold in just one state.[36] While there is some evidence that patients who receive antibiotics for colds are less likely to return for a second visit in the next month, the difference (17 percent for people who do not receive antibiotics versus 15 percent for those who do) is very small.[51] The same estimates indicate that physicians would have to treat 59 adults or 30 children with an antibiotic to prevent one patient with a cold from making a follow-up visit. So antibiotics are neither cheap nor very

effective at keeping patients from returning for unresolved symptoms.

Finally, some physicians justify their use of antibiotics for colds by suggesting that this strategy will reduce the likelihood of a complication such as sinusitis or otitis media. However, there is no evidence that early treatment of a cold with antibiotics prevents development of otitis media, sinusitis, or other complications.[39] In fact, the overuse of antibiotics for upper respiratory infections that are presumably caused by viruses has been linked to the development of drug-resistant bacteria. In regions that have successfully reduced the use of antibiotics for viral respiratory conditions, the rates of resistance of *Streptococcus pneumoniae* have been reduced.[52,53]

Alternatives to Antibiotics

DECONGESTANTS

A variety of alternatives to antibiotics for colds have been investigated and have their advocates, if not strong evidence of their effectiveness. Currently, the most effective symptomatic treatments are over-the-counter decongestants.[55] The most popular decongestants include pseudoephedrine hydrochloride and phenylpropanolamine. However, the Food and Drug Administration recently asked companies to voluntarily pull phenylpropanolamine off the market because of studies suggesting a link between its use and hemorrhagic strokes, especially in young women.

Also beneficial are topical nasal decongestants. These agents contain vasoconstrictors that reduce nasal edema and discharge. Unfortunately, long-term use of these agents can result in rebound edema and discharge (rhinitis medicamentosa). However, their use for a few days can bring relief to those whose most troublesome cold symptom is nasal congestion.

ANTIHISTAMINES

Antihistamines, with a few exceptions, have not been shown to be effective treatments.

Therefore, the use of over-the-counter antihistamines such as diphenhydramine and chlorpheniramine should not be recommended for treating the common cold.[4,54,55] There are also a number of over-the-counter medications that contain a mix of decongestants, cough suppressants, and pain relievers. Again, the use of these preparations will not cure the common cold, but it will provide symptomatic relief.

ANTICHOLINERGICS

Ipratropium bromide nasal spray also has been shown to reduce nasal discharge in patients with colds. In a double-blinded study using nasal ipratropium spray or saline, patients in the ipratropium group had less rhinorrhea and sneezing, although they had similar amounts of congestion.[56] The higher strength of ipratropium (0.06%) is indicated for use with colds, while the lower strength (0.03%) is used for allergic rhinitis. The lower strength is approved for children as well as adults, but the higher strength used for colds is approved only for ages 12 and up. In addition, ipratropium should be avoided or used with caution in patients who are likely to experience complications from anticholinergic therapy, such as those with narrow-angle glaucoma or those at risk for urinary retention.

VITAMINS AND MINERAL SUPPLEMENTS

Vitamins and minerals have also been suggested as a remedy for the common cold. Systematic reviews of the literature provide only weak support for the effectiveness of vitamin C.[57] However, many people (including the late Nobel laureate Linus Pauling) advocate the use of vitamin C as a stimulant for the immune system. As for minerals, zinc gluconate lozenges are available without a prescription and have been suggested as effective in decreasing the duration of the common cold.[58] However, a meta-analysis that combined 15 previous studies on zinc concluded that zinc lozenges were not effective in reducing the duration of cold symptoms.[59,60]

HERBAL MEDICINES

Some herbal medicines are also useful for treatment of the common cold. Echinacea, also known as the American coneflower, has been purported to reduce the duration of the common cold by stimulating the immune system. The evidence for its use, however, is mixed. A systematic review of 16 studies conducted prior to 1998 indicated that the majority of available studies report positive results of echinacea.[61] However, three randomized placebo-controlled trials that were published subsequent to that article showed no benefit from echinacea.[62–64] If one considers using echinacea, it should be used only for a period of 2 to 3 weeks to avoid liver damage and other possible side effects that have been reported with the long-term use of this herb.

Another herbal remedy that is useful in treating the symptoms of the common cold is ephedra, also known as ma huang. This herb has decongestant properties that make it similar to pseudoephedrine. However, ephedra is more likely than pseudoephedrine to cause increased blood pressure and tachyarrhythmias. This is especially true if it is used in conjunction with caffeine.

Other herbal remedies that have been suggested to be useful in treatment of the common cold include goldenseal, yarrow, eyebright, and elderflower. However, no systematic evidence supports the use of these herbs for the common cold.

HOMEOPATHIC REMEDIES

There are also homeopathic remedies that can be used to reduce the duration and severity of URIs. The most common of these is *Zincum Gluconicum.* Preliminary studies suggest that patients who used this preparation resolved their symptoms faster than those on a placebo.

A commonly used nutritional therapy for URIs that has been the focus of discussions both in scientific communities and around dinner tables is chicken soup. A recent study suggests that chicken soup inhibits neutrophil chemotaxis, a physiological activity associated with URIs.[65] The mild anti-inflammatory effect of chicken soup may make it an effective treatment for URIs.

Complications

The primary complications from upper respiratory tract infection are otitis media and sinusitis. As noted in other chapters, these conditions arise from closure of the middle ear space or sinuses as a result of edema in the nasal passages. Accumulation of fluid can give rise to bacterial infections in the middle ear or sinuses. Treatment of these infections with antibiotics is common, but the vast majority of them clear without antibiotic therapy.

One misconception is that these complications can be prevented by using antibiotics during the acute phase of a cold. Evidence shows that using antibiotics during a cold does not reduce the incidence of sinusitis or otitis media.

Prevention

As stated previously, the mechanisms of transmission suggest that colds can be spread through contact with inanimate surfaces,[10] but that the primary transmission mechanism appears to be hand-to-hand contact.[11] Attention to removing viruses from the hands is supported by observations that children in day care or school settings have been shown to reduce school absences from colds through the use of antiseptic hand wipes throughout the day.[66] Rather than focusing on treatment, physicians can have a big impact on the spread of colds by encouraging patients to wash their hands frequently.

References

1. Tenover FC, Hughes JM: The challenge of emerging infectious diseases: development and spread of multiply resistant bacterial pathogens. *JAMA* 275:300–304, 1996.
2. Carroll K, Reimer L: Microbiology and laboratory diagnosis of upper respiratory tract infections. *Clin Infect Dis* 23:442–448, 1996.
3. McCaig LF, Hughes JM: Trends in antimicrobial drug prescribing among office-based physicians in the United States. *JAMA* 273:214–219, 1995.
4. Smith MBH, Feldman W: Over-the-counter cold medications: a critical review of clinical trials between 1950 and 1991. *JAMA* 269:2258–2263, 1993.
5. Kogan MD, Pappas G, Yu SM, Kotelchuck M: Over-the-counter medication use among US preschool-age children. *JAMA* 272:1025–1030, 1994.
6. Hueston WJ, Mainous AG III, Dacus EN, Hopper JE: Does acute bronchitis really exist? A reconceptualization of acute viral respiratory infections. *J Fam Pract* 49:401–406, 2000.
7. Croughan-Minihane MS, Petitti DB, Rodnick JE, Eliaser G: Clinical trial examining effectiveness of three cough syrups. *J Am Board Fam Pract* 6:109–115, 1993.
8. Sperber SJ, Levine PA, Sorrentino JV, et al: Ineffectiveness of recombinant interferon-beta serine nasal drops for prophylaxis of natural colds. *J Infect Dis* 160:700–705, 1989.
9. Adams PF, Hendershot GE, Marano MA: Current estimates from the National Health Interview Survey, 1996. National Center for Health Statistics. *Vital Health Stat* [10] 200, 1999.
10. Sattar SA, Jacobsen H, Springthorpe VS, et al: Chemical disinfection to interrupt transfer of rhinovirus type 14 from environmental surfaces to hands. *Appl Environ Microbiol* 59:1579–1585, 1993.
11. Ansari SA, Springthorpe VS, Sattar SA, et al: Potential role of hands in the spread of respiratory viral infections: studies with human parainfluenza virus 3 and rhinovirus 14. *J Clin Microbiol* 29:2115–2119, 1991.
12. Warshauer DM, Dick EC, Mandel AD, et al: Rhinovirus infections in an isolated Antarctic station. Transmission of the viruses and susceptibility of the population. *Am J Epidemiol* 129:319–340, 1989.

13. Makela MJ, Puhakka T, Ruuskanen O, et al: Viruses and bacteria in the etiology of the common cold. *J Clin Microbiol* 36:539–542, 1998.

14. Glezen WP, Greenberg SB, Atmar RL, et al: Impact of respiratory virus infections on persons with chronic underlying conditions. *JAMA* 283:499–505, 2000.

15. Koch A, Melbye M, Sorensen P, et al: Acute respiratory tract infections and mannose-binding lectin insufficiency during early childhood. *JAMA* 285:1316–1321, 2001.

16. Adam P, Stiffman M, Blake RL: A clinical trial of hypertonic saline nasal spray in subjects with the common cold or rhinosinusitis. *Arch Fam Med* 7:39–43, 1998.

17. Williams JW, Simel DL: Does this patient have sinusitis: diagnosing acute sinusitis by history and physical examination. *JAMA* 270:1242–1246, 1993.

18. Gordon M, Lovell S, Dugdale AE: The value of antibiotics in minor respiratory illness in children. *Med J Aust* 1:304–306, 1974.

19. Stott NC, West RR: Randomized controlled trial of antibiotics in patients with cough and purulent sputum. *Br Med J* 2:556–559, 1976.

20. Mainous AG III, Zoorob RJ, Oler MJ, Haynes DM: Patient knowledge of colds: implications for antibiotic expectations and unnecessary utilization. *J Fam Pract* 45:75–83, 1997.

21. Mainous AG III, Hueston WJ, Eberlein C: Color of respiratory discharges and antibiotic use. *Lancet* 350:1077, 1997.

22. Manning SC, Biavati MJ, Phillips DL: Correlation of clinical sinusitis signs and symptoms to imaging findings in pediatric patients. *Int J Pediatr Otorhinolaryngol* 37:65–74, 1996.

23. Lindbaek M, Hjortdahl P, Johnsen UL-F: Use of symptoms, signs, and blood tests to diagnose acute sinus infections in primary care: comparison with computer tomography. *Fam Med* 28:183–188, 1996.

24. Lindbaek M, Hjortdahl P, Johnsen UL-F: Randomized, double blind, placebo controlled trial of penicillin V and amoxycillin in treatment of acute sinus infection in adults. *Br Med J* 313:325–329, 1996.

25. Van Buchem FL, Knottnerus JA, Schrijnemaekers VJJ, Peeters MF: Primary-care-based randomized placebo-controlled trial of antibiotic treatment in acute maxillary sinusitis. *Lancet* 349:683–687, 1997.

26. Wald ER, Chiponis D, Ledesma-Medina J: Comparative effectiveness of amoxicillin and amoxicillin-clavulanate potassium in acute paranasal sinus infection in children: a double-blinded, placebo controlled trial. *Pediatrics* 77:795–800, 1986.

27. Hansen JG, Schmidt H, Rosborg J, Lung E: Predicting acute maxillary sinusitis in a general practice population. *Br Med J* 311:233–236, 1995.

28. Hueston WJ, Eberlein C, Johnson D, Mainous AG III: Criteria used by clinicians to differentiate sinusitis from viral upper respiratory tract infection. *J Fam Pract* 46:487–492, 1998.

29. Little DR, Mann BL, Godbout CJ: How family physicians distinguish acute sinusitis from upper respiratory tract infection: a retrospective analysis. *J Am Board Fam Pract* 13:101–106, 2000.

30. Oeffinger KC, Snell LM, Foster BM, et al: Diagnosis of acute bronchitis in adults: a national survey of family physicians. *J Fam Pract* 45:402–409, 1997.

31. Verheij JM, Hermans J, Kaptein AA, et al: Acute bronchitis: general practitioners' views regarding diagnosis and treatments. *Fam Pract* 7:175–180, 1990.

32. Hueston WJ: A comparison of albuterol and erythromycin for the treatment of acute bronchitis. *J Fam Pract* 3:476–480, 1991.

33. Hueston WJ: Albuterol delivered by metered-dose inhaler to treat acute bronchitis. *J Fam Pract* 39:437–440, 1994.

34. Littenberg B, Wheeler M, Smith DS: A randomized controlled trial of oral albuterol in acute cough. *J Fam Pract* 42:49–53, 1996.

35. Vingilis E, Brown U, Hennen B: Common colds. Reported patterns of self-care and health care use. *Can Fam Physician* 45:2644–2646, 1999.

36. Mainous AG III, Hueston WJ, Clark JR: Antibiotics and upper respiratory infection: do some folks think there is a cure for the common cold? *J Fam Pract* 42:357–361, 1996.

37. Gonzales R, Steiner JF, Sande MA: Antibiotic prescribing for adults with colds, upper respiratory tract infections, and bronchitis by ambulatory care physicians. *JAMA* 278:901–904, 1997.

38. Townsend EH: Chemoprophylaxis during respiratory infections in a private pediatric practice. *J Dis Child* 99:566–573, 1960.

39. Townsend EH, Radebaugh JF: Prevention of complications of respiratory illnesses in pediatric practice. *N Engl J Med* 266:683–689, 1962.

40. Lexomboon U, Duangmani C, Kusalasai V, et al: Evaluation of orally administered antibiotics for treatment of upper respiratory infections in Thai children. *J Pediatr* 78:772–778, 1971.

41. Taylor B, Abbott GD, Kerr MM, Fergusson DM: Amoxycillin and co-trimoxazole in presumed viral respiratory infections of childhood: placebo-controlled trial. *Br Med J* 2:552–554, 1977.

42. Arroll B, Kenealy T: Antibiotics for the common cold. *Cochrane Database Syst Rev* 2:CD000247, 2000.

43. Davey PG, Bax RP, Newey J, et al: Growth in the use of antibiotics in the community in England and Scotland in 1980–93. *Br Med J* 312:613, 1996.

44. MacFarlane J, Lewis SA, MacFarlane R, Holmes W: Contemporary use of antibiotics in 1089 adults presenting with acute lower respiratory tract illness in general practice in the UK: implications for developing management guidelines. *Respir Med* 91:427–434, 1997.

45. McIsaac WJ, Levine N, Goel V: Visits by adults to family physicians for the common cold. *J Fam Pract* 47:366–369, 1998.

46. Braun BL, Fowles JB: Characteristics and experiences of parents and adults who want antibiotics for cold symptoms. *Arch Fam Med* 9:589–595, 2000.

47. Hamm RM, Hicks RJ, Bemben DA: Antibiotics and respiratory infections: are patients more satisfied when expectations are met? *J Fam Pract* 43:56–62, 1996.

48. Holmes WF, MacFarlane JT, MacFarlane RM, Lewis S: The influence of antibiotics and other factors on reconsultation for acute lower respiratory tract illness in primary care. *Br J Gen Pract* 47:815–818, 1997.

49. Couchman GR, Rasco TG, Forjuoh SN: Back-up antibiotic prescription for common respiratory symptoms. *J Fam Pract* 49:907–913, 2000.

50. Mainous AG III, Hueston WJ: The cost of antibiotics in treating upper respiratory tract infections in a Medicaid population. *Arch Fam Med* 7:45–49, 1998.

51. Hueston WJ, Mainous AG III, Ornstein S, et al: Antibiotics for upper respiratory tract infections: follow-up utilization and antibiotic use. *Arch Fam Med* 8:426–430, 1999.

52. Arason VA, Kristinsson KG, Sigurdsson JA, et al: Do antimicrobials increase the carriage rate of penicillin resistant pneumococci in children? Cross sectional prevalence study. *Br Med J* 313:387–391, 1996.

53. Seppala H, Klaukka T, Vuopio-Varkila J, et al: The effect of changes in the consumption of macrolide antibiotics on erythromycin resistance in group A streptococci in Finland. *N Engl J Med* 337:441–446, 1997.

54. Luks D, Anderson MR: Antihistamines and the common cold: a review and critique of the literature. *J Gen Intern Med* 11:240–244, 1996.

55. Gwaltney JM Jr, Park J, Paul RA, et al: Randomized controlled trial of clemastine fumarate for treatment of experimental rhinovirus colds. *Clin Infect Dis* 22:656–662, 1996.

56. Hayden FG, Diamond L, Wood PB, et al: Effectiveness and safety of intranasal ipratropium bromide in common colds. *Ann Intern Med* 125:89–97, 1996.

57. Hemila H: Does vitamin C alleviate the symptoms of the common cold? A review of current evidence. *Scand J Infect Dis* 26:1–6, 1994.

58. Mossad SB, Macknin ML, Medendorp SV, Mason P: Zinc gluconate lozenges for treating the common cold: a randomized, double-blind, placebo-controlled study. *Ann Intern Med* 125:81–88, 1996.

59. Jackson JL, Lesho E, Peterson C: Zinc and the common cold: a meta-analysis revisited. *J Nutr* 130(5S Suppl):1512S–1515S, 2000.

60. Marshall I: Zinc for the common cold. *Cochrane Database Syst Rev* 2:CD001364, 2000.

61. Melchart D, Linde K, Fischer P, Kaesmayr J: Echinacea for preventing and treating the common cold. *Cochrane Database Syst Rev* 2:CD00530, 2000.

62. Turner RB, Riker DK, Gangemi JD: Ineffectiveness of echinacea for prevention of experimental rhinovirus colds. *Antimicrob Agents Chemother* 44:1708–1709, 2000.

63. Grimm W, Muller HH: A randomized controlled trial of the effect of fluid extract of *Echinacea purpurea* on the incidence and severity of colds and respiratory infections. *Am J Med* 106:138–143, 1999.

64. Melchart D, Walther E, Linde K, et al: Echinacea root extracts for the prevention of upper respiratory tract infections: a double-blind, placebo-controlled randomized trial. *Arch Fam Med* 7:541–545, 1998.

65. Rennard BO, Ertl RF, Gossman GL, et al: Chicken soup inhibits neutrophil chemotaxis in vitro. *Chest* 118:1150–1157, 2000.
66. Falsey AR, Criddle MM, Kolassa JE, et al: Evaluation of a handwashing intervention to reduce respiratory illness rates in senior day-care centers. *Infect Control Hosp Epidemiol* 20:200–202, 1999.

Jonathan L. Temte

Pharyngitis

A well-known adage regarding carpentry suggests, "If one has only a hammer, all the world looks like a nail." Throughout primary care practices, such an observation has some truth with regard to sore throats, group A beta-hemolytic *Streptococcus pyogenes*, and penicillin. This commonly applied monocular view too often results in a dichotomous diagnostic conclusion: streptococcal pharyngitis or viral pharyngitis. But the pharynx is more complex than that.

The term *pharynx* is derived from the Greek word for *gulf* or *chasm*, and it is that chasm that is the point of entry for air; food- and water-borne pathogens; and occasional sexually transmitted agents, chemicals, and physical agents. Moreover, disorders resulting in pharyngitis, or inflammation of the pharynx, which range from life-threatening complications to benign conditions, have become "medicalized," thus contributing to great overuse of antibiotic medications.

Better understanding of this common primary care diagnosis is needed for appropriate, evidence-based approaches to care. This chapter reviews the common primary entities of pharyngitis, tonsillitis, and laryngitis.

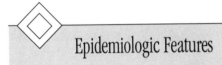

Epidemiologic Features

Frequency in Primary Care Medical Practice

Sore throats are very common in primary care practice. At the University of Wisconsin Department of Family Medicine's (UW-DFM) outpatient clinics, the diagnoses of viral pharyngitis and streptococcal pharyngitis, when taken together, represent the sixth most common pathologic diagnosis.[1] On a national scale, symptoms referable to the throat account for approximately 17.3 million ambulatory patient visits annually, or 2.4 percent of the total office visits in the United States.[2] The distribution of "pharyngitis" across primary care disciplines accounts for 4.3 percent of family practice visits, 2.4 percent of internal medicine visits, and 5.0 percent of pediatric visits.[2]

The overwhelming majority of clinically defined cases of pharyngitis seen in primary care represent nonstreptococcal pharyngitis.[3–8] Streptococcal involvement is reported in only 10 to 30 percent of cases. The overall distribution of diagnostic categories is illustrated by data on 12,018 cases of "sore throat" within the clinical practices of the UW-DFM (Fig. 5-1).[1]

Demographics of Pharyngitis Visits

There are few data available regarding the overall demographics, in terms of age and gender, of patients who have pharyngitis, tonsillitis, and laryngitis in primary care practices. Evaluation of data from the Wisconsin clinics demonstrates some trends in the occurrence of these disorders (Table 5-1).

Streptococcal pharyngitis due to group A beta-hemolytic *Streptococcus pyogenes* (GABHS) peaks in children aged 5 to 9 years and exhibits a secondary peak in females of childbearing age (Fig. 5-2). It becomes relatively uncommon after the age of 50, with only 2 percent of cases occurring in older adults. Overall, 60 percent of reported cases were in female patients. Nonstreptococcal pharyngitis (NSP) (Fig. 5-3) shows some similar demographic trends, but the condition appears in slightly older patients. Peak occurrence is during the teen years, with a secondary peak in females of childbearing age. Only 4 percent of cases are reported after age 50. As with GABHS cases, a high percentage of patients (64 percent) are female.

Acute tonsillitis is uncommon in primary care, representing only 3 percent of total cases. The age and sex distributions are similar to those of GABHS, with this diagnosis occurring rarely in older adults.

Figure 5-1

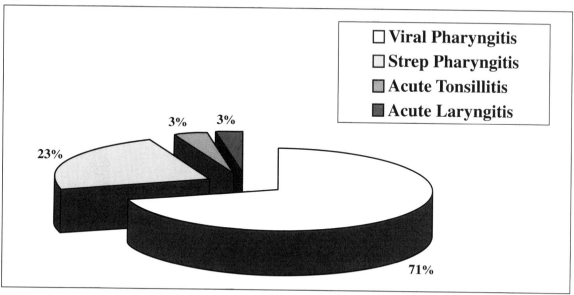

Frequency of occurrence of pharyngeal diagnoses in family practice settings. Data based upon the result of 12,018 encounters.

Table 5-1

Demographic Trends in Primary Care Visits for Sore Throats

DIAGNOSIS	DISTRIBUTION OF CASES, %	GENDER, %	AGE RANGE, YEARS	MEAN AGE, YEARS
Streptococcal pharyngitis	23	F: 59.8 M: 40.2	0–98	15.2
Nonstreptococcal pharyngitis	71	F: 63.8 M: 36.2	0–98	16.8
Acute tonsillitis	3	F: 61.4 M: 38.6	1–80	15.3
Acute laryngitis	3	F: 70.8 M: 29.2	0–87	34.8

Acute laryngitis disorder spans all ages; the age-sex distribution is significantly different from that for other complaints of the upper airway. Most patients who seek care are middle-aged women. It is uncommon, accounting for about 3 percent of total cases.

Seasonality and Other Temporal Trends

Complaints of sore throat have long been recognized to have strong seasonality, with most cases occurring during the cooler months and coinciding with the respiratory virus season.[8] Similar

Figure 5-2

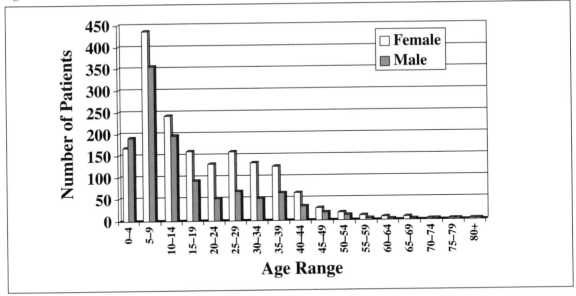

Age and gender of patients diagnosed with streptococcal pharyngitis (IDC-9: 034.0). Data based upon the results of 2819 encounters.

Figure 5-3

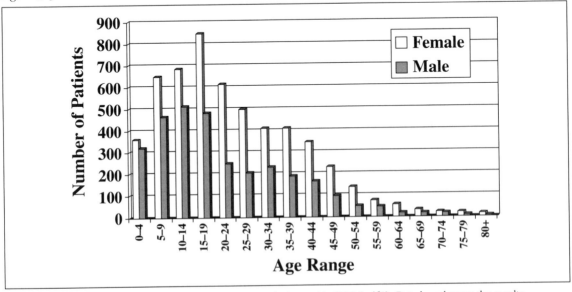

Age and gender of patients diagnosed with nonstreptococcal pharyngitis (IDC-9: 462). Data based upon the results of 8441 encounters.

trends are nicely demonstrated by the Wisconsin clinics data. The lowest number of cases presenting to primary care clinicians for evaluation occurs in August, followed by a gradual but steady rise to a peak incidence in February (Fig. 5-4). The amplitude of the seasonal trend demonstrates an approximately twofold difference in patient visits between peak and nadir.

Closer inspection of temporal trends indicates a more complex pattern than a simple sinusoidal path across the seasons. A three-year study of weekly prevalence of NSP at one clinic[9] illustrated 14 separate peaks and notable clustering of cases. The pattern reflected the prevalence of respiratory viruses known to cause pharyngitis.

Two significant and relatively predictable seasonal trends are worthy of note. In North America, influenza tends to peak in January and February,[10] as does respiratory syncytial virus (RSV).[11] Both of these respiratory viruses are associated with pharyngitis. In addition, some seasonality in host susceptibility may exist, thus further contributing to seasonal trends.[12]

Etiologic Agents of Pharyngitis

Causes of acute throat complaints are many and varied, fitting into a number of categories. Clinicians usually, and correctly, consider bacteria and viruses in their differential diagnoses, but other agents such as chemical exposures, physical factors, autoimmune conditions, cancers, parasites, and fungal infections should be considered as well.

A number of chemicals have been reported as contributing to complaints of acute pharyngitis, including fluorinated hydrocarbons,[13] wood dust,[14] and swimming pool products.[15] Gastric acid irritation due to gastroesophageal reflux is a common cause of chronic laryngitis.[16]

Physical factors such as exposure to dry air can act as upper airway irritants, especially when

Figure 5-4

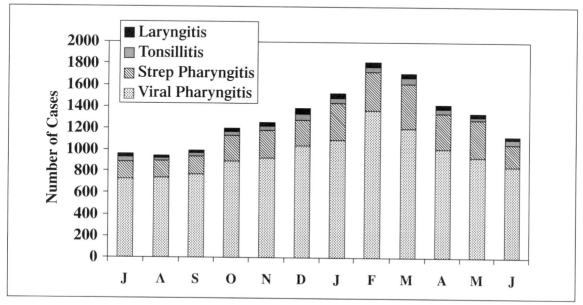

Seasonal occurrence of pharyngeal disorders, demonstrating peak in late winter. Data based upon 12,018 encounters.

coupled with the increased minute ventilation accompanying high altitudes. Additionally, superheated air, such as occurs with the smoking of cigarettes, marijuana,[17] or crack cocaine,[18] can cause thermal injury to the pharynx. Postoperative sore throats occur in about 90 percent of intubated patients, probably as a result of pressure exerted upon the airway.[19] Radiation associated with cancer therapy can also induce cellular damage resulting in pharyngitis.[20] Direct trauma due to foreign bodies, such as fishbones,[21] can be an unusual cause of pharyngitis with significant complications.

Medical conditions such as Kawasaki syndrome,[22] Still's disease,[23] severe combined immunodeficiency syndrome (SCIDS),[24] psoriasis,[25] and leukemia[26] can be associated with pharyngeal symptoms. Periodic fever, aphthous stomatitis, pharyngitis, and cervical adenopathy (PFAPA) is a recently described syndrome that affects infants and children and has no known cause.[27,28]

Rare reports have been made of parasitic etiologies of pharyngitis.[29] More common are cases due to fungal infections in patients with neutropenia[30] or advanced human immunodeficiency virus (HIV) or associated with the use of steroid sprays.[31]

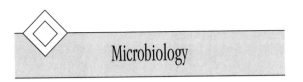

Microbiology

Viruses and bacteria are the most common causes of acute pharyngitis presenting to the primary care clinician (Table 5-2). Until recently, however, ambulatory practice behavior has been biased by the ability to directly diagnose only GABHS in patients presenting with pharyngitis. The development and availability of rapid diagnostic testing for viruses is likely to shift our understanding of the causative agents of pharyngitis.

Viruses

Most episodes of pharyngitis are due to acute respiratory virus infections. From estimates of the frequency of causative agents (Table 5-2) and similar demographic trends,[52] one can correctly surmise that approximately 70 to 80 percent of pharyngitis episodes evaluated in primary care are virally induced. Brief descriptions of the more common viral pathogens involved with acute pharyngitis syndromes are provided here.

RHINOVIRUS

Human rhinoviruses are probably the leading cause of sore throats seen in primary care practices. These viruses are ubiquitous and include more than 100 serotypes.[53] Complaints of sore throat will occur in up to 50 percent of infections and typically last 3 to 4 days.[54] These infections usually occur in the spring and fall and have associated nasal symptoms and/or cough.

INFLUENZA

Influenza is a very important respiratory pathogen characterized by high attack rates and considerable morbidity and mortality. Both influenza A and influenza B strains circulate in annual wintertime epidemics in the United States.[10] The standard definition of an influenza-like illness is a fever of 100°F or higher accompanied by a cough or a sore throat.[10] The sore throat associated with influenza typically lasts 2 to 3 days.[55]

RESPIRATORY SYNCYTIAL VIRUS

RSV is usually considered a childhood infection, but it is also a common pathogen in older children and adults and can be cultured from patients with sore throats. Infections are almost always associated with nasal discharge and cough and demonstrate distinct seasonality, with more infections occurring in the winter months.[11]

Table 5-2

Microbial Agents Associated with Acute Pharyngitis

MICROBE	ESTIMATED PREVALENCE	SOURCE
VIRUSES		
Rhinoviruses	30%	32
Respiratory syncytial virus	? (elderly)	33
Adenoviruses	10%	34
Enteroviruses	8%	34
Influenza viruses types A, B	1–7%	33, 35
Parainfluenza viruses types 1–4	6% (elderly)	33
Herpes simplex	5.7% (college students)	35
Epstein-Barr virus	?	36, 37
Coronavirus	1%	32
HIV	Rare	38
BACTERIA		
Group A beta-hemolytic streptococcus	8–44%	39–42
Group C beta-hemolytic streptococcus	4–6%	43, 44
Arcanobacterium haemolyticum	2.5%	45
Pseudomonas pseudomallei	Rare	46
Corynebacterium pseudodiphtheriticum	Rare	47
Neisseria gonorrhoeae	1%	48
Treponema pallidum	Rare	49
ATYPICALS		
Mycoplasma pneumoniae	2.3–13%	35, 50
Chlamydia pneumoniae	?	51

ADENOVIRUS

Pharyngitis along with fever is a common presentation of adenovirus in children and military recruits.[56] Another presentation, pharyngoconjunctival fever, is characterized by pharyngitis, which may be exudative, conjunctivitis, and spiking fever.

ENTEROVIRUSES

Sore throat symptoms with the appearance of small vesicles, which progress to small white ulcers, on the soft palate and tonsillar pillars are suggestive of herpangina, a condition caused by coxsackieviruses. Other enteroviruses are associated with mild respiratory symptoms, including pharyngitis.[57]

EPSTEIN-BARR VIRUS

Tonsillitis occurs in between 70 and 80 percent of children with mononucleosis. Because of the similarities in presenting symptoms with streptococcal pharyngitis, infectious mononucleosis can be mistaken for a GABHS infection early in the course of illness. Clinical characteristics of infectious mononucleosis include an exudative tonsillitis/pharyngitis, cervical lymph node enlargement, fever, malaise, and hepatospleno-megaly. Fever and lymphadenopathy are the most common symptoms of infectious mononucleosis and occur in over 90 percent of children with this infection.[58]

Bacteria

Pharyngeal infections attributable to GABHS have been the driving force for a significant and costly component of primary medical care. The ability to accurately diagnose a bacterial illness in ambulatory settings, coupled with the availability of effective antibiotic prophylaxis of rheumatic fever, has contributed to much confusion about the appropriate management of pharyngitis. Bacterial pathogens are less common, but nonetheless significant factors in pharyngitis. More important, bacterial infections are associated with most of the known complications of acute pharyngitis.

GROUP A BETA-HEMOLYTIC STREPTOCOCCUS PYOGENES

Typical findings associated with GABHS pharyngitis can vary, but may include severe pharyngeal pain, difficulty swallowing, cervical lymphadenopathy, and fever. Posterior pharyngeal or tonsillar exudates can be found in about 50 percent of children 3 years of age or older with GABHS, and almost 75 percent of children with exudates are culture-positive for this organism.[59] Systemic symptoms may include myalgia, headache, nausea, and emesis.[60] Although cough and runny nose are more consistent with viral infections, coryza is not uncommon in young children with GABHS.[59] Of significance is the association of GABHS with scarlet fever,[61] rheumatic fever,[62] severe invasive infections,[61] and glomerulonephritis.[63]

The pathogenesis of GABHS in pharyngotonsillitis appears to be a response to tonsillar crypt and pharyngeal surface infection.[64] Bacteria penetrate the pharyngeal mucosa, adhere to the sur-face epithelium, and are internalized, setting off a cascade of cytokine release and inflammatory response.[65] Not surprisingly, recurrent pharyngotonsillitis with the same serotype of GABHS is associated with reduced symptoms.[66]

GROUP C BETA-HEMOLYTIC STREPTOCOCCUS

Infections with GCBHS tend to be somewhat milder, but can have essentially the same clinical presentation as GABHS pharyngitis.[8,44]

Nonstreptococcal Bacterial Pharyngitis

Symptomatic gonococcal pharyngeal infections are rare. When they do occur, they usually result in mild pharyngitis.[48]

Other bacteria associated with pharyngitis include *Mycoplasma pneumoniae* and *Chlamydia pneumoniae*. Both of these atypically cause acute respiratory tract infections, with associated mild pharyngitis. Compared to other NSP cases, pharyngitis attributable to mycoplasma is more likely to include hoarseness and less likely to include postnasal drip.[50] Chlamydial infections are associated with chronic pharyngitis.[51]

Mode of Transmission

The mode of transmission becomes important when considering the etiologic agents of pharyngitis. The most frequent mode of transmission is through inhalation of airborne pathogens. Accordingly, highly evolved respiratory viruses and some enteroviruses are easily transmitted. GABHS and GCBHS are also frequently transmitted through respiratory droplets.[67]

Other modes of transmission can occur. Explosive epidemics of streptococcal disease have been traced to ingestion of contaminated food.[68] Coxsackie and other enteroviruses can be spread via fecal-oral transmission.[67] Transmission of HIV, herpes simplex II, *N. gonorrhoeae*, and *Treponema pallidum*, all associated with pharyngitis, occur sexually.

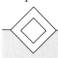

Patient Evaluation and Laboratory Testing

The goal of initial patient evaluation is to establish a rational differential diagnosis and to appropriately use discriminating or confirmatory laboratory tests. Several clues to identifying the causative agent can be determined efficiently in the patient encounter through a history and physical examination. Based upon the diagnostic impression, laboratory support, available in most ambulatory clinics, can narrow the pool, or possibly confirm the etiologic agent.

History

A complete history for pharyngitis will focus on the characteristics of the sore throat, associated respiratory and systemic symptoms, and possible risks and exposures (Table 5-3). The initial history helps to identify syndromes that need immediate attention, referral, or hospitalization, such as epiglottitis, retropharyngeal abscess, and palatal cellulitis.[61] Difficulty in swallowing, trismus, neck swelling, and drooling are all indications of significant pathology.

The presence of additional respiratory tract symptoms, especially cough in the winter, can help to exclude GABHS. Oral ulcers may be more suggestive of herpes or coxsackieviruses. Conjunctivitis with pharyngitis occurs with adenovirus infection. A complete immunization history is essential for children, especially concerning diphtheria and infections associated with *Haemophilus influenzae* B.

Because of the ease of transmission of many of the agents causing pharyngitis, knowing whether the patient has been exposed to others with similar symptoms can be helpful. Most respiratory viruses and GABHS have incubation periods of 1 to 3 days.[67] On the other hand, mycoplasma and chlamydia tend to have much

Table 5-3

Suggested Components of a Complete Pharyngitis History

Specific Symptoms of a Sore Throat
  Date/time of onset
  Duration of symptoms
  Intensity of throat pain
  Difficulty in swallowing
  Use of analgesics or other agents
    to reduce pain
  Presence of trismus
  Presence of foul breath odor
  Neck swelling
  Change in voice or hoarseness
  Drooling
  Enlarged or painful lymph nodes in neck

Associated Respiratory Tract or Systemic Symptoms
  Runny nose or nasal congestion
  Cough
  Fever
  Nausea and/or vomiting
  Rash
  Oral ulcers
  Fatigue
  Conjunctivitis

Risks and Exposures
  Age
  Presence of acute respiratory illnesses in
    family, school, or workplace
  Immunization history (especially diphtheria
    and *Haemophilus influenzae* B)
  Incubation time (i.e., from possible exposure
    to symptoms)
  Season of year
  Circulating viruses (based upon surveillance
    systems)
  Epidemic pharyngitis in the community

longer periods of incubation. Making use of public health–based infectious disease surveillance systems (e.g., CDC's U.S. Influenza Sentinel Physician Surveillance Network, National Respiratory Virus and Enterovirus Surveillance

System[10]) allows clinicians to make clinical decisions based upon knowledge of the prevalence of specific pathogens such as influenza.[69]

Physical Examination

A directed physical examination provides additional evidence of causative agents. In addition to observation of vital signs, a complete examination of the head, eyes, ears, nose, oral cavity and pharynx, neck, heart, lungs, and skin should be performed.[60] The physical examination can help to identify GABHS infections, suggested by tonsillar or posterior pharyngeal exudates, fever, erythematous pharynx, palatal petechiae, and anterior cervical adenopathy. Coryza, especially in older children and adults, is less consistent with GABHS.[59] A sandpaper-like rash on the trunk characterizes scarlet fever, a cutaneous manifestation of GABHS.

Laboratory Testing

The ambulatory clinical laboratory is on the verge of explosive change. The currently available tools to identify infectious agents causing pharyngitis include throat culture on blood agar plates, rapid streptococcal testing, rapid antigen testing for influenza and RSV, complete blood cell counts, erythrocyte sedimentation rate (ESR), MonoSpot testing, and Antistreptolysin-O (ASO) titers.[8,59,70] Throat culture, rapid streptococcal testing, and ASO titers are used primarily for the detection of GABHS. Rapid antigen detection for specific viruses and the MonoSpot are useful if positive, but need to be used in context and are not advocated for general use in pharyngitis diagnosis. Complete blood counts and ESR are of little diagnostic value for most cases of pharyngitis, but can be of use if significant infections, such as peritonsillar abscess, are suspected.

Three types of tests are specifically aimed at GABHS. A twofold rise in ASO titer, between acute and convalescent sera, is the gold standard test for acute streptococcal pharyngitis.[70] This test, however, is of almost no value in a primary care setting, since it requires 2 weeks for the titers to rise. More recently, antigen detection tests have come into prominence for detection of GABHS.[71] Most of these offer acceptable sensitivities and specificities.[71–74] The overall performance of antigen detection tests, however, depends not only upon their sensitivity and specificity, but also upon the prevalence of GABHS in the testing population and specimen collection techniques.[75] In addition, lab error and detection of colonized GABHS can produce false results (Table 5-4). Finally, the standard throat culture is available to detect GABHS. Like that of the antigen detection tests, the sensitivity of the throat culture is dependent upon obtaining a suitable sample from the posterior pharynx. Also, the test will detect asymptomatic carriers as well as infected individuals, which reduces its specificity.

To help guide clinicians in selecting the most appropriate way to evaluate patients with suspected GABHS, a recent decision analysis[76] evaluated several strategies currently in use for the diagnosis and treatment of GABHS pharyngitis. In most situations, an approach using a highly sensitive rapid test without culture confirmation of all negatives was found to be the most cost-effective approach in which a diagnostic test was used. Treating all suspect patients was associated with antibiotic resistance and high numbers of allergic reactions.

Scoring Systems for GABHS

Prediction rules for assessing the probability of GABHS have recently been systematically reviewed.[77] Such rules allow combinations of individual clinical signs and symptoms that, when taken alone, have little predictive value. When combined, these clinical parameters can assist the clinician in assessing the risk of strep throat and determining whether to treat empirically (high risk), not test or treat (low risk), or

Table 5-4

Outcomes of Rapid Antigen Tests for GABHS

	GABHS INFECTION	No GABHS INFECTION
Rapid Test Positive	**True Positive**	**False Positive** GABHS carrier Lab error Nonspecific test (Low prevalence)
Rapid Test Negative	**False Negative** Poor specimen collection Lab error Low test sensitivity (High prevalence)	**True Negative**

treat depending upon the outcome of an appropriate diagnostic test (moderate risk).

A reasonable protocol for inclusion in primary care practice is McIsaac's modification of the Centor strep score.[78] This prediction rule has been validated within primary care populations for both adults and children (Table 5-5).

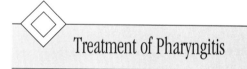

Treatment of Pharyngitis

The management of pharyngitis can be divided into symptomatic treatments and antimicrobial interventions.

Symptomatic Care

There is very little evidence-based information on non-antimicrobial treatments for pharyngitis.[79] Whereas recommendations exist for warm salt water gargle and dyclonine hydrochloride (Sucrets lozenges),[80] there is little evidence to support their use or disuse. Dye studies have demonstrated that sprays reach the pharynx better than do gargles.[81]

Analgesics such as viscous lidocaine and narcotic preparations are in common use for severe pharyngeal pain. Nonsteroidal anti-inflammatory drugs such as ibuprofen and flurbiprofen have been shown to be effective in relieving sore throat pain.[79,82] Intramuscular injection of betamethasone has also been shown to be an effective adjuvant therapy in the treatment of GABHS pharyngitis.[83]

Antibiotic Treatment for GABHS

Antibiotic treatment of acute pharyngitis is directed toward the eradication of the infecting organism, reduction of associated suppurative and nonsuppurative complications, and reduction of symptoms. An excellent overview of existing evidence is provided in the report of Del Mar et al.[84]

Del Mar's review[84] found a 70 percent reduction in the risk for acute rheumatic fever with antibiotic treatment in acute GABHS pharyngitis, along with possible reductions in acute glomerulonephritis. Moreover, suppurative complications such as sinusitis, otitis media, and peritonsillar abscess were reduced by levels of 54 percent, 78 percent, and 82 percent, respectively. Modest

Table 5-5

Modified Centor Strep Score

SYMPTOM OR SIGN	POINTS IF "YES"
History of fever or measured temperature > 38°C (100.4°F)	1
Absence of cough	1
Tender anterior cervical lymph nodes	1
Tonsillar swelling or exudates	1
Age less than 15 years	1
Age greater or equal to 45 years	−1
Sum of sign/symptom points	(−1 to 5)

RISK OF GABHS	
TOTAL POINTS	PERCENT OF PATIENTS WITH GABHS
−1 or 0	1 (low risk)
1	10 (moderate risk)
2	17 (moderate risk)
3	35 (moderate risk)
4 or 5	51 (high risk)

SOURCE: Adapted from Ebell et al[77] and McIsaac et al, with permission.[78]

benefits in symptomatic relief and reduced duration of 8 h overall are associated with antibiotic treatment.

Multiple antibiotics have been demonstrated to provide effective treatment for GABHS. These include penicillin, ampicillin, and amoxicillin, as well as cephalosporins, macrolides, and clindamycin. Penicillin is preferred because of its efficacy, low risk, narrow spectrum, and low cost.[85] Current guidelines, based upon extensive study,[85,86] recommend twice daily to three times daily dosing of oral penicillin for 10 days (Table 5-6). Longer courses (7 days) of penicillin were found to be more effective for symptom relief in GABHS than shorter (3 days) courses.[87] A single dose of intramuscular benzathine penicillin G is an appropriate alternative for patients who are unlikely or unable to complete a 10-day course of oral antibiotics. Erythromycin is appropriate for penicillin-allergic patients. Other approaches include once daily dosing of amoxicillin 750 mg for 10 days.[88] Clindamycin or amoxicillin/clavu-

lanate are recommended for patients with multiply-treated, recurrent episodes of symptomatic GABHS.[85] Whereas the period of transmissibility can last for 21 days in uncomplicated and untreated GABHS pharyngitis, patients are no longer considered contagious 24 h after initiation of treatment.[67]

Drug failure rates, defined as a persistently positive culture, occur in 11 to 45 percent of patients with GABHS treated with penicillin. A single daily dose of amoxicillin for acute GABHS given at a dose of 40 mg/kg/day for 10 days appears to be very successful, resulting in excellent clinical responses and low posttreatment carrier rates (5 to 10 percent). However, amoxicillin therapy frequently results in a rash in patients with mononucleosis who are mistakenly diagnosed as having GABHS. Treatment with other agents such as azithromycin and clarithromycin produces no better results than amoxicillin or penicillin V, but at much greater expense.

Table 5-6

Antibiotic Regimens for Group A Beta-Hemolytic Streptococcal Infections

ANTIBIOTIC	DOSE	TIMING	DURATION
Children			
Penicillin V	250 mg	b.i.d. to t.i.d.	10 days
Benzathine penicillin G	0.6 million units	1	
Amoxicillin	750 mg	Daily	10 days
Erythromycin estolate	20–40 mg/kg/day	b.i.d. to t.i.d.	10 days
Erythromycin ethyl succinate	40 mg/kg/day	b.i.d. to t.i.d.	10 days
Amoxicillin/clavulanate	40 mg/kg/day	t.i.d.	10 days
Clindamycin	20–30 mg/kg/day	t.i.d. to q.i.d.	10 days
Adults			
Penicillin V	500 mg	b.i.d.	10 days
Benzathine penicillin G	1.2 million units	1	
Erythromycin estolate	250 mg	q.i.d.	10 days
Erythromycin ethyl succinate	400 mg	t.i.d.	10 days
Amoxicillin/clavulanate	250 mg	t.i.d.	10 days
Clindamycin	300 mg	b.i.d.	10 days

RECURRENCE AND CARRIAGE OF GABHS

Recurrent infections with GABHS are not uncommon and occur as a result of nonadherence to the full antibiotic regimen, reexposure to GABHS, eradication of normal flora, and antibiotic resistance.[89,90] There can also be some reexposure as a result of the use of removable dental appliances.[91] In addition, evidence exists that intracellular GABHS can serve as a reservoir for reinfection.[92] Rates of recurrent infection appear to be increasing, and recurrence is more common in children under 8 years of age.[93] Along with searching for the source of the reinfection, retreatment with a course of penicillin at the same dosing regimen used for the initial infection is adequate for treating recurrences.

Healthy carriers of GABHS also can serve as a source for reinfection. Furthermore, carriers with a viral pharyngitis will test positive on antigen testing and culture, leading to a false positive diagnosis of strep pharyngitis (Table 5-4). The carrier state has been documented in 2 to 21 percent of children and 2 to 4 percent of adults.[39,93] A regimen of intramuscular penicillin V plus oral rifampin has been shown to reverse the carrier status in 93 percent of patients treated.

Treatment of Non-EBV Viral Infections

Several new antiviral medications are available or are being developed for the treatment of other pathogens associated with pharyngitis. Amantadine, rimantadine, oseltamivir, and zanamivir can reduce symptoms of influenza, but they need to be started within 36 to 48 h of symptom onset.[10] Similarly, pleconaril is an oral antiviral under development that is effective against human rhinoviruses and enterovirus infections.[53] Like other viral agents, to be effective it must be started early. Currently, pleconaril has not been approved for use in the United States or in Europe, but it is expected to be available in 2002.[94] Although some small studies have suggested that erythromycin therapy can be beneficial for patients with NSP,[95] the effects are relatively small and this treatment is not recommended.[96]

Prevention offers an additional modality for the control of pharyngitis. Immunization with the trivalent influenza vaccine is highly effective in preventing this infection.[10] The encouragement of hygienic practices and hand washing[97] may help to decrease the burden of both respiratory and fecal-oral transmissions.

Treatment of Mononucleosis

EBV-associated infectious mononucleosis is a self-limited condition that usually resolves over several weeks. Fever, often the earliest manifestation of illness, usually abates after 1 or 2 weeks, but malaise and hepatosplenomegaly may take 4 to 6 weeks to resolve. During this time, activities that could result in splenic trauma, such as contact sports, should be avoided. Although the exact time for return to full activities is predicated on the degree of splenic swelling and the absence of other complications, a minimum of 1 month's time to recuperate is suggested before patients resume contact sports.[98]

Some patients with infectious mononucleosis experience severe tonsillitis, with potential compromise of their airway. In these patients, administration of corticosteroids should be considered.[99] If airway obstruction is severe and life-threatening, an artificial airway should be provided. Installation of an airway is preferable over emergency tonsillectomy.

Finally, acyclovir has been evaluated as a potential therapy for infectious mononucleosis. However, acyclovir in doses of 600 mg for 10 days did not appear to reduce clinical symptoms, although it did reduce viral shedding.[100] Combining acyclovir with steroids did not appear to produce any clinical benefit, either.[101]

Tonsillectomy for Pharyngitis

Recommendations for tonsillectomy should be made only for patients meeting the following criteria: (1) The sore throat is due to tonsillitis, (2) there are five or more episodes per year, (3) symptoms have occurred for at least 1 year, and (4) the episodes of sore throat are disabling and prevent normal functioning.[102] A randomized controlled trial of tonsillectomy demonstrated modest benefit from this surgical procedure, but also provided support for nonsurgical management.[103]

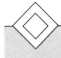

Complications of Pharyngitis

Acute pharyngitis is usually a self-limited condition. Nevertheless, significant complications occur and have contributed much to our current approach to clinical management. Complications such as scarlet fever, rheumatic fever, and glomerulonephritis are commonly associated with GABHS. Peritonsillar abscess also occurs with GABHS, but can occur with other infectious agents as well.[104]

Overall, the risk of serious complications from GABHS is low. Antibiotic therapy lowers this risk, but does not completely eliminate complications. Information on the risks of suppurative complications, such as peritonsillar abscesses, was reviewed in a cost-effectiveness analysis[76] and estimated at between 1 and 5.1 percent for untreated patients and between 0.5 and 2 percent for treated patients.

Scarlet fever is a GABHS with a strain that secretes an erythrogenic toxin. The toxin causes red cell lysis, producing an erythematous blush to the skin with a superimposed sandpapery papular rash. Scarlet fever was considered a relatively benign condition until the onset of an epidemic in Dublin, Ireland, in 1831 that caused significant mortality. After that, clusters of cases across the United States and Europe were associated with case fatality rates as high as 30 percent until the mid-1880s. At that point, although it was decades before the development of antibiotics, the death rate from scarlet fever fell precipitously.[62,105]

Acute rheumatic fever (ARF) resulted in a crude death rate of 7 per 100,000 in the United States in 1910 and of 10 to 12 per 100,000 in Canada in the 1940s. When injections of penicillin were first given to military recruits with exudative pharyngotonsillitis in the 1950s, dramatic declines in ARF were noted.[62,106] The prevalence of ARF tends to change over time and geography, resulting in sporadic epidemics. At present, the risk for developing ARF with untreated GABHS is estimated to be 0.3 to 4 per 1000.[76,107]

Acute poststreptococcal glomerulonephritis is associated with GABHS infections.[63] Previous reports have stated that there appears to be no significant effect on risk reduction with antibiotic treatment.[106] However, more recent analyses of controlled trials by Del Mar and colleagues[84] suggest that there may be a small protective effect against glomerulonephritis with antibiotic use in GABHS.

Peritonsillar abscess is a more common complication of streptococcal pharyngitis. These infections result from invasion of bacteria through the tonsillar capsule. Infection is most common in adolescents and young adults. Patients present with increased sore throat, fever, and difficulty swallowing and speaking. The affected tonsil is large and usually displaces the palate. Visualization of the uvula deviated to the contralateral side is a useful indicator of peritonsillar abscess. Treatment includes draining the infection, usually with an 18-gauge needle inserted into the tonsil, along with antibiotic therapy. Single aspiration with antibiotic therapy has been shown to result in cure rates of 92 per-

cent, which compare favorably with more aggressive surgical management.[108] Without therapy, peritonsillar abscesses may invade the head and neck, with fatal consequences.

Lemierre's syndrome or postanginal septicemia, characterized by thrombophlebitis of the internal jugular vein and spread of infection to the lung or other sites, rarely occurs as a complication of pharyngeal infections. When it does occur, healthy teens and young adults are most commonly affected. *Fusobacterium necrophorum* is the causative agent.[8,109]

References

1. University of Wisconsin Department of Family Medicine, Clinical Data Warehouse.
2. Nelson C, Woodwell D: National ambulatory medical care survey: 1993 summary. Data from the National Health Survey. *Vital Health Stat* [13] 136: 1–99, 1998.
3. Hayes CS, Williamson H Jr: Management of group A beta-hemolytic streptococcal pharyngitis. *Am Fam Physician* 63:1557–1564, 2001.
4. Bisno AL: Acute pharyngitis. *N Engl J Med* 344: 205–211, 2001.
5. Richardson MA: Sore throat, tonsillitis, and adenoiditis. *Med Clin North Am* 83:75–83, 1999.
6. Dowell SF, Schwartz B, Phillips WR: Appropriate use of antibiotics for URIs in children. Part II. Cough, pharyngitis and the common cold. The Pediatric URI Consensus Team. *Am Fam Physician* 58:1335–1342, 1998.
7. Pichichero ME: Group A beta-hemolytic streptococcal infections. *Pediatr Rev* 19:291–302, 1998.
8. Gwaltney JM Jr: Pharyngitis, in Mandell GL, Bennett JE, Dolin R (eds.): *Principles and Practice of Infectious Diseases*, 4th ed. Philadelphia, Churchill Livingstone, 1995; pp 566–572.
9. Yusef-Safavi Y, Temte JL: Symptoms associated with non-streptococcal pharyngitis: the role of viral disease in the community. *Wis Med J* 97:46, 1998.
10. Advisory Council for Immunization Practices: Prevention and control of influenza. *MMWR* 50(RR04):1–44, 2001.

11. Respiratory syncytial virus activity—United States, 1999–2000 season. *MMWR* 49:1091–1093, 2000.

12. Dowell SF: Seasonal variation in host susceptibility and cycle of certain infectious diseases. *Emerg Infect Dis* 7:369–374, 2001.

13. Lyons RA, Wright D, Fielder HM, et al: Investigation of an acute chemical incident: exposure to fluorinated hydrocarbons. *Occup Environ Med* 57:577–581, 2000.

14. Bohadana AB, Massin N, Wild P, et al: Symptoms, airway responsiveness, and exposure to dust in beech and oak wood workers. *Occup Environ Med* 57:268–273, 2000.

15. Massin N, Bohadana AB, Wild P, et al: Respiratory symptoms and bronchial responsiveness in lifeguards exposed to nitrogen trichloride in indoor swimming pools. *Occup Environ Med* 55:258–263, 1998.

16. Hanson DG, Jiang JJ: Diagnosis and management of chronic laryngitis associated with reflux. *Am J Med* 108(Suppl 4a):112S–119S, 2000.

17. Guarisco JL, Cheney ML, LeJeune FE Jr, Reed HT: Isolated uvulitis secondary to marijuana use. *Laryngoscope* 98:1309–1312, 1988.

18. Meleca RJ, Burgio DL, Carr RM, Lolachi CM: Mucosal injuries of the upper aerodigestive tract after smoking crack or freebase cocaine. *Laryngoscope* 107:620–625, 1997.

19. Porter NE, Sidou V, Husson J: Postoperative sore throat: incidence and severity after the use of lidocaine, saline, or air to inflate the endotracheal tube cuff. *AANAJ* 67(1):49–52, 1999.

20. Cengiz M, Ozyar E, Ozturk D, et al: Sucralfate in the prevention of radiation-induced oral mucositis. *J Clin Gastroenterol* 28:40–43, 1999.

21. Matsuki M, Matsuo M, Kaji Y, Okada N: An adult case of retropharyngeal cellulitis: diagnosis by magnetic resonance imaging. *Radiat Med* 16(4):289–291, 1998.

22. Chatterjee A, Leonard J, Awadallah S, Matsuda J: Kawasaki disease: a diagnostic challenge. *S D J Med* 53:527–530, 2000.

23. Mok CC, Lau CS, Wong RW: Clinical characteristics, treatment, and outcome of adult onset Still's disease in southern Chinese. *J Rheumatol* 25:2345–2351, 1998.

24. Stocks RM, Thompson JW, Church JA, et al: Severe combined immunodeficiency: otolaryngological presentation and management. *Ann Otol Rhinol Laryngol* 108:403–407, 1999.

25. Naldi L, Peli L, Parazzini F, Carrel CF: Family history of psoriasis, stressful life events, and recent infectious disease are risk factors for a first episode of acute guttate psoriasis: results of a case-control study. *J Am Acad Dermatol* 44:433–438, 2001.

26. Hou GL, Huang JS, Tsai CC: Analysis of oral manifestations of leukemia: a retrospective study. *Oral Dis* 3:31–38, 1997.

27. Rogers RS III: Recurrent aphthous stomatitis: clinical characteristics and associated systemic disorders. *Sem Cutaneous Med Surg* 16:278–283, 1997.

28. Padeh S, Brezniak N, Zemer D, et al: Periodic fever, aphthous stomatitis, pharyngitis, and adenopathy syndrome: clinical characteristics and outcome. *J Pediatr* 135:98–101, 1999.

29. Chung DI, Moon CH, Kong HH, et al: The first human case of *Clinostomum complanatum* (Trematoda: Clinostomidae) infection in Korea. *Korean J Parasitol* 33:219–223, 1995.

30. Krcmery V Jr, Koza I, Hornikova M, et al: Fluconazole in the treatment of mycotic oropharyngeal stomatitis and esophagitis in neutropenic cancer patients. *Chemotherapy* 37:343–345, 1991.

31. Kyrmizakis DE, Papadakis CE, Lohuis PJ, et al: Acute candidiasis of the oro- and hypopharynx as the result of topical intranasal steroids administration. *Rhinology* 38:87–89, 2000.

32. Arruda E, Pitkaranta A, Witek TJ Jr, et al: Frequency and natural history of rhinovirus infections in adults during autumn. *J Clin Microbiol* 35:2864–2868, 1997.

33. Falsey AR, Treanor JJ, Betts RF, Walsh EE: Viral respiratory infections in the institutionalized elderly: clinical and epidemiologic findings. *J Am Geriatr Soc* 40:115–119, 1992.

34. Sharland M, Hodgson J, Davies EG, et al: Enteroviral pharyngitis diagnosed by reverse transcriptase-polymerase chain reaction. *Arch Dis Child* 74:462–463, 1996.

35. McMillan JA, Weiner LB, Higgins AM, Lamparella VJ: Pharyngitis associated with herpes simplex virus in college students. *Pediatr Infect Dis J* 12:280–284, 1993.

36. Rea TD, Russo JE, Katon W, et al: Prospective study of the natural history of infectious mononucleosis caused by Epstein-Barr virus. *J Am Board Fam Pract* 14:234–242, 2001.

37. Yoda K, Sata T, Kurata T, Aramaki H: Oropharyngotonsillitis associated with nonprimary Epstein-

Barr virus infection. *Arch Otolaryngol Head Neck Surg* 126:185–193, 2000.

38. Vanhems P, Dassa C, Lambert J, et al: Comprehensive classification of symptoms and signs reported among 218 patients with acute HIV-1 infection. *J AIDS* 21:99–106, 1999.

39. Gunnarsson RK, Holm SE, Soderstrom M: The prevalence of beta-haemolytic streptococci in throat specimens from healthy children and adults. Implications for the clinical value of throat cultures. *Scand J Prim Health Care* 15:149–155, 1997.

40. Woods WA, Carter CT, Schlager TA: Detection of group A streptococci in children under 3 years of age with pharyngitis. *Pediatr Emerg Care* 15:338–340, 1999.

41. Woods WA, Carter CT, Stack M, et al: Group A streptococcal pharyngitis in adults 30 to 65 years of age. *South Med J* 92:491–492, 1999.

42. Nussinovitch M, Finkelstein Y, Amir J, Varsano I: Group A beta-hemolytic streptococcal pharyngitis in preschool children aged 3 months to 5 years. *Clin Pediatr* 38:357–360, 1999.

43. Lewis RF, Balfour AE: Group C streptococci isolated from throat swabs: a laboratory and clinical study. *J Clin Pathol* 52:264–266, 1999.

44. Meier FA, Centor RM, Graham L Jr, Dalton HP: Clinical and microbiological evidence for endemic pharyngitis among adults due to group C streptococci. *Arch Intern Med* 150:825–829, 1990.

45. Mackenzie A, Fuite LA, Chan FT, et al: Incidence and pathogenicity of *Arcanobacterium haemolyticum* during a 2-year study in Ottawa. *Clin Infect Dis* 21:177–181, 1995.

46. Tan NG, Sethi DS: An unusual case of sore throat: nasopharyngeal melioidosis. *Singapore Med J* 38:223–225, 1997.

47. Izurieta HS, Strebel PM, Youngblood T, et al: Exudative pharyngitis possibly due to *Corynebacterium pseudodiphtheriticum*, a new challenge in the differential diagnosis of diphtheria. *Emerg Infect Dis* 3:65–68, 1997.

48. Komaroff AL, Aronson MD, Pass TM, Ervin CT: Prevalence of pharyngeal gonorrhea in general medical patients with sore throats. *Sex Transm Dis* 7:116–119, 1980.

49. Chapel TA: The signs and symptoms of secondary syphilis. *Sex Transm Dis* 7:161–164, 1980.

50. Williams WC, Williamson HA Jr, LeFevre ML: The prevalence of *Mycoplasma pneumoniae* in ambulatory patients with nonstreptococcal sore throat. *Fam Med* 23:117–121, 1991.

51. Falck G, Engstrand I, Gad A, et al: Demonstration of *Chlamydia pneumoniae* in patients with chronic pharyngitis. *Scand J Infect Dis* 29:585–589, 1997.

52. Monto AS: Viral respiratory infections in the community: epidemiology, agents, and interventions. *Am J Med* 99 (suppl 6B):24S–27S, 1995.

53. Robart HA, Hayden FG: Picornavirus infections: a primer for the practitioner. *Arch Fam Med* 9:913–920, 2000.

54. Gwaltney JM, Hendley O, Simon G, Jordan WS Jr: Rhinovirus infections in an industrial population. II. Characteristics of illness and antibody response. *JAMA* 202:158–164, 1967.

55. Dolin R: Influenza: current concepts. *Am Fam Physician* 14:72–77, 1976.

56. Foy HM: Adenovirus, in Evans AS, Kaslow RA (eds.): *Viral Infections of Humans*, 4th ed. New York, Plenum, 1997; pp 119–138.

57. Melnick JL: Polio and other enteroviruses, in Evans AS, Kaslow RA (eds.): *Viral Infections of Humans*, 4th ed. New York, Plenum, 1997; pp 583–663.

58. Sumaya CV, Ench Y: Ebstein-Barr virus infection in children: I. Clinical and general laboratory findings. *Pediatrics* 75:1003–1010, 1985.

59. Kaplan EL, Top FH Jr, Dudding BA, Wannamaker LW: Diagnosis of streptococcal pharyngitis: differentiation of active infection from the carrier state in the symptomatic child. *J Infect Dis* 123:490–501, 1971.

60. Perkins A: An approach to diagnosing the acute sore throat. *Am Fam Physician* 55:131–138, 1997.

61. American Academy of Pediatrics: Severe invasive group A streptococcal infections: a subject review. *Pediatrics* 101:136–140, 1998.

62. Denny FW Jr: A 45-year perspective on the streptococcus and rheumatic fever: the Edward H. Kass lecture in infectious disease history. *Clin Infect Dis* 19:1110–1122, 1994.

63. Mori K, Ito Y, Kamikawaji N, Sasazuki T: Elevated IgG titer against the C region of streptococcal M protein and its immunodeterminants in patients with poststreptococcal acute glomerulonephritis. *J Pediatr* 131: 293–299, 1997.

64. Ebenfelt A, Ericson LE, Lundberg C: Acute pharyngotonsillitis is an infection restricted to the crypt and surface secretion. *Acta Otolaryngol* 118: 264–271, 1998.

65. Lilja M, Silvola J, Raisanen S, Stenfors LE: Where are the receptors for *Streptococcus pyogenes* located on the tonsillar surface epithelium? *Int J Pediatr Otorhinolaryngol* 50:37–43, 1999.

66. Lee LH, Ayoub E, Pichichero ME: Fewer symptoms occur in same-serotype recurrent streptococcal tonsillopharyngitis. *Arch Otolaryngol Head Neck Surg* 26:1359–1362, 2000.

67. Chin J: *Control of Communicable Diseases Manual,* 17th ed. Washington, DC, American Public Health Association, 2000.

68. Decker MD, Lavely GB, Hutcheson RH Jr, Schaffner W: Food-borne streptococcal pharyngitis in a hospital pediatrics clinic. *JAMA* 253: 679–681, 1985.

69. Temte JL, Shult PA, Kirk CJ, Amspaugh J: Effects of viral disease education and surveillance on antibiotic prescribing. *Fam Med* 31:101–106, 1999.

70. Kline JA, Runge JW: Streptococcal pharyngitis: a review of pathophysiology, diagnosis and management. *J Emerg Med* 12:665–680, 1994.

71. Roddey OF Jr, Clegg HW, Martin ES, et al: Comparison of throat culture methods for the recovery of group A streptococci in a pediatric office setting. *JAMA* 274:1863–1865, 1995.

72. Roosevelt GE, Kulkarni MS, Shulman ST: Critical evaluation of a CLIA-waived streptococcal antigen detection test in the emergency department. *Ann Emerg Med* 37:377–381, 2001.

73. Kuhn S, Davies HD, Katzko G, et al: Evaluation of the Strep A OIA assay versus culture methods: ability to detect different quantities of group A streptococcus. *Diagn Microbiol Infect Dis* 34:275–280, 1999.

74. Hart AP, Buck LL, Morgan S, et al: A comparison of the BioStar Strep A OIA rapid antigen assay, group A Selective Strep Agar (ssA), and Todd-Hewitt broth cultures for the detection of group A streptococcus in an outpatient family practice setting. *Diagn Microbiol Infect Dis* 29:139–145, 1997.

75. Kurtz B, Kurtz M, Roe M, Todd J: Importance of inoculum size and sampling effect in rapid antigen detection for diagnosis of *Streptococcus pyogenes* pharyngitis. *J Clin Microbiol* 38:279–281, 2001.

76. Webb KH: Does culture confirmation of high-sensitivity rapid streptococcal tests make sense? A medical decision analysis. *Pediatrics* 101(2):E2, 1998.

77. Ebell MH, Smith MA, Barry HC, et al: The rational clinical examination. Does this patient have strep throat? *JAMA* 284:2912–2918, 2000.

78. McIsaac WJ, Goel V, To T, Low DE: The validity of a sore throat score in family practice. *Can Med Assoc J* 163:811–815, 2000.

79. Thomas M, Del Mar C, Glasziou P: How effective are treatments other than antibiotics for acute sore throat? *Brit J Gen Pract* 50:817–820, 2000.

80. Shaughnessy AF: Treating the common cold. *Fam Pract Recertification* 17:15–19, 1995.

81. Patel SK, Ghufoor K, Jayaraj SM, et al: Pictorial assessment of the delivery of oropharyngeal rinse versus oropharyngeal spray. *J Laryngol Otol* 13:1092–1094, 1999.

82. Watson N, Nimmo WS, Christian J, et al: Relief of sore throat with the anti-inflammatory throat lozenge flurbiprofen 8.75 mg: a randomised, double-blind, placebo-controlled study of efficacy and safety. *Int J Clin Pract* 54:490–496, 2000.

83. Marvez-Valls EG, Ernst AA, Gray J, Johnson WD: The role of betamethasone in the treatment of acute exudative pharyngitis. *Acad Emerg Med* 5:567–572, 1998.

84. Del Mar CB, Glasziou PP, Spinks AB: Antibiotics for sore throat. *Cochrane Database of Systematic Reviews* 2:CD000023, 2000.

85. Bisno AL, Gerber MA, Gwaltney JM Jr, et al: Diagnosis and management of group A streptococcal pharyngitis: a practice guideline. *Clin Infect Dis* 25:574–583, 1997.

86. Lan AJ, Colford JM, Colford JM Jr: The impact of dosing frequency on the efficacy of 10-day penicillin or amoxicillin therapy for streptococcal tonsillopharyngitis: a meta-analysis. *Pediatrics* 105(2): E19, 2000.

87. Zwart S, Sachs AP, Ruijs GJ, et al: Penicillin for acute sore throat: randomised double blind trial of seven days versus three days treatment or placebo in adults. *Br Med J* 320:150–154, 2000.

88. Feder HM Jr, Gerber MA, Randolph MF, et al: Once-daily therapy for streptococcal pharyngitis with amoxicillin. *Pediatrics* 103:47–51, 1999.

89. Pichichero ME, Casey JR, Mayes T, et al: Penicillin failure in streptococcal tonsillopharyngitis: causes and remedies. *Pediatr Infect Dis J* 19:917–923, 2000.

90. Brook I: Microbial factors leading to recurrent upper respiratory tract infections. *Pediatr Infect Dis J* 17(8 Suppl):S62–S67, 1998.

91. Brook I, Gober AE: Persistence of group A beta-hemolytic streptococci in toothbrushes and removable orthodontic appliances following treatment of pharyngotonsillitis. *Arch Otolaryngol Head Neck Surg* 124:993–995, 1998.

92. Osterlund A, Popa R, Nikkila T, et al: Intracellular reservoir of *Streptococcus pyogenes* in vivo: a possible explanation for recurrent pharyngotonsillitis. *Laryngoscope* 107:640–647, 1997.

93. Pichichero ME, Green JL, Francis AB, et al: Recurrent group A streptococcal tonsillopharyngitis. *Pediatr Infect Dis J* 17:809–815, 1998.

94. Billich A: Pleconaril Sanofi Synthelabo/ViroPharma. *Curr Opin Invest Drugs* 1:303–307, 2000.

95. Marlow RA, Torrez AJ Jr, Haxby D: The treatment of nonstreptococcal pharyngitis with erythromycin: a preliminary study. *Fam Med* 21:425–427, 1989.

96. Petersen K, Phillips RS, Soukup J, et al: The effect of erythromycin on resolution of symptoms among adults with pharyngitis not caused by group A streptococcus. *J Gen Intern Med* 12:95–101, 1997.

97. Master D, Longe SH, Dickson H: Scheduled hand washing in an elementary school population. *Fam Med* 29:336–339, 1997.

98. Haines JD Jr: When to resume sports after infectious mononucleosis. How soon is safe? *Postgrad Med* 81:331–333, 1987.

99. Peter J, Ray CG: Infectious mononucleosis. *Pediatr Rev* 19:276–279, 1998.

100. van der Horst C, Joncas J, Ahronheim G, et al: Lack of effect of peroral acyclovir for the treatment of acute infectious mononucleosis. *J Infect Dis* 164:788–792, 1991.

101. Tynell E, Aurelius E, Brandell A, et al: Acyclovir and prednisolone treatment of acute infectious mononucleosis: a multicenter, double-blind, placebo-controlled study. *J Infect Dis* 174:324–331, 1996.

102. Management of sore throat and indications for tonsillectomy. A national clinical guideline. Edinburgh (UK), Scottish Intercollegiate Guidelines Network, Scottish Cancer Therapy Network, 1999.

103. Paradise JL, Bluestone CD, Bachman RZ, et al: Efficacy of tonsillectomy for recurrent throat infection in severely affected children. Results of parallel randomized and nonrandomized clinical trials. *N Engl J Med* 310:674–683, 1984.

104. Gooch WM III: Potential infectious disease complications of upper respiratory tract infections. *Pediatr Infect Dis J* 17(8 Suppl):S79–S82, 1998.

105. Quinn RW: Comprehensive review of morbidity and mortality for rheumatic fever, streptococcal disease and scarlet fever: the decline of rheumatic fever. *Rev Infect Dis* 11:928–953, 1989.

106. McIsaac WJ, Goel V, Slaughter PM, et al: Reconsidering sore throats: Part 1: problems with current clinical practice. *Can Fam Physician* 43:485–493, 1997.

107. American Academy of Pediatrics: Report of the Committee on Infectious Diseases, 22d ed. Elk Grove Village, IL, American Academy of Pediatrics, 1991.

108. Ophir D, Bawnik J, Poria Y, et al: Peritonsillar abscess. A prospective evaluation of outpatient management by needle aspiration. *Arch Otolaryngol Head Neck Surg* 114:661–663, 1988.

109. Shaham D, Sklair-Levy M, Weinberger G, Gomori JM: Lemierre's syndrome presenting as multiple lung abscesses. *Clin Imaging* 4:197–199, 2000.

Morten Lindbaek
John M. Hickner

Chapter 6

Sinusitis

The first modern description of bacterial sinusitis was published in 1889, when Dr. J. H. Bryan, an ear-nose-and-throat surgeon, described four classical cases of "abscess of the antrum."[1] Bryan listed the causes of sinusitis in his day: (1) "traumatism," which was acute infectious diseases such as measles, scarlet fever, or smallpox, (2) syphilis, (3) extension of inflammation from the lining membrane of the nose, and (4) extension of suppurative infection from dental caries. He also described the clinical findings associated with sinusitis: focal facial or dental pain and "discharge of fetid pus from the nose, generally unilateral and of long standing." In addition, he noted that some patients have focal tenderness with pressure over the affected sinus. Our knowledge of sinus infections has advanced significantly during the past 110 years, but his clinical descriptions, especially regarding the symptoms and signs of abscess of the antrum, bacterial sinusitis, have stood the test of time.

One must be cautious, however, in the diagnosis and treatment of sinusitis. Today, acute bacterial sinusitis is overdiagnosed and overtreated in primary care practice. In this chapter we will discuss in detail and present evidence for the following key points. First, most cases of acute sinusitis are caused by viral infections and resolve without antibiotic treatment. Second, the clinical diagnosis of acute bacterial sinusitis is difficult in primary care practice. In clinical trials of antibiotic treatment, only about half of patients diagnosed with acute bacterial sinusitis by experienced primary care physicians actually have a bacterial sinus infection. Third, antibiotic treatment of acute sinusitis is indicated only in patients with severe symptoms of sinusitis or in patients with moderate symptoms of duration greater than 7 days. Symptomatic treatment is sufficient in patients with mild symptoms. Fourth, sinus imaging studies are not recommended in routine diagnosis and may be helpful only in selected cases. Finally, other than pain medication, there is no evidence that use of adjunctive treatments such as decongestants is effective in symptom relief.

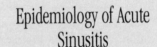

Epidemiology of Acute Sinusitis

Estimates of the incidence of acute sinusitis vary widely, depending on the source of the information. Sinusitis is one of the ten most common diagnoses in ambulatory practice, accounting for an estimated 25 million U.S. physician office visits in 1995.[2] Data from the 1995 National Ambulatory Medical Care Survey (NAMCS) estimated that of the 700 million visits made to nonfederally employed physicians in office-based practices, about 3 million of these (0.4 percent) were for acute sinusitis. Comparing these data with data from the same survey in 1990, the frequency with which sinusitis was diagnosed appears to have doubled between 1990 and 1995 (from 0.2 percent of visits to 0.4 percent). It is not clear whether this trend represents an actual increase in disease prevalence or changes in physicians' diagnoses or patients' care-seeking behavior.[3]

Some 14 percent of Americans claim to have had a prior diagnosis of sinusitis,[4] but the term *sinusitis* typically has a different meaning for patients and for primary care physicians.[5] When patients say, "I have sinus trouble," they usually describe acute or chronic symptoms such as headache, facial pain, nasal congestion, or rhinorrhea, each of which may have a variety of causes. Primary care physicians usually think of sinusitis as an acute bacterial infection for which they prescribe an antibiotic.[6]

The best data on the incidence of sinus infections requiring medical care come from Europe. Studies from several countries give estimates of the frequency of sinusitis based on diagnosis in general practice. In Larvik, Norway, which has 31,000 adult inhabitants, 1138 cases of acute sinusitis were diagnosed in primary care offices during a 1-year period, an incidence of approximately 3.5 per 100 adults per year.[7] About 7 percent of the patients had two episodes during the

12-month recording period, and 0.5 percent had three or more episodes. There was significant seasonal variation, with the highest frequency being in the winter months and the lowest in the summer and autumn.[7] In a Swedish general practice study, sinusitis was the diagnosis in 2 percent of patients seeking medical care.[8] In studies in British and Dutch general practice where the diagnoses were based on clinical examination only, an incidence of 2.1 to 2.5 episodes of acute sinusitis per 100 patient visits per year was found.[9] Van Duijn and colleagues' study from Holland demonstrated a frequency of confirmed sinusitis of 1.6 per 100 adults per year, of whom 9 percent had recurrent episodes.[9] Taken together, it appears that the incidence of sinusitis-like illness severe enough to prompt a visit to a clinician is between 1.6 and 3.5 episodes per 100 adults per year.

We know little about people with sinus infections who do not seek medical care. Since studies examining treatment strategies for sinusitis have demonstrated that acute sinusitis is a self-limiting disease in many cases,[10–12] it is likely that many patients with sinusitis never seek medical care. From community-based studies in the United States, it has been estimated that adults have two to three common colds each year and that 0.5 to 2 percent of those with a common cold develop acute bacterial sinusitis.[13–15] Based on the incidence numbers for colds and sinusitis, one would expect 1000 to 2000 cases of acute sinusitis per year in the Larvik, Norway, study, and 1138 episodes were diagnosed.[7] However, in a phone survey in Canada, during a 2-week period only 15 percent of people with acute respiratory infection symptoms sought medical care.[16]

Gender Differences in Acute Sinusitis

Acute sinusitis is diagnosed more often in women than in men.[7,9] This difference is not due entirely to differences in health care-seeking behavior. In a large Norwegian study that

included 250,000 patients in primary care, the proportion of women diagnosed with acute sinusitis was 0.68 compared to 0.58 for other acute respiratory illnesses.[17] Two reasonable explanations exist that can account for a higher incidence of sinusitis in women than in men. First, because of child care duties, women aged 20 to 39 are exposed to upper respiratory tract infections (URIs) in children more often and more intimately than are men. Second, menstruating women have increased mucosal thickening due to estrogen exposure, and this may lead to a greater likelihood of ostial obstruction and subsequent sinus infection.[7]

Frequency of Sinusitis in Children

The incidence of acute sinusitis in children has not been carefully documented. Children experience six to eight common colds per year,[13] and one author estimates that 7 to 10 percent of these respiratory infections in children are complicated by acute sinusitis.[18] In a study of children in a primary care practice, acute sinusitis accounted for 9.3 percent of visits overall and 17.3 percent of visits for patients presenting with cold and cough symptoms.[19]

In summary, high-quality evidence on the prevalence and incidence of acute bacterial sinusitis in the general population and in primary care practices is lacking. Estimating the prevalence of bacterial, viral, and fungal sinusitis requires the use of more specific diagnostic criteria in epidemiologic studies.

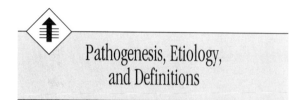

Pathogenesis, Etiology, and Definitions

Sinusitis means inflammation of the mucosa of the paranasal sinuses, irrespective of the cause.

Because sinusitis is invariably accompanied by inflammation of the contiguous nasal mucosa, some prefer the broader term *rhinosinusitis*. Most cases of sinusitis involve more than one of the paranasal sinuses, most commonly the maxillary and ethmoid sinuses.

Sinusitis can be categorized as acute, subacute, and chronic. Acute sinusitis usually lasts for less than 30 days, whereas subacute sinusitis lasts from 1 to 3 months and chronic sinusitis denotes a problem present for more than 3 months.[4]

Predisposing Factors

In primary care settings, the most common predisposing factor is URIs like the common cold and influenza.[12] Allergic rhinitis, which is very common in patients with chronic sinusitis, is assumed to be a predisposing factor for acute sinusitis, but research data are conflicting.[12] URIs and allergic rhinitis can lead to mucosal edema, ostial narrowing, increased secretion, and decreased mucociliary activity. Anatomic malformations, polyps, septal deviation, foreign bodies, and tumors may cause ostial obstruction leading to sinusitis.[20] In 5 to 10 percent of cases, sinusitis is caused by an upper tooth infection that spreads directly to the maxillary sinus.[12]

Research during the last decade has demonstrated the importance for the health of the sinuses and adjacent tissues of having a well-functioning mucociliary transport system.[21] A protective blanket of mucus covers the respiratory cilia of the sinuses and is moved constantly along predetermined pathways to the ostia. In the normal maxillary sinus, mucus is moved from the floor of the sinus radially up the walls and superiorly to the ostium.[21] Dysfunction of the mucociliary system can lead to higher risk for sinus infections. An understanding of the importance of the mucociliary function has been vital for the development of modern functional endoscopic sinus surgery (FESS) for patients with chronic sinusitis.

A less common predisposing factor for sinus infections is an immunocompromised state, as in patients with diabetes mellitus[4] or HIV infection. Chronic sinusitis has been associated with depressed immunoglobulin levels, low IgG subclass levels, and decreased vaccine responsiveness.[4] These immune defects have not been studied systematically in adults, but they have been found in 30 percent of pediatric patients with chronic or recurrent sinus infections.[4]

Pathogenesis

Our knowledge of the pathogenesis of sinusitis is based on studies of the maxillary sinus. It is presumed that the same mechanisms cause sinusitis in the other paranasal sinuses. The common cold causes mucosal thickening and secretion, resulting in obstruction of the ostium. Obstruction of the narrow sinus passages is crucial in the pathogenesis of sinusitis.[12]

Recent research on sinusitis has concentrated on discovering where in the nose and paranasal sinuses the pathologic processes start. Attention has to a great extent been focused on the infundibulum area and the anterior group of ethmoidal cells.[22] It is assumed that this is a key area for occlusion of the ostium and blockage of the drainage of secretions from the main sinus systems. This is the basis for FESS, which aims to reestablish functional drainage of the sinuses through an operation in the infundibulum area.[22]

Viral (Serous) Sinusitis

Viral infections cause mucosal thickening, which may narrow or close the ostium. The closing of the ostium leads to a change in the sinus environment. The concentration of oxygen decreases and the concentration of carbon dioxide increases while the normal drainage through the ostium is obstructed.[23] This leads to the formation of a serous secretion in the sinus. This condition is called *serous sinusitis* and may give modest symptoms of facial pressure. The prognosis is good, and most cases resolve regardless of treatment.[24]

Maxillary sinus radiographs of young adults with typical viral URIs showed mucosal abnormalities in 39 percent of cases on the seventh day of illness,[25] and computed tomographic (CT) scans were abnormal in 87 percent of similar cases.[26] These studies demonstrate that some degree of inflammation of the sinus mucosa is very common in viral URIs, but rarely progresses to a more serious illness such as bacterial sinusitis.

Bacterial (Purulent) Sinusitis

Acute bacterial sinusitis is usually a secondary infection resulting from obstruction of the sinus ostia and/or impaired mucus clearance mechanisms caused by an acute viral URI.[12] A healthy sinus is sterile or nearly so. A prerequisite for development of a mucopurulent sinusitis is the presence of bacteria in the sinuses. Nose blowing may create pressure differentials that cause the deposition of bacteria-containing nasal secretions in the sinus.[12] If bacteria enter the sinus via the ostium, and if serous secretion and good growth conditions are present, rapid growth of bacteria may result.[12] The body responds with an inflammatory reaction, and polymorphonuclear leukocytes (PMNs) are mobilized, resulting in pus formation.

The development of purulent secretions indicates that the defense system of the body has been mobilized. The PMNs phagocytize and kill the bacteria. In this phase, the pus is mucopurulent. This is the usual situation in *acute mucopurulent sinusitis*, as it appears in general practice. In immunocompetent people, the infection is usually successfully contained, accounting for the spontaneous resolution of acute bacterial sinusitis in the majority of patients presenting to primary care practices.

Occasionally the inflammatory system of the body is not able to limit bacterial growth. The process progresses, and the pus becomes thinner and more fluid-like, homogeneous, and sometimes foul smelling. If such findings occur, there is greater risk of irreversible damage to the sinus mucosa. There is also a risk of serious sinus complications in this category of patients. The best way to cure these patients is puncture and lavage of the sinus to flush out the infected material, along with antibiotic treatment. Fortunately, these cases are rare in primary care practice.

Table 6-1 shows the typical etiologic agents associated with acute maxillary sinusitis.[12] The most common bacterial pathogens are *Streptococcus pneumoniae* and *Haemophilus influenzae*. *Moraxella catarrhalis* is the next most likely organism and often produces beta-lactamase. The role of this species in the pathogenesis of sinusitis is still not clarified. Some anaerobes, most of them beta-lactamase-producing, have been found as etiologic agents. *Haemophilus* spp. and staphylococci that are resistant to penicillin are common pathogens cultured from sinus aspirates of patients who fail to improve on treatment with penicillin.[27]

Investigators have explored the relationship between acute bacterial sinusitis and bacterial growth in the nasal cavity. Table 6-2 gives the results of nasal bacterial cultures in patients with acute respiratory infections, some of whom had sinusitis and some of whom did not, as diagnosed by CT scan.[28] *S. pneumoniae and H. influenzae* were the dominant nasal airway pathogens in this group of patients with acute sinusitis. This corresponds well with previous studies, based both on sinus puncture[29,30] and on specimens from the nasopharynx.[31] One investigator found that in patients with acute sinusitis who underwent sinus puncture, the same pathogen was found in the sinus aspirate and the nasal sample in 91 percent of the cases. The predictive value of a pathogen-positive nasal finding was highest for group A streptococcus (94 percent), followed by *H. influenzae* (78 percent) and *S. pneumoniae* (69 percent) cases.[31] This indicates that in patients with

Table 6-1

Viral and Bacterial Etiology of Acute Maxillary Sinusitis Based on Sinus Puncture

	MEAN % OF CASES INVOLVING	
ETIOLOGIC AGENTS	ADULTS	CHILDREN
Viruses*		
Rhinovirus	15	—
Influenza virus	5	—
Parainfluenza virus	3	2
Adenovirus	—	2
Bacteria (range)		
Streptococcus pneumoniae	31 (20–35)	36
Haemophilus influenzae (unencapsulated)	21 (6–26)	23
S. pneumoniae and *H. influenzae*	5 (1–9)	—
Anaerobic bacteria		
(e.g., *Bacteroides, Peptostreptococcus,* or *Fusobacterium* species)	6 (0–10)	—
Moraxella catarrhalis	2 (2–10)	19
Staphylococcus aureus	4 (0–8)	—
Streptococcus pyogenes	2 (1–3)	2
Gram-negative bacteria[†]	9 (0–24)	2

*Data are from [13].
†One study had a 24 percent rate of isolation of gram-negative bacteria, but in four other studies the recovery rate was < 5 percent. Gram-negative bacteria recovered included *Pseudomonas aeruginosa, Klebsiella pneumoniae,* and *Escherichia coli.*
SOURCE: From Gwaltney,[15] with permission.

Table 6-2

Bacteriologic Findings in Nasopharyngeal Specimens from 427 Patients with a Diagnosis of Acute Sinusitis
by Computed Tomography (CT) in Vestfold, Norway, Winter Seasons 1993–1995

	CT RESULTS			
	POSITIVE N = 252 (%)	NEGATIVE N = 175 (%)	TOTAL	P-VALUES
Streptococcus pneumoniae	67 (27)	6 (3)	73 (17)	0.0001
Haemophilus influenzae	25 (10)	4 (2)	29 (8)	0.002
Moraxella catarrhalis	8 (3)	8 (5)	16 (4)	0.45
Gram-negative bacteria	4 (2)	4 (2)	8 (2)	0.60
Beta-hemolytic streptococcus group A	6 (2)	3 (2)	9 (2)	0.64
Staphylococcus aureus	29 (12)	31 (18)	60 (14)	0.07
Normal nasal flora/no growth	113 (45)	119 (62)	232 (54)	0.0001
Total	252 (100)	175 (100)	427 (100)	

SOURCE: From Lindbaek,[28] with permission.

suspected acute sinusitis, the same pathogen that is in the affected sinus can usually be found on nasopharyngeal specimens. Potentially, nasal cultures could guide antibiotic therapy, although this has not been tested in clinical practice.

Unfortunately, a great proportion of the nasal specimens of patients with bacterial sinusitis show no bacterial findings or "normal nasal flora." Therefore, bacterial culture of the nasal cavity is of limited value in the routine management of bacterial sinusitis in primary care settings.

Sinuses Involved in Acute Infections

Table 6-3[32] shows the CT results for each sinus system evaluated separately in 201 patients with bacterial sinusitis. The diagnostic standard for these data is fluid level or total opacification, which has a positive predictive value of 90 percent for bacterial sinusitis. The ethmoid sinuses were most frequently affected, followed by the maxillary sinuses. Table 6-4[32] shows the results of CT findings from the same study for each individual patient. The maxillary sinuses showed evidence of infection in 84 patients

(42 percent), and the small sinuses—ethmoid, sphenoid, and frontal—showed evidence of infection without involvement of the maxillary sinuses in 43 patients (21 percent).

New Research on Nitrogen Monoxide

During the last decade, researchers have found that nitrogen monoxide (NO) in the sinuses seems to be an important defense against infection.[33] NO is a unique molecule, a free radical that is a potent vasodilator that inhibits bacterial growth. Large quantities of NO are produced continuously in the human sinuses, and the high local concentrations can be of great importance in the first-line immune defense in these sensitive cavities.

Furthermore, NO from the sinuses passes down to the lungs along with the inspiratory air and contributes to increased oxygenation of the blood and lowered resistance in the pulmonary blood vessels. This may be part of the explanation for the purpose of paranasal sinuses in humans, which has puzzled researchers for many years.[33]

Table 6-3

Computed Tomographic (CT) Findings in Each Sinus System Evaluated Separately in 201 Patients with Suspected Acute Sinusitis, Vestfold, Norway, 1993

	MAXILLARY		ETHMOID		FRONTAL		SPHENOID	
	N	%	N	%	N	%	N	%
Negative CT, no mucosal thickening	36	18	42	21	74	37	124	62
Negative CT, mucosal thickening < 5 mm	30	15	44	22	58	29	36	18
Mucosal thickening ≥ 5 mm	51	25	—	—	51	25	31	15
Fluid level	73	36	4	2	8	4	3	1
Total opacification	11	6	111	55	10	5	7	4
	201	100	201	100	201	100	201	100

SOURCE: From Lindbaek,[33] with permission.

Table 6-4

Overall Computed Tomographic (CT) Assessment of Sinuses Affected in 201 Patients with Clinically Suspected
Acute Sinusitis from Larvik, Norway, 1993

GROUP	SINUSES INVOLVED		N	%
1	Negative CT		49	24
2	Mucosal thickening ≥ 5 mm in either sinus, no opacification/fluid		25	13
3a	Fluid level or total opacification in			
	Ethmoid alone	30		
	Frontal alone	2		
	Sphenoid alone	2		
	Ethmoid + sphenoid	1		
	Ethmoid + frontal	6		
	Ethmoid + sphenoid + frontal	2	43	21
3b	Fluid level or total opacification in			
	Maxillary alone	5		
	Maxillary + ethmoid	64		
	Maxillary + sphenoid	1		
	Maxillary + ethmoid + frontal	9		
	Maxillary + ethmoid + sphenoid	2		
	Maxillary + ethmoid + sphenoid + frontal	3	84	42
Total			201	100

SOURCE: From Lindbaek,[32] with permission.

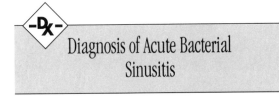

Diagnosis of Acute Bacterial Sinusitis

The best diagnostic standard for bacterial sinusitis is sinus puncture and aspiration of purulent secretions that grow ≥ 10^4 organisms per milliliter; however, this test is not practical in the primary care setting.[12] The diagnosis of sinusitis in primary care practice is difficult because of the lack of specific clinical features that distinguish it from nonbacterial upper respiratory tract infections.

Primary care doctors overdiagnose acute bacterial sinusitis. Relying on overall clinical impressions, primary care doctors who classify patients as highly likely to have bacterial sinusitis are correct in approximately 40 to 50 percent of cases.[13,26,34] Plain radiographs are not generally indicated because of their low positive predictive value, and CT scans, though more accurate, are of limited value because of their expense and limited availability.

Clinical Findings that Predict Acute Bacterial Sinusitis

Four studies from primary care practice provide useful information on symptoms, signs, and blood tests that help discriminate bacterial sinusitis from viral upper respiratory infections.[9,30,34,35] (Table 6-5). Purulent rhinorrhea as a symptom and the finding of purulent secretions in the nasal cavity were associated with bacterial sinusitis in three of the four studies.

Table 6-5

Symptoms, Signs, and Blood Tests Independently Associated with a Confirmed Diagnosis of Acute Sinusitis in Four Studies from General Practice

Author Reference Standard Number of patients	Hansen[30] Puncture N = 174	Lindbaek[32] CT sinus N = 201	Williams[35] X-ray N = 247	van Duijn[9] Ultrasound N = 441	Total*
Symptoms					
Purulent rhinorrhea	−	+	+	−	2+, 2−
Pain in teeth	−	−	+	+	2+, 2−
Start with URI	−	−	−	+	1+, 3−
Unilateral maxillary pain	−	−	−	+	1+, 3−
Two phases in history	0	+	0	0	1+
No response to nasal decongestant	0	0	+	0	1+
Signs					
Purulent secretion in nares	−	+	+	+	3+, 1−
Pain at bending forward	−	−	−	+	1+, 3−
Transillumination of sinus	0	0	+	0	1+
Blood tests					
ESR > 10/20 mm/h	+	+	0	0	2+
CRP > 10g/L	+	−	0	0	1+, 1−

ABBREVIATIONS: CT, computed tomography; URI, upper respiratory tract infection; ESR, erythrocyte sedimentation rate; CPR, C-reactive protein.
* + means association, − means no association demonstrated, 0 means not investigated.
SOURCE: From Lindbaek, unpublished.

Tooth pain was associated with bacterial infection in two. Other findings were less consistent predictors of bacterial sinusitis. A biphasic history with worsening following initial improvement (so-called double sickening) and lack of effect of decongestants were associated in one study each and were not investigated in the others. An erythrocyte sedimentation rate (ESR) > 10 for men and > 20 for women was associated in the two studies in which it was investigated, while C-reactive protein (CRP) > 10 was associated in one, but not in the other in which it was investigated.

All these studies, however, are limited by the use of imperfect diagnostic standards. None used the best criterion for diagnosing bacterial sinusitis, aspiration of purulent secretions that grow ≥ 10^4 organisms per milliliter of a likely respiratory pathogen on culture. No single sign or symptom had strong diagnostic value in any study.

EVALUATION OF CLINICAL PREDICTORS IN PRIMARY CARE STUDIES

Unfortunately, the one study that did rely on the culture of aspirated material from the sinuses did not show any clinical signs or symptoms as having predictive value in diagnosing sinusitis.[30] In Hansen and colleagues' study of 172 patients with suspected bacterial sinusitis referred from general practitioners in Denmark, 53 percent of patients had pus or mucopurulent fluid on sinus aspiration, and three-fourths of this group had positive bacterial cultures. In initial bivariate analysis, unilateral maxillary pain, maxillary toothache, unilateral tenderness of the maxillary sinus, and mucopurulent nasal discharge were statistically more likely in patients with positive sinus aspirates, but the magnitude of association was small (odds ratios ranging from 1.9 to 2.5). However, when a logistic regression was performed, only elevated ESR and CRP were independently associated with bacterial infection; none of the clinical findings was found to be a significant predictor of bacterial sinus infection.

Other studies have not used aspiration samples as the gold standard, but have relied on imaging studies to establish probable bacterial sinusitis cases. Air-fluid levels or complete sinus opacification on CT sinus radiography can be considered an intermediate sign of bacterial sinusitis, since these findings have approximately a 90 percent positive predictive value for purulent or mucopurulent secretions on sinus aspiration. In one study using these imaging criteria to define sinusitis, Lindbaek and colleagues[34] found worsening of URI symptoms after initial improvement, purulent rhinorrhea, and purulent secretions in the nasal cavities to be the best independent clinical predictors of acute sinusitis. This study also found that an elevated ESR was associated with likely bacterial sinusitis.

Using plain radiographs as the diagnostic standard, Williams and Simel[35] identified five independent predictors of acute bacterial sinusitis in a study of men with suspected sinusitis in a Veterans Administration outpatient clinic: history of colored nasal discharge, purulent nasal secretions on examination, poor response to decongestants, maxillary toothache, and abnormal transillumination. In a Dutch study that used ultrasound as the standard for diagnosing sinusitis, preceding URI, purulent rhinorrhea, facial pain on bending forward, unilateral maxillary pain, and tooth pain were significantly associated with suspected sinusitis.[9] However, these results should be interpreted with caution, since studies that rely on plain sinus radiography or ultrasonography as the diagnostic standard may overestimate the presence of bacterial infection by as much as 50 percent, giving a large opportunity for misclassification.[36]

Furthermore, a number of clinical signs and symptoms that have been suggested to predict sinusitis have not been demonstrated to be of value in primary care–based studies. In particular, bilateral pain over the maxillary sinuses, pain over the frontal sinuses, headache, allergy, malaise, cough, anosmia and cacosmia (the sensation that something smells bad), nasal congestion, fever $> 38°C$, tenderness over the maxillary and frontal sinuses, purulent pharyngeal discharge, and swelling over the maxillary sinuses do not appear to be useful in predicting the presence of a bacterial sinusitis. Although many of these symptoms may be frequent in patients with acute sinusitis, they are equally common in patients with viral URIs. A prior diagnosis of sinusitis does not appear to be a useful predictor of bacterial sinusitis either.[30]

STUDIES FROM SPECIALTY PRACTICE

Two older studies of clinical predictors of bacterial sinusitis have been performed in otorhinolaryngology practices.[37,38] Berg and colleagues studied patients with sinusitis symptoms of under 3 months' duration using sinus aspiration of purulent secretions as the diagnostic standard. Four findings were associated with bacterial sinusitis: history of purulent nasal discharge with unilateral predominance, history of bilateral purulent nasal discharge, history of facial pain with unilateral predominance, and pus in the nasal cavity on physical examination. When two or more of these findings were present, 67 to 85 percent of patients had bacterial sinusitis. If one or none were present, less than 10 percent had a bacterial infection. Because the diagnostic standard was the finding of sinus empyema, which is the most serious type of bacterial sinusitis, the patients in this study may have been sicker on average than those encountered in primary care practice. Moreover, the relevance of Berg and colleagues' findings to patients with acute sinusitis in primary care is limited by the inclusion of patients with symptom duration greater than 30 days. Nonetheless, his results are consistent with the findings in the studies from primary care. Axelsson and Runze used sinus x-ray as the diagnostic standard and found that purulent rhinorrhea, preceding URI, cough, hyposmia, and malaise were predictors of bacterial sinusitis.[38]

IMPORTANCE OF DURATION OF SYMPTOMS

Because acute bacterial sinusitis usually develops as a complication of a viral URI, experts have proposed that duration of illness of less than 7 days be used as a negative diagnostic criterion. But in clinical trials of diagnosis and treatment of sinusitis, duration of illness alone did not reliably distinguish prolonged viral infection from bacterial sinusitis. Two studies by Lindbaek and colleagues provide useful information regarding the predictive value of duration of illness.[24,34] In these studies, using a duration of symptoms greater than 7 days as a diagnostic test for bacterial sinusitis was 80 percent sensitive and 30 percent specific. The positive predictive value was 60 percent, and the negative predictive value was 51 percent. In other words, of patients in general practice presenting with sinusitis symptoms of more than 7 days' duration, about 60 percent will have bacterial sinus-

itis and 40 percent will have prolonged viral respiratory infections. On the other hand, of patients presenting with sinusitis symptoms of 7 days' or less duration, half will have bacterial sinusitis and half will have viral upper respiratory tract infections. Overall, the duration of symptoms is a poor single predictor of acute bacterial sinusitis.

CONCLUSIONS REGARDING CLINICAL PREDICTORS

Of possible clinical symptoms and signs, purulent rhinorrhea and the finding of purulent secretions in the nasal cavity on physical examination are the best predictors of acute bacterial sinusitis. Tooth pain, a biphasic history with worsening of symptoms following an initial improvement, a lack of effect of decongestants, and an elevated ESR are supportive evidence of bacterial infection, although they are weaker predictors. Patients with less than 7 days' duration of sinusitis-like symptoms are slightly less likely to have a bacterial infection.

Use of Radiography and Ultrasound

Table 6-6[36] shows the sensitivity and specificity of sinus radiographs and ultrasound in diagnosing

Table 6-6

Results of a Meta-analysis of Diagnostic Tests with Sinus Puncture and Sinus Radiograph as the Diagnostic Standards.

DIAGNOSTIC STANDARD	STUDIES/ COMPARISONS	SENSITIVITY (95% CI)	SPECIFICITY (95% CI)
Sinus puncture	—	Reference test	
Sinus radiograph: fluid or opacity[7–9,12–14]	6/10	75%(62%–86%)	79%(63%–89%)
Sinus radiograph: fluid, opacity, or thickening[7–9,12–14]	6/10	90%(68%–97%)	61%(20%–91%)
Sinus radiograph: opacity only[7–9,12–14]	6/10	85%(76%–91%)	41%(33%–49%)
Ultrasonogram[7–9,12,14]	5/10	84%(75%–90%)	69%(57%–79%)
Clinical examination[15]	1/5	Inconclusive	
Sinus radiograph	—	Reference test	
Clinical examination[10,16,17]	3/11	57%(37%–74%)	76%(60%–87%)
Ultrasonogram[18–20]	3/5	Inconclusive	

ABBREVIATION: CI, confidence interval.
From Benninger,[36] with permission.

sinusitis as compared to sinus puncture (as the gold standard). When using fluid or opacity the criterion for bacterial sinusitis, the sensitivity and specificity of x-ray are 76 percent and 79 percent, respectively. A completely normal sinus radiograph with no fluid level, opacification, or mucosal thickening is quite reliable in ruling out sinusitis, as the sensitivity is 90 percent. For ultrasonography, the test characteristics vary considerably from study to study. The specificity is low, 69 percent, giving a high proportion of false positive cases. A recent study demonstrated both low sensitivity and low specificity of ultrasonography compared with sinus puncture when general practitioners performed the procedure.[39]

Sinus CT appears to have a high specificity when fluid level and total opacification are used as the criteria for acute sinusitis. This assertion is based on the finding of a high positive predictive value of 90 percent from Hansen's study on CT compared with puncture of the sinus.[30] CT also has the advantage of providing a good evaluation of the small sinuses, which, as noted previously, are frequently involved in sinus infections, especially the ethmoid sinuses.[32]

Differential Diagnosis

A viral respiratory infection with predominant symptoms of nasal discharge and head congestion is the condition most often confused with acute bacterial sinusitis.[26] A number of pain conditions such as atypical migraine, tension headache, trigeminal neuralgia, and dysfunction of the mandibular joint are important conditions to consider in the differential diagnosis.[27] These are all conditions associated with recurring facial pain and are easily confused with recurrent sinusitis. In patients with recurrent episodes of facial pain and no other signs or symptoms of sinus infection, a negative x-ray or ultrasonography will exclude bacterial sinusitis as the cause. A combination of one of these pain conditions and a common cold can be very difficult to distinguish from a bacterial sinusitis. In such cases,

a positive x-ray or ultrasound might give a false positive for bacterial sinusitis, although a negative test will rule out sinusitis.

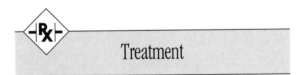

Symptomatic Treatment

Patients with mild to moderate symptoms consistent with acute sinusitis should be given symptomatic treatment only, as most of them will recover fully within 10 days without antibiotic treatment.

While symptomatic treatments can be offered to all patients, there is no evidence that any of these therapies shorten the duration of illness. Options for symptomatic treatment of sinusitis include decongestants and nonprescription pain relievers. Nasal irrigation with saline has also been suggested, especially by ear, nose, and throat specialists.[21]

The results of eight randomized trials of various symptomatic treatments of sinusitis symptoms in adults have been inconclusive.[40–47] Topically or orally administered alpha-adrenergic agents (decongestants), proteolytic enzymes, mucolytic agents, antihistamines, and corticosteroids have been used. Theoretically, agents that encourage the drainage of sinus secretions may be of value. Topical and oral decongestants may ameliorate some of the nasal symptoms and promote mucus clearance. Decongestants reduce the mucosal edema of the ostia, thus potentially improving the drainage from the sinuses. Studies have shown that oral decongestants improve the function of the sinus ostium and reduce the nasal airway resistance, but a significant clinical effect on acute sinusitis has not been documented.[48] Well-designed placebo-controlled trials of these ancillary treatments are needed to determine their effectiveness in treating acute sinusitis. They can be offered to patients with mild symptoms as an alternative to an antibiotic. Pain control is always important, as over 50 percent of patients with acute bacterial sinusitis complain of facial pain.[30,34]

No controlled trial of systemic steroid therapy for acute sinusitis has been performed. In three studies, topical steroids were given in addition to antibiotic treatment.[21] In one of these studies, inclusion of steroids was found to be useful. Since steroids take a long time to exert their effect, an episode of acute sinusitis may resolve before the beneficial effects of steroids are noticed.[21] Topical steroids are highly effective for treatment of allergic rhinitis, which may be misdiagnosed as bacterial sinusitis. Theoretically, chronic use of topical steroids in patients with allergic rhinitis may prevent recurrent sinusitis and assist in control of chronic sinusitis symptoms, but at this time there are no controlled trials to support these assertions.

Antibiotic Treatment

Symptomatic treatment and reassurance is the preferred initial management strategy for patients with mild symptoms. Antibiotic therapy should be reserved for patients with moderate to severe symptoms of purulent nasal discharge and unilateral facial pain. Patients with worsening sinusitis-like symptoms after initial improvement are more likely to have a bacterial infection, and antibiotic treatment is indicated. Patients with a duration of illness greater than 7 days are somewhat more likely to have a bacterial infection, so it is reasonable to be more aggressive with antibiotic treatment even though many do not require it. Conversely, bacterial infection is somewhat less likely with a shorter duration of symptoms, so watchful waiting is reasonable and is well accepted by some patients. Because antibiotic treatment is only marginally effective in most cases of clinically diagnosed sinusitis, shared decision making with the patient is always appropriate. Initial treatment should be with the most narrow-spectrum agent that is active against the likely pathogens, *S. pneumoniae* and *H. influenzae*.

Randomized, double-blind, placebo-controlled trials of antibiotic treatment of acute bacterial sinusitis using pretreatment and posttreatment culture of sinus aspirates have not been performed. However, nonrandomized treatment trials have shown appropriate antibiotics to be highly effective in eradicating or substantially reducing bacterial growth in the sinuses.[12]

The evidence on the clinical effectiveness of antibiotics in sinusitis is less compelling. Five randomized double-blinded clinical trials have compared antibiotic with placebo treatment of acute sinusitis in adults.[14–16,49,50] Three meta-analyses have been published.[51–53] All three conclude that although antibiotics are statistically more effective than placebo in reducing or eliminating symptoms at 10 and 14 days, the amount of benefit (the effect size) is relatively small and the majority of placebo-treated patients improve without antibiotic therapy.

The specific findings of each of these five trials have been well summarized by Williams et al.[51] One study used clinical clues for inclusion,[16] three used plain radiographs for diagnosis of sinusitis,[15,49,50] and one used CT criteria.[14] When considered in the aggregate, 47 percent of the antibiotic-treated subjects and 32 percent of the control subjects were considered cured at 10 to 14 days follow-up, while 81 percent of antibiotic-treated patients and 66 percent of controls were responders (with clinical findings of either cure or improvement).[51] This is an absolute benefit of 15 percent, giving a number needed to treat (NNT) of 7.

However, the two placebo-controlled trials of acute sinusitis in primary care failed to find a significant clinical effect of antibiotic treatment. Stalman et al[12] studied the effectiveness of doxycycline compared to placebo in general practice patients with symptoms of bacterial sinusitis. The inclusion criteria were based on guidelines of the Dutch College of General Practitioners: three main symptoms (complaints after a common cold or influenza, purulent nasal discharge, and pain in the maxillary sinuses on bending forward) or two main symptoms and one other symptom (predominately unilateral maxillary pain, toothache, or pain when chewing). There was no significant difference in time to resolution of facial pain and return to normal activities. Using radiographs for the diagnostic standard, van Buchem and colleagues[11] found no significant advantage of a 7-day course of amoxicillin over placebo at 14 days. Symptoms were substantially improved or resolved in 83 percent of patients on amoxicillin and 77 percent of patients on placebo.

The one modern placebo-controlled trial in a primary care population that showed a positive treatment effect for amoxicillin or penicillin used CT scanning for diagnosis and eligibility for the study.[14] Only patients with an air-fluid level or complete opacification of a sinus were eligible for inclusion. At day 10 of treatment, 56 percent of patients treated with placebo, 82 percent of those treated with penicillin, and 89 percent of those treated with amoxicillin were substantially better.

A recent study from Denmark has been published that was not included in the meta-analyses. This study included 133 patients from general practice with clinically diagnosed acute sinusitis who had maxillary pain and an elevated ESR and/or CRP.[54] The patients were treated with penicillin or placebo. After 10 days, 71 percent of patients in the penicillin-treated group were cured compared to 37 percent in the placebo group. However, the treatment effect was confined to those patients with severe or moderately severe facial pain.

One reason that clinical trials as a whole show antibiotic treatment of sinusitis to be less effective than one might predict from the bacteriologic studies can be explained by the "Pollyanna" phenomenon.[55] Because the clinical and radiologic diagnosis of acute bacterial sinusitis is inaccurate, the measured effect of antibiotic treatment for the entire treatment group is diluted by the cases that do not truly have a bacterial infection. When studies use a diagnostic criterion with a low specificity for sinusitis, such as x-ray opacification, a large number of patients without sinusitis are included in the trial. As a result, treatment for sinusitis is

less likely to be found to be beneficial. However, when treatment trials have used a more specific diagnostic standard, such as a positive CT scan, more of the patients actually have sinusitis and a significant benefit from antibiotics is more likely to be found.

Taking into consideration the 40 to 50 percent prevalence of bacterial sinusitis in patients diagnosed by signs and symptoms and the modest effectiveness of antibiotic treatment, a cost-effectiveness model favored antibiotic treatment for patients with moderate to severe symptoms and symptomatic treatment for those with mild symptoms.[56] In a cost-effectiveness analysis, de Bock et al calculated that in patients presenting with a clinical diagnosis of acute sinusitis, postponing antibiotics for 1 week is the most cost-effective strategy.[57]

Once it is decided to use an antibiotic for sinusitis, antibiotic selection and duration of therapy are important issues. Three meta-analyses have concluded that newer and broad-spectrum antibiotics are not significantly more effective than narrow-spectrum agents such as penicillin, amoxicillin, trimethoprim-sulfamethoxazole, or erythromycin.[36,51,52] In addition to the cost benefits of using less expensive narrow-spectrum agents, there is additional societal value in using these agents rather than newer, broad-spectrum antibiotics to reduce the rate of development of resistant microorganisms in the community.[51] However, because of the rapid increase in antibiotic resistance of *S. pneumoniae* and *H. influenzae*, treatment must take into account current recommendations for treating infections due to these organisms. If patients fail to respond to treatment within 72 h and/or are seriously ill, a trial of a fluoroquinolone or sinus puncture to obtain a specimen for culture and sensitivity may be indicated.

Sinus Puncture

The indication for sinus puncture and irrigation of the sinuses is sinus empyema when there is no natural drainage from the affected sinus and antibiotic treatment has produced no clinical improvement. In this situation, there is danger of serious complications. In these cases antibiotics have low penetration and the mucosal concentration does not reach bactericidal levels, even with high antibiotic dosages. Puncture should thus be performed as often as every second day until improvement results.[27] Some primary care physicians have been trained to perform sinus puncture, but if the primary care physician has not been so trained, these patients should be referred to an otolaryngologist for treatment and follow-up.

Fortunately, the need for puncture in the treatment of acute bacterial sinusitis in primary care seems to be rare. In two of the studies in which the need for puncture was reported, only 1 to 2 percent of the patients needed puncture to have resolution of the symptoms.[7,15] Both these studies were in patients with a confirmed sinusitis.

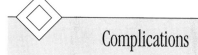

Complications

Serious complications of sinusitis such as meningitis, brain abscess, and periorbital cellulitis are rare, and good data regarding the frequency of these events in antibiotic-treated compared to untreated patients with sinusitis are not available.[3] In our review of 27 trials that included more than 2700 patients, we found no mention of any of these serious complications. In addition, data from large referral hospitals show that these events are rarely reported.[54] An estimated 1 out of 95,000 hospital discharges in the United States is for brain abscess; given the large number of sinusitis cases in the general population, the risk of developing a brain abscess from a case of sinusitis is negligible.

Among the studies on diagnosis and treatment that have been performed in general practice, only one case of serious complication, meningitis secondary to bacterial sinusitis, has been reported. The 60-year-old woman was hospitalized and recovered from her meningitis with no sequelae after intravenous antibiotic treatment.[7] To our knowledge, there are no data to suggest that the use of newer, more expensive antibiotics would reduce the rate of these rare complications.

Nevertheless, it should be emphasized that these data apply to patients with uncomplicated, community-acquired acute sinusitis. Rarely, patients with acute bacterial sinusitis present with dramatic symptoms of severe unilateral maxillary pain, swelling, and fever. These patients must be treated promptly with an appropriate antibiotic and may require early surgical referral for sinus drainage. Patients with complicated sinusitis and those who are severely ill with sinusitis or with important underlying diseases might merit initial treatment with broad-spectrum antibiotics.[51]

Another important complication is the development of chronic sinusitis from inadequately treated acute sinusitis. However, this risk has not been studied extensively. Van Buchem et al found that after 1 year, 5 of 488 patients with suspected sinusitis had developed chronic complaints.[11] Lindbaek et al found that in their population study, 5 of 386 patients with acute sinusitis developed chronic complaints.[7] From these two studies, one may conclude that 1 to 2 percent of patients with acute sinusitis may develop chronic sinusitis.

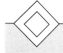

Recurrent Sinusitis

Patients with recurrent sinusitis constitute 7 to 9 percent of all patients with acute sinusitis.[7,9] They may have an underlying physiologic or anatomic abnormality. The most common is allergic rhinitis, which may respond well to a variety of treatments, of which the first choice should be topical steroids. Effective treatment for allergic rhinitis decreases mucosal edema and may lessen the chance of bacterial sinusitis by providing improved sinus drainage.[4] If allergic rhinitis is not present, other predisposing factors should be considered. Recurrent sinusitis can be a manifestation of immune compromise or an underlying anatomic abnormality. Nasal polyps or abnormalities in the ostiomeatal complex producing reduced drainage of the sinuses may be present. Patients with more than three episodes of acute sinusitis per year should be evaluated by a specialist for possible FESS.

Chronic Sinusitis

Chronic sinusitis is diagnosed when patients have symptoms of sinusitis for a minimum of 12 weeks. Chronic sinusitis differs in many ways from acute sinusitis. In acute sinusitis, the trigger is usually a viral URI. Chronic sinusitis, however, is associated more often with allergic rhinitis, asthma, anatomic abnormalities of the nasal cavity, immunocompromised states such as acquired immunodeficiency syndrome (AIDS) and diabetes mellitus, and a number of underlying diseases, most notably cystic fibrosis.[20,58] Other rare conditions associated with chronic sinusitis include Wegener's granulomatosis, Kartagener's syndrome, immotile cilia syndrome, and tumors. Chronic sinusitis may also result from untreated or insufficiently treated acute bacterial sinusitis.

Histologically, chronic sinusitis is a proliferative process with fibrosis of the lamina propria. There is infiltration with lymphocytes, plasma cells, and eosinophils. Bony changes may occur. There may be polyp formation and granulomas. A chronic smoldering bacterial or fungal infection may be present. Acute exacerbations may be due to a flare-up of infection and usually require a prolonged course of the appropriate antimicrobial agent.[58]

Patients with chronic sinusitis are often infected with the same bacterial pathogens as those with acute sinusitis, such as *S. pneumoniae, H. influenzae,* and *M. catarrhalis.* In addition to these, *Pseudomonas aeruginosa*, group A streptococcus, *Staphylococcus aureus*, and anaerobes such as *Bacteroides* species and fusobacteria may be involved.

Aspergillus fumigatus is the organism most often associated with fungal sinusitis in immunocompetent individuals. Allergic fungal sinusitis may be caused by a variety of other fungi as well.[59] Patients with diabetes mellitus, leukemia, or solid malignancies; those on high-dose steroid therapy; and those with severely impaired cell-mediated immunity are most likely to get fungal sinusitis. *Aspergillus* species are the most common infecting organisms.

Treatment of chronic sinusitis requires recognition and treatment of the underlying predisposing factors and diseases.[20,60] Nasal cytology to diagnose allergic disorders, sweat chloride to test for cystic fibrosis, and tests for immunodeficiency, such as quantitative immunoglobulins, antibody tests, serum IgE, and complement components, may be helpful if an underlying immunodeficiency is suspected. Patients with chronic sinusitis usually benefit from consultation with an otorhinolaryngologist for a more detailed anatomic and histologic evaluation than is feasible in primary care. For example, sinus mucosa biopsy may be necessary for culture of unusual organisms. Referral to an allergist may be of benefit as well. Intravenous immunoglobulin therapy has been used with some success in patients with immunodeficiency syndromes, but no randomized trials are available.

Treatment of chronic sinusitis is directed at control of infection, reduction of tissue edema, and facilitation of the drainage of sinus secretions. Both medical and surgical therapies are used to treat chronic sinusitis, but selection of the optimal treatment strategy is hampered by the lack of controlled trials comparing treatments.[60] In addition to medical therapy, FESS has become a popular surgical approach that focuses on restoring the drainage to the maxillary and ethmoid sinuses at the middle ostiomeatal complex and ethmoid cells.

Sinusitis in Children

There are few well-designed studies that have examined the diagnosis and treatment of sinus infections in children. Much of the research on sinusitis in adults applies to children, so this section will highlight some differences and similarities in the diagnosis and treatment of sinusitis in children.

The paranasal sinuses are a very common site of infection in children. Children have on average six to eight URIs per year. Most of these are viral infections, and, as previously noted, these infections usually involve the sinus mucosa as well as the nasopharynx. It is estimated that 5 to 13 percent of these infections may result in a secondary bacterial sinusitis, which is a higher frequency than estimates in adults.[19]

As in adults, the diagnosis of acute bacterial sinusitis in children should be based on the clinical presentation rather than on imaging studies. However, symptoms in children are less specific. Bacterial sinusitis should be suspected in children with persistent or severe sinusitis-like symptoms lasting greater than 10 to 14 days. Symptoms suggesting bacterial sinusitis are persistent nasal or postnasal discharge of any quality and persistent daytime cough that is not explained by asthma or allergic disease.[61]

Concurrent symptoms of high fever for 3 to 4 days accompanied by facial pain and/or purulent nasal discharge suggest severe sinusitis that needs urgent management. Facial pain and tenderness, however, is not a frequent finding in children with bacterial sinusitis.[61]

Because some children may have a second viral respiratory infection following soon after a previous one, the clinician must be careful to determine if there was a symptom-free period during the illness. A symptom-free period is strong evidence of a second viral infection rather than bacterial sinusitis.

Imaging studies are occasionally helpful in children with sinusitis-like complaints. In a study of children ages 2 to 16, positive bacterial cultures were obtained on sinus puncture in 70 to 75 percent of children with persistent or severe sinusitis-like symptoms and abnormal sinus radiographs (complete opacification, mucosal thickening of at least 4 mm, or an air-fluid level).[62] However, persistent unimproved symptoms for greater than 10 days predicts abnormal sinus radiographs in 80 percent of cases, so radiographs add little predictive value to diagnosis over and above clinical presentation.[61] As in adults, sinus radiographs are most helpful in ruling out bacterial sinusitis. A completely normal sinus radiograph is strong evidence against bacterial sinusitis.[63]

Antibiotic treatment is recommended for children with bacterial sinusitis for a more rapid cure.[64] One double-blind placebo-controlled trial of children with acute sinusitis diagnosed by clinical and radiographic findings demonstrated improvement at 3 and 10 days for the groups treated with amoxicillin and amoxicillin-clavulanic acid compared to placebo.[65] On the third day, 83 percent of children on the antibiotics were cured or improved, compared to 51 percent in the placebo group. At day 10, 79 percent of those treated with an antibiotic and 60 percent of those receiving placebo were cured or improved. However, in a recent study in which children were included based on clinically diagnosed acute sinusitis only, neither amoxicillin nor amoxicillin-clavulanate offered any clinical benefit compared with placebo.[66] This demonstrates the same problem as for adults. Sinusitis diagnosed on clinical symptoms and signs alone does not show a benefit of antibiotic treatment compared to placebo because at least 50 percent of cases that are clinically diagnosed may not have bacterial sinusitis. Sinusitis diagnosed more accurately with imaging studies, especially CT scan, is more likely to show benefit from antibiotic treatment because patients are more likely to have a bacterial infection.

S. pneumoniae and *H. influenzae* are the most common pathogens in children as well as in adults. *M. catarrhalis* is the next most likely bacterial organism. Amoxicillin remains the first-line drug of choice in 2001, but this may change as a result of the increasing resistance of these organisms to penicillins and other narrow-spectrum agents. Antibiotic therapy must be guided by local resistance patterns.

References

1. Bryan JH: Landmark article, Oct 5, 1889: Diagnosis and treatment of abscess of the antrum. By J. H. Bryan. *JAMA* 250(3):395–399, 1983.
2. Shappert S: *Ambulatory Care Visits to Physician's Offices, Hospital Outpatient Departments and Emergency Departments.* National Center for Health Statistics, series 13, no 134, 1998.
3. Zucher D, Balk E, Engels E, et al: *Diagnosis and Treatment of Acute Bacterial Sinusitis.* Agency for Health Care Policy and Research publication no 99-E016: Evidence report/ Technology assessment no 9, 1999.
4. Willett LR, Carson JL, Williams JW Jr: Current diagnosis and management of sinusitis. *J Gen Intern Med* 9(1):38–45, 1994.
5. Hickner JM: Acute sinusitis: a diagnostic and therapeutic challenge. *J Fam Pract* 50(1):38–40, 2001.
6. Gonzales R, Bartlett JG, Besser RE, et al: Principles of appropriate antibiotic use for treatment of acute respiratory tract infections in adults: background, specific aims, and methods. *Ann Intern Med* 134(6):479–486, 2001.
7. Lindbaek M, Hjortdahl P, Holth V: Acute sinusitis in Norwegian general practice—incidence, complications, referral to ear-nose-throat specialist and economic costs. *Eur J Gen Pract* 3:7–11, 1997.
8. Hovelius B, Widäng K: *Common Cold or Sinusitis.* Mårdh PH. Infektioner i primärvård. Stockholm, Almquist & Wiksell, 1986; pp 75–79.
9. van Duijn NP, Brouwer HJ, Lamberts H: Use of symptoms and signs to diagnose maxillary sinusitis in general practice: comparison with ultrasonography. *Br Med J* 305(6855): 684–687, 1992.
10. Lindbaek M, Hjortdahl P, Johnsen UL: Randomised, double blind, placebo controlled trial of penicillin V and amoxicillin in treatment of acute sinus infections in adults. *Br Med J* 313(7053): 325–329, 1996.
11. van Buchem FL, Knottnerus JA, Schrijnemaekers VJ, et al: Primary-care-based randomised placebo-controlled trial of antibiotic treatment in acute maxillary sinusitis. *Lancet* 349 (9053):683–687, 1997.
12. Stalman W, van Essen GA, van der Graaf Y, et al: The end of antibiotic treatment in adults with acute sinusitis-like complaints in general practice? A placebo-controlled double-blind randomized doxycycline trial. *Br J Gen Pract* 47(425):794–799, 1997.
13. Dingle J, Badger G, Jordan WS Jr: *Illnesses in a Group of Cleveland Families.* Cleveland, OH, Western Reserve University, 1964.
14. Berg O, Carenfelt C, Kronvall G: Bacteriology of maxillary sinusitis in relation to character of inflammation and prior treatment. *Scand J Infect Dis* 20(5):511–516, 1988.
15. Gwaltney JM Jr: Acute community-acquired sinusitis. *Clin Infect Dis* 23(6):1209–1223; quiz 1224–1225, 1996.
16. McIsaac WJ, Levine N, Goel V: Visits by adults to family physicians for the common cold. *J Fam Pract* 47(5):366–369, 1998.
17. Mellbye H: *Lunger og luftveier (Lungs and Airways).* Oslo, Gyldendal-Ad Notam, 1997.
18. Wald ER: Sinusitis in children. *Isr J Med Sci* 30 (5–6):403–407, 1994.
19. Aitken M, Taylor JA: Prevalence of clinical sinusitis in young children followed up by primary care pediatricians. *Arch Pediatr Adolesc Med* 152(3): 244–248, 1998.
20. Evans KL: Diagnosis and management of sinusitis. *Br Med J* 309(6966):1415–1422, 1994.
21. Low DE, Desrosiers M, McSherry J, et al: A practical guide for the diagnosis and treatment of acute sinusitis. *Can Med Assoc J* 156 (Suppl 6):S1–S14, 1997.

22. Stammberger HR, Kennedy DW: Paranasal sinuses: anatomic terminology and nomenclature. The Anatomic Terminology Group. *Ann Otol Rhinol Laryngol Suppl* 167:7–16, 1995.

23. Carenfelt C, Lundberg C, Nord CE, et al: Bacteriology of maxillary sinusitis in relation to quality of the retained secretion. *Acta Otolaryngol* 86(3–4):298–302, 1978.

24. Lindbaek M, Kaastad E, Dolvik S, et al: Antibiotic treatment of patients with mucosal thickening in the paranasal sinuses, and validation of cut-off points in sinus CT. *Rhinology* 36(1):7–11, 1998.

25. Puhakka T, Makela MJ, Alanen A, et al: Sinusitis in the common cold. *J Allergy Clin Immunol* 102(3):403–408, 1998.

26. Gwaltney JM Jr, Phillips CD, Miller RD, et al: Computed tomographic study of the common cold. *N Engl J Med* 330(1):25–30, 1994.

27. Engquist S, Lundberg C: Akut sinuit—nar, hur och av vem bor den behandlas? (Acute sinusitis—when, how and by whom should it be treated?). *Lakartidningen* 83(38):3112–3114, 1986.

28. Lindbaek M, Melby K, Schøyen R, et al: Bacteriological findings in nasopharynx specimens from patients with a clinical diagnosis of acute sinusitis. *Scand J Prim Health Care* 2:126–130, 2001.

29. Ylikoski J, Savolainen S, Jousimies-Somer H: The bacteriology of acute maxillary sinusitis. *ORL J Otorhinolaryngol Relat Spec* 51(3):175–181, 1989.

30. Hansen JG, Schmidt H, Rosborg J, et al: Predicting acute maxillary sinusitis in a general practice population. *Br Med J* 311(6999): 233–236, 1995.

31. Jousimies-Somer HR, Savolainen S, Ylikoski JS: Comparison of the nasal bacterial floras in two groups of healthy subjects and in patients with acute maxillary sinusitis. *J Clin Microbiol* 27(12):2736–2743, 1989.

32. Lindbaek M, Johnsen UL, Kaastad E, et al: CT findings in general practice patients with suspected acute sinusitis. *Acta Radiol* 37(5):708–713, 1996.

33. Djupesland PG, Chatkin JM, Qian W, et al: Nitrogenmonoksid i nese og bihuler—luftveienes fysiologi i et nytt perspektiv. *Tidsskr Nor Laegeforen* 119(27):4070–4072, 1999.

34. Lindbaek M, Hjortdahl P, Johnsen UL: Use of symptoms, signs, and blood tests to diagnose acute sinus infections in primary care: comparison with computed tomography. *Fam Med* 28(3):183–188, 1996.

35. Williams JW Jr, Simel DL: Does this patient have sinusitis? Diagnosing acute sinusitis by history and physical examination. *JAMA* 270(10):1242–1246, 1993.

36. Benninger MS, Sedory Holzer SE, Lau J: Diagnosis and treatment of uncomplicated acute bacterial sinusitis: summary of the Agency for Health Care Policy and Research evidence-based report. *Otolaryngol Head Neck Surg* 122(1):1–7, 2000.

37. Berg O, Bergstedt H, Carenfelt C, et al: Discrimination of purulent from nonpurulent maxillary sinusitis. Clinical and radiographic diagnosis. *Ann Otol Rhinol Laryngol* 90(3 Pt 1):272–275, 1981.

38. Axelsson A, Runze U: Comparison of subjective and radiological findings during the course of acute maxillary sinusitis. *Ann Otol Rhinol Laryngol* 92(1 Pt 1):75–77, 1983.

39. Laine K, Maatta T, Varonen H, et al: Diagnosing acute maxillary sinusitis in primary care: a comparison of ultrasound, clinical examination and radiography. *Rhinology* 36(1):2–6, 1998.

40. Braun JJ, Alabert JP, Michel FB, et al: Adjunct effect of loratadine in the treatment of acute sinusitis in patients with allergic rhinitis. *Allergy* 52(6):650–655, 1997.

41. Taub SJ: The use of bromelains in sinusitis: a double-blind clinical evaluation. *Eye, Ear, Nose & Throat Monthly* 46(3):361–362 passim, 1967.

42. Ryan RE: A double-blind clinical evaluation of bromelains in the treatment of acute sinusitis. *Headache* 7(1):13–17, 1967.

43. Seltzer AP: Adjunctive use of bromelains in sinusitis: a controlled study. *Eye, Ear, Nose & Throat Monthly* 46(10):1281–1288, 1967.

44. Lewison E: Comparison of the effectiveness of topical and oral nasal decongestants. *Eye, Ear, Nose & Throat Monthly* 49(1):16–18, 1970.

45. Wiklund L, Stierna P, Berglund R, et al: The efficacy of oxymetazoline administered with a nasal bellows container and combined with oral phenoxymethyl-penicillin in the treatment of acute maxillary sinusitis. *Acta Otolaryngol Suppl* 515:57–64, 1994.

46. Harris PG: A comparison of bisolvomycin and oxytetracycline in the treatment of acute infective sinusitis. *Scand J Respir Dis Suppl* 90:87–88, 1974.

47. Meltzer EO, Orgel HA, Backhaus JW, et al: Intranasal flunisolide spray as an adjunct to oral antibiotic therapy for sinusitis. *J Allergy Clin Immunol* 92(6):812–823, 1993.

48. Melen I, Friberg B, Andreasson L, et al: Effects of phenylpropanolamine on ostial and nasal patency in patients treated for chronic maxillary sinusitis. *Acta Otolaryngol* 101(5–6):494–500, 1986.

49. Axelsson A, Chidekel N, Grebelius N, et al: Treatment of acute maxillary sinusitis. A comparison of four different methods. *Acta Otolaryngol* 70(1): 71–76, 1970.

50. Gananca M, Trabulsi LR: The therapeutic effects of cyclacillin in acute sinusitis: in vitro and in vivo correlations in a placebo-controlled study. *Curr Med Res Opin* 1(6):362–368, 1973.

51. Williams JW Jr, Aguilar C, Makela M, et al: Antibiotics for acute maxillary sinusitis. *Cochrane Database of Systematic Reviews* [computer file] 2:CD000243, 2000.

52. de Bock GH, Dekker FW, Stolk J, et al: Antimicrobial treatment in acute maxillary sinusitis: a meta-analysis. *J Clin Epidemiol* 50(8):881–890, 1997.

53. de Ferranti SD, Ioannidis JP, Lau J, et al: Are amoxycillin and folate inhibitors as effective as other antibiotics for acute sinusitis? A meta-analysis. *Br Med J* 317(7159):632–637, 1983.

54. Hansen JG, Schmidt H, Grinsted P: Randomised, double blind, placebo controlled trial of penicillin V in the treatment of acute maxillary sinusitis in adults in general practice. *Scand J Prim Health Care* 18(1):44–47, 2000.

55. Marchant CD, Carlin SA, Johnson CE, et al: Measuring the comparative efficacy of antibacterial agents for acute otitis media: the "Pollyanna phenomenon." *J Pediatr* 120(1):72–77, 1992.

56. Balk E, Zucher D, Engels E, et al: Strategies for diagnosing and treating acute bacterial sinusitis: a cost-effectiveness analysis. (Submitted for publication), 2001.

57. de Bock G, van Erkel A, Springer M, et al: Antibiotic prescription for acute sinusitis in otherwise healthy adults. Clinical cure in relation to costs. *Scand J Prim Health Care* 1:58–63, 2001.

58. Lanza DC, Kennedy DW: Adult sinusitis defined. *Otolaryngol Head Neck Surg* 117(3 Pt 2):S1–S7, 1997.

59. Cody DT 2d, Neel HB 3d, Ferreiro JA, et al: Allergic fungal sinusitis: the Mayo Clinic experience. *Laryngoscope* 104(9):1074–1079, 1994.

60. Mirza N, Lanza DC: Diagnosis and management of sinusitis before scheduled immunosuppression: a schematic approach to the prevention of acute fungal sinusitis. *Otolaryngol Clin North Am* 33(2): 313–321, 2000.

61. Wald ER: Diagnosis and management of sinusitis in children. *Adv Pediatr Infect Dis* 12:1–20, 1996.

62. Wald ER, Reilly JS, Casselbrant M, et al: Treatment of acute maxillary sinusitis in childhood: a comparative study of amoxicillin and cefaclor. *J Pediatr* 104:297–302, 1984.

63. Kovatch AL, Wald ER, Ledesma-Medina J, et al: Maxillary sinus radiographs in children with nonrespiratory complaints. *Pediatrics* 73:306–308, 1984.

64. O'Brien K, Cowell S, Schwartz B: Acute sinusitis—principles of judicious use of antimicrobial agents. *Pediatrics* 101:174–177, 1998.

65. Wald ER, Chiponis D, Ledesma-Medina J: Comparative effectiveness of amoxicillin and amoxicillin-clavulanate potassium in acute paranasal sinus infections in children: a double-blind, placebo-controlled trial. *Pediatrics* 77:795–800, 1986.

66. Garbutt J, Goldstein M, Gellman E, et al: A randomized, placebo-controlled trial of antimicrobial treatment for children with clinically diagnosed acute sinusitis. *Pediatrics* 107:619–625, 2001.

Terrence E. Steyer
William J. Hueston

Chapter 7

Otitis Media and Otitis Externa

Otitis media and otitis externa are two of the most common reasons why patients visit primary care clinicians. It is estimated that in 1999 there were over 13 million visits to physicians for ear infections and ear pain.[1] It is estimated that during the same year, over $3.8 billion was spent to treat this condition.[2] Infections of the ear are especially common in children, with over two-thirds of all children having been diagnosed with at least one ear infection prior to the age of 2 years.[3]

Differential Diagnosis of Ear Problems

While this chapter focuses on otitis media and otitis externa, when a patient presents with ear discomfort, it is important not to overlook other problems that can cause ear pain. Common causes of ear discomfort are shown in Table 7-1.

Table 7-1

Causes of Ear Pain

| Otitis media |
| Otitis externa |
| Cerumen impaction |
| Referred pain from throat or temporal bone |
| Acoustic trauma |
| External ear dermatitis |
| Perichondritis |
| Foreign body in the canal |
| Furunculosis |
| Mastoiditis |
| Ear tumors (eosinophilic granulomas, rhabdosarcomas) |

Cerumen Impaction and Foreign Bodies

Noninfectious causes of inflammation in the outer ear and ear canal can cause pain that can mimic an ear infection. Pain may be the result of insertion of foreign bodies into the external ear or of impaction with excessive cerumen. Generally, cerumen impaction or foreign body presence does not produce pain, but rather results in hearing loss. However, with excessive pressure in the auditory canal, mucosal irritation may occur, which can result in pain. Another possible source of pain with foreign body presence is penetration of the thin skin of the auditory canal by insects such as ticks.

Referred Pain

Pain referred to the ear is another problem that can be misinterpreted as an ear infection. In particular, problems in the lateral and posterior pharynx can be referred to the ear because the middle ear receives its neural innervation through branches of the glossopharyngeal nerve (the ninth cranial nerve). Since this nerve also innervates the throat and tongue, it is common for problems such as streptococcal pharyngitis or a peritonsillar abscess to be referred to the middle ear.

Dental Problems

It is important to ask about dental problems, pain with chewing, throat pain, or other problems that are affecting the throat and jaw. Referred pain to the ear is common, and other sources of the problem should be sought. Patients with temporomandibular disorders are particularly prone to pain radiating to the ear.[4] In patients with temporomandibular disorders, the prevalence of otalgia without infection varied between 12 and 16 percent.[5] Patients with suspected temporomandibular disorders should be referred to a dentist or an oral surgeon for further assessment and treatment.

Outer Ear Infections

Infections or other inflammatory problems (e.g., Waldenström's macroglobulinemia) of the outer ear also can cause ear pain and may be mistaken for otitis externa. External ear infection (perichondritis) is generally located in the body of the auricle and spares the noncartilagenous lobule. Involvement of the lobule of the auricle, which does not contain cartilage, is an ominous sign that suggests a more virulent infection, such as erysipelas. If the lobule is involved in infection, rapid initiation of antistreptococcal antibiotics is imperative to keep the infection from rapidly progressing into the surrounding neck tissue.

Mastoiditis

Another infection adjacent to the ear that may cause pain that is mistaken for otitis media or otitis externa is mastoiditis. This usually accompanies otitis media, but it may be seen after an apparent otitis is cleared. The hallmark of this infection is tenderness over the mastoid process of the temporal bone. Treatment of mastoiditis usually requires surgical debridement of the mastoid bone.

Tumors

Among the primary ear problems that can cause pain and/or hearing loss and can be confused with an ear infection are tumors that impinge upon the ear canal or eighth nerve. Tumors can erode into the middle ear, causing an ulcerated or nonhealing lesion in the canal. If this type of lesion is seen, a biopsy of the ulcerated or nonhealing area is indicated. Rhabdomyosarcomas can occur in the middle ear and cause pain or a chronic otitis media. A seventh nerve palsy can result from an enlarging tumor and is a red flag that further evaluation of the middle ear is indicated.

Otitis Media

Definition

Otitis media is defined as inflammation of the middle ear mucosa. Acute inflammation associated with an infection in the middle ear space is called *acute otitis media*. Otitis media may or may not be accompanied by an effusion, which is a collection of fluid in the middle ear secondary to obstruction of the eustachian tube. When effusion is present, the condition is called *otitis media with effusion* or *secretory otitis media*.

Epidemiology

Otitis media is most commonly diagnosed in children. In the United States, the peak incidence occurs in the first 2 years of life, typically between 6 and 18 months. The peak is somewhat later in European countries, probably because of later entry of European children into child care settings.[2] Other risk factors associated with otitis media are shown in Table 7-2.

Otitis media is a seasonal problem. More cases of otitis media occur in the winter and spring than at other times of year. This is true in both the northern and southern hemispheres.[6]

Table 7-2

Risk Factors for the Development of Otitis Media

Age less than 2 years
Winter and spring seasonal variation
Socioeconomic status
Male sex
Exposure to children in day care settings
Passive smoke exposure
Formula feeding

The importance of demographic risk factors, such as sex and race, is more controversial. Some studies show that more males than females are affected by otitis media, whereas other studies do not show this.[2,6] Some studies suggest that Hispanics and non-Hispanic whites are more likely to develop otitis media than African Americans,[2,7] but other studies suggest that there is no racial difference.[8,9] Some researchers believe that racial differences in prevalence rates are due to socioeconomic and environmental factors.

The environmental factor that places a child at highest risk for the development of otitis media is exposure to other children in child care settings outside of the home. One meta-analysis has shown that the risk for developing otitis media increases 2.5 times for children in child care outside of the home.[10]

Another important environmental factor is exposure to passive, or secondhand, smoke. Two meta-analyses showed that the risk for developing otitis media in children exposed to tobacco smoke was 1.2 to 1.7 times that of children who were not so exposed.[10,11] However, studies of passive smoking often underestimate the amount of tobacco consumed because they rely on self-report of cigarette use. Therefore, this may actually be an underestimate of the effect of passive smoking as a risk factor for otitis media.

A final factor associated with an increased risk for the development of otitis media is bottle feeding. While many studies have shown that breast feeding is protective, these protective effects are seen only in infants who are exclusively breast-fed during the first 3 to 6 months of life. A meta-analysis showed that breast feeding of this duration led to a 13 percent reduction in the prevalence of otitis media.[10] The hypotheses for why breast-fed babies have fewer cases of otitis media are varied. Some suggest that antibodies in the breast milk protect infants from developing infection. Others suggest that the position of the baby while feeding accounts for the difference; breast-fed babies may be positioned such that aspiration of oral contents into the eustachian tubes is less common. Still others suggest that a detection bias exists, as bottle-feeding mothers are more likely to take their children to physicians than breast-feeding mothers.[2] More research in this area is needed to help determine the mechanism by which breast feeding protects against otitis media.

Pathophysiology

Three bacteria cause the majority of cases of otitis media. *Streptococcus pneumoniae* is the predominant cause of acute otitis media in the United States. It is estimated that 40 to 50 percent of otitis media infections are caused by this organism.[12] The two other bacteria responsible for large numbers of cases of otitis media are *Haemophilus influenzae* and *Moraxella catarrhalis*. These agents cause 25 and 15 percent of otitis media cases, respectively.[12] The remainder of cases are caused by a wide variety of bacteria and viruses. Otitis media with effusion is more likely to be caused by viruses, but because of its confusion with acute otitis media, it is often treated as a bacterial infection.[13]

Diagnosis

HISTORY

Since many of the patients who present with acute otitis media are very young, it is often difficult to obtain a detailed history. For example, the true duration of symptoms and the quality of the pain frequently cannot be ascertained. Instead, nonspecific signs of infection such as fussiness or a fever are the only clues that the child has anything more ominous than a common cold.

Therefore, physicians must rely on the attentiveness of parents when acute otitis media is suspected. The development of a new fever in a child who has had a cold for several days may be one sign that acute otitis media has developed. The presence of an earache along with night restlessness and a fever increases the likelihood of an acute otitis media.[14] On the other hand, children may not exhibit any symptoms or signs of infection and may not be suspected of having otitis media until the tympanic membrane ruptures and a purulent discharge appears in the ear canal. Additionally, parents can misinterpret a child's actions as indicating an ear infection when otitis media is not present. For example, cues such as a child pulling at the ears can lead parents to suspect otitis. However, ear pulling is not associated with ear infections.

In older patients with acute otitis media, the most useful history in ear pain is the location of the pain, the type of pain, and actions that make the pain worse. Outer ear infections are sensitive to touch of the ear. Otitis externa and furunculosis occur in the auditory canal and are worsened by moving the ear. Acute otitis media causes a deeper pain that is unaffected by movement of the outer ear.

Hearing impairment is common in acute otitis media, but total hearing loss rarely occurs. Patients usually report a muffled or dull sense of hearing, sometimes described as like "hearing under water." Complete hearing loss in the presence of acute otitis media suggests a rupture of the tympanic membranes or complete obstruction of the external auditory canal with purulent material.

Otitis media with effusion is more difficult to diagnose based on history, especially in younger children. Otitis media with effusion generally arises from a persistent effusion following an acute otitis media. Illnesses that prolong obstruction of the eustachian tube, such as allergic rhinitis, make clearance of the effusion more difficult. In younger children, the only history that might suggest a persistent effusion is delayed or abnormal speech development. Older children often will report a sensation of pressure in the ear or decreased hearing on the affected side. Pain is

not present, and usually there is no tinnitus involved either.

PHYSICAL EXAMINATION

In patients who present with ear pain associated with acute otitis media, the first step in the physical examination is localizing the source of the pain. Manipulation of the external ear will exacerbate most pain located in the external ear or the auditory canal. However, referred pain and middle ear pain will be unaffected by this maneuver. Inspection of the outer ear and auditory canal will confirm the presence of foreign bodies or inflammation.

If manipulation of the outer ear fails to reproduce or worsen the pain, the source is more likely to be the middle ear or referred pain. The next step in the evaluation is visualization of the tympanic membrane plus possible ancillary testing such as pneumatic otoscopy and tympanometry to determine if the membrane is mobile. A mobile tympanic membrane suggests that no fluid is present in the middle ear, making acute otitis media unlikely.

Unfortunately, visualization of fluid behind the tympanic membrane is a fairly insensitive and nonspecific test for the diagnosis of acute otitis media. In a classic acute otitis media, the tympanic membrane will be bulging and red, with evident cloudy fluid and decreased mobility. Perforations may exist, in which case purulent material will be exuded into the auditory canal. The combination of a cloudy effusion, bulging membrane, and loss of mobility has a predictive value for otitis media in the area of 95 percent.[15]

A classic presentation of acute otitis media is rare. In one study, practicing primary care doctors admitted that in over 40 percent of the patients that they diagnosed with otitis media, they were not really certain of their diagnosis.[16] Other investigations have shown significant disagreement between expert examiners on the presence of effusion.[17] When clinical otoscopy was compared to myringotomy in a study of 226 children, the sensitivity of clinical examination was only 74 percent and the specificity was 60 percent.[18] The presence of erythema without a bulging or cloudy tympanic membrane is even less helpful; the positive predictive value of erythema alone in predicting acute otitis media was found to be only 65 percent when compared to myringotomy.[19]

To improve diagnostic accuracy, pneumatic otoscopy has been advocated as an adjunctive maneuver to simple visualization. In this test, air is introduced into the auditory canal while the tympanic membrane is visualized. Movement of the tympanic membrane with increased air pressure is believed to indicate a mobile tympanic membrane and no middle ear effusion. However, this test does not improve positive predictive value significantly.[19]

In otitis media with effusion, visualization of the tympanic membrane usually shows a cloudy or opaque fluid behind the eardrum rather than erythema as in acute otitis media. Pneumatic otoscopy shows decreased movement of the membrane as well. Because of the presence of fluid and lack of tympanic membrane movement, otitis media with effusion can be misdiagnosed as acute otitis media or as an unresolved acute otitis media. Fluid in the middle ear can take up to 6 weeks to resolve following an episode of acute otitis media, so it is important to differentiate persistent fluid from resistant infection.

DIAGNOSTIC TESTING

Diagnostic testing for otitis media includes tests that examine the mobility of the tympanic membrane (tympanometry and acoustic reflectometry) and those that sample the fluid in the middle ear (myringotomy and needle tympanostomy). Tests that examine only movement of the tympanic membrane are not sensitive in differentiating acute otitis media from otitis media with effusion. Sampling of the fluid can be helpful in determining if an infection is present, but patients with otitis media with effusion can har-

bor some bacteria in the middle ear. Aspiration of fluid at the time of surgery in children having tympanostomy tubes placed for persistent otitis media with effusion but no sign of infection showed that 7 percent were positive for *S. pneumoniae* and that half of these were penicillin-resistant.[3]

MYRINGOTOMY AND TYMPANOSTOMY Myringotomy involves making a small puncture in the tympanic membrane to allow middle ear fluid to drain, much as one would incise and drain an abscess elsewhere. Aspiration of the fluid that exudes from the middle ear space can provide identification of the causative agent. Myringotomy also is valuable because it provides venting of the closed space, making it therapeutic as well as diagnostic. However, in practice myringotomy is rarely performed. A similar but less invasive procedure called needle tympanostomy allows for sampling of the middle ear fluid, but does not provide a drainage tract to decompress the ear. The value of needle tympanostomy is for identification of the organisms that are causing the infection and determination of drug sensitivities. It is used primarily for research protocols that require identification and culture of organisms and for public health surveillance of antibiotic resistance.

TYMPANOMETRY Tympanometry does not diagnose infection, but rather is helpful in indicating the presence of a middle ear effusion. The addition of tympanometry to pneumatic otoscopy has been shown to improve the sensitivity and specificity of the diagnosis of middle ear effusion. Tympanometry measures the amount of a test sound that traverses the tympanic membrane at given positive and negative auditory canal pressures. The tympanometer forms an airtight seal around the auditory canal, and a sound wave is introduced by pushing a button on the instrument. The machine monitors the amount of the sound reflected back from the tympanic membrane. This procedure is repeated as various positive and negative pressures are applied, and the results are plotted based on the amount of sound transmitted. In a series of studies evaluating this test, the sensitivity of tympanometry compared to myringotomy has ranged from 79 to 95 percent, with a corresponding specificity of 57 to 93 percent.[15] However, the patient's level of cooperation influences the reliability of the test. In poorly cooperative children, the predictive value drops substantially.[20]

ACOUSTIC REFLECTOMETRY Acoustic reflectometry is another adjunctive test in which sound reflected off the tympanic membrane is measured. The amount of sound reflected is measured in decibels. However, the most appropriate cutoff value for a positive test is still controversial. Studies of acoustic reflectometry have used either tympanometry or clinical examination as the gold standard, which limits their application. Even given these weak gold standards, positive and negative predictive values of acoustic reflectometry are in the 80 percent range.[14] Acoustic reflectometry appears to have higher specificity than tympanometry, but this is balanced by lower sensitivity. The overall accuracy of the test appears to be no better than that of tympanostomy.[21]

Treatment

ACUTE OTITIS MEDIA

Despite extensive clinical experience in the management of acute otitis media and recommendations from various professional organizations, there is no worldwide consensus regarding which antibiotics are most appropriate for initial or recurrent therapy, the optimal duration of therapy, or even whether antibiotics are of any significant benefit at all. The variation in the management of acute otitis media is typified by an examination of the management of acute otitis media in nine countries in the mid-1980s.[16] In this study, the use of antibiotics varied over a wide range (31 to 98 percent of episodes), with

considerable variation in the types of antibiotics used and duration of therapy.

ACUTE EPISODES In the United States, routine use of antibiotics for acute otitis media has been the customary mode of care. Recently, the Centers for Disease Control and Prevention have issued guidelines for treatment of otitis media (Table 7-3). However, little evidence exists to suggest that routine antibiotic treatment is better than other strategies.[22] In other countries, most notably the Netherlands, antibiotic use for acute otitis media is provided only to high-risk children between the ages of 6 months and 2 years. Data from two meta-analyses showed that the routine use of amoxicillin is associated with only a 12.3 to 13.7 percent lower failure rate than observation (or placebo).[22,23] This translates into needing to treat six children with otitis media to prevent one

Table 7-3

Centers for Disease Control and Prevention Guidelines for Antibiotic Therapy in Otitis Media

—Amoxicillin should be the first-line drug used for otitis media.
—The initial dose of amoxicillin should be 80–90 mg/kg/day (double the previous standard dosage).
—Patients at low risk for penicillin-resistant streptococcal pneumonia infection can still be treated with 40–45 mg/kg/day of amoxicillin.
—Tympanocentesis should be considered in treatment failures to identify the organism and pattern of resistance.
—If no clinical response occurs in 3 days, consideration should be given to changing to one of the following agents: amoxicillin-clavulanic acid, cefuroxime, or intramuscular ceftriaxone.
—Surveillance mechanisms should be developed to monitor for drug resistance.

SOURCE: From Dowell et al,[12] with permission.

case of failure in a patient not treated with antibiotics.

A guide to antibiotic use in otitis media is shown in Table 7-4. When the effectiveness of these antibiotics in treating suppurative acute otitis media was compared, there appeared to be no benefit from any one drug over any other. When used for 5 days only, antibiotics showed equal effectiveness with therapy of longer durations.[24] One study has suggested, however, that 2 days of therapy with oral antibiotics is as effective as treatment for 7 days.[22] In addition to the cost benefit of a shorter duration of therapy, reports have noted fewer drug-related side effects in patients taking short courses of antibiotics. One study estimated that the number that needed to be treated with short-duration therapy to avoid one gastrointestinal adverse effect was eight children. In addition to comparing short-duration therapy to long-duration therapy with oral antibiotics, the study showed that a single intramuscular dose of ceftriaxone was just as effective as a longer-duration course of other antibiotics.

Table 7-4

Antibiotic Therapy for Acute Otitis Media

Drug	Contraindications/ Cautions	Dosage	Adverse Effects
Initial therapy			
Amoxicillin	Penicillin allergy	40 mg/kg split b.i.d. for 5 days	Diarrhea (~2%)
Sulfamethoxazole-trimethoprim	Sulfa allergy; avoid in patients with glucose-6-phosphatase deficiency; avoid in folate deficiency	8 mg sulfa/40 mg trimethoprim per day in 2 equal doses	Light sensitivity, skin reactions (2%; severe in < 0.1%); may cause bone marrow suppression with chronic use
Ceftriaxone	Cross-reactivity with penicillin allergy	50 mg/kg up to 1 g	Pain at injection site, diarrhea (5–6%)
Amoxicillin-clavulanate	Penicillin allergy; history of jaundice	20–45 mg/day of amoxicillin component in 2 or 3 doses	Diarrhea (up to 40%)
Azithromycin	Macrolide allergy	10 mg/kg on day 1 followed by 5 mg/kg for 5 days	Diarrhea (~5%), nausea (~3%), abdominal pain (~3%)
Second- or third-generation cephalosporin (cefaclor, cefuroxime, cefixime)	Caution in penicillin allergy	Varies with drug	Diarrhea (3–5%), rash
Prophylaxis for Recurrent Acute Otitis Media			
Amoxicillin	Penicillin allergy	20 mg/kg at bedtime	Diarrhea (2%)
Sulfamethoxazole	Sulfa allergy	8 mg/kg at bedtime	Skin reactions (2%, severe in < 0.1%)

Because of the emergence of multiple-drug-resistant strains of *S. pneumoniae*, there has been some concern that standard doses of medications might not be sufficient to cover strains that are intermediately resistant to common antibiotics. Some studies have shown that the bacteriologic clearance rate in cases of resistant *S. pneumoniae* and *H. influenzae* is only 80 to 85 percent.[25] Children who are younger, who attend day care, or who have been hospitalized recently are at highest risk for harboring a resistant organism.[25] To provide better antibiotic coverage for these resistant organisms, higher-dose regimens of amoxicillin-clavulanate have been suggested. However, in two controlled studies, high-dose amoxicillin-clavulanate has shown no greater clinical effectiveness than standard dosing regimens.

RECURRENCES The treatment of recurrent acute otitis media after a previous resistant episode is another area of controversy. Some physicians treat recurrent infection with a second-line drug in order to avoid a treatment failure in the new episode after a previous treatment. However, recurrences several weeks after an initial episode are usually produced by a new organism and do not necessarily have the same resistance pattern as previous infections. One nonrandomized study that investigated the effectiveness of a second-line drug versus a first-line agent (amoxicillin or trimethoprim-sulfamethoxazole) showed no benefit from the broader-spectrum second-line agent in a recurrent infection following a previously resistant episode.[26] To reduce the development of resistance, new episodes should be treated with narrower-spectrum agents.

In children with multiple episodes of acute otitis media, prevention of recurrent infections may be necessary. Recurrent otitis is defined as three or more episodes in a 6-month period or four episodes in a year, with a normal examination documented between each two episodes of infection.[27] The first approach in preventing recurrences is to identify conditions that predispose children to eustachian tube dysfunction.

Most commonly, this is an upper respiratory infection that cannot be prevented. However, some children have chronic allergic rhinitis that results in eustachian tube dysfunction. Treatment of these children with antihistamines or nasal steroids may reduce the risk of a recurrent infection.

For children with no evidence of allergic rhinitis, options include long-term antibiotic prophylaxis or surgical ventilation of the inner ear through the placement of tubes. Tympanostomy tubes and antibiotic prophylaxis have nearly equal effectiveness for the prevention of recurrence,[27,28] but medication use is associated with fewer side effects. Antibiotic prophylaxis can be achieved with either amoxicillin or sulfamethoxazole given as a single dose at bedtime. The usual prophylactic dose is one-half the customary daily dose used for acute otitis media. For children who continue to have episodes of acute otitis media despite antibiotic prophylaxis, the insertion of tympanostomy tubes may reduce the frequency of future infections. If antibiotic prophylaxis does fail, it is most likely to fail in the first 6 months, so a short trial of antibiotic suppression is probably indicated in most patients.[27] An exception to this may be in children who already have language delay and recurrent infections complicated by persistent serous otitis media, for whom tympanostomy tubes are indicated as initial therapy.[28]

FOLLOW-UP Follow-up of patients with acute otitis media is routine, but has not been proven to be beneficial. Since an effusion can persist for several weeks after an acute otitis media, the finding of an effusion in the first few weeks after an acute otitis episode has little prognostic value. Therefore, routine follow-up to identify children with persistent acute otitis media is of questionable value. In a study of 181 patients who returned for routine follow-up 1 to 3 weeks after an acute otitis media, it was found that 97 percent of the parents could tell whether the child had resolved or not based on their own observations.[29] It is unclear whether a further examination by their physician provided any additional benefit to these families.

PATIENT EDUCATION Finally, patient education is important in the treatment of acute otitis media. Ear pain is very common in childhood. The symptoms experienced by children with ear disorders may create a great deal of anxiety in parents, in addition to causing them sleepless nights and requiring days off from work. When encountering the family of a young child who has ear pain, clinicians should recognize the stress that this illness places on the family and try to dispel myths that may have arisen regarding treatment of the problem.

Some of the issues about which clinicians should be prepared to counsel families include the following:

- Antibiotic therapy may not change outcomes in children but can cause adverse effects. Parents are accustomed to receiving antibiotics, so challenging this long-held assumption can be difficult. In addition, parents often focus on short-term successes ("Will it help me get some sleep tonight?") as opposed to long-term consequences.
- A treatment failure in one infection does not indicate that a second-line antibiotic must be used for all subsequent infections. Many parents assume that because amoxicillin did not work the last time, it is not going to work this time. This can lead to the unnecessary use of broader-spectrum, more expensive agents and speed the development of drug resistance. When treatment failures occur, physicians should emphasize that the use of a different drug this time should not influence the treatment if the child should get another infection in the future.

OTITIS MEDIA WITH EFFUSION

Otitis media with effusion, also known as secretory or serous otitis media, is not a dangerous condition in itself, but is of concern because of the observed impact on speech development in young children (< 4 years old). Based on a cohort of 205 children who were followed from birth to 3 years of age, children who experienced frequent effusions in the first 6 to 12 months of life experienced the greatest decline in speech and language scores when tested at age 3.[30] In addition, effects on educational attainment and socialization also have been associated with effusions. In a large study of over 1500 children, otitis media with effusion was found to be associated with a lower level of attention in school and decreased social behaviors in children between the ages of 2 and 6.[31] However, a cohort study that followed children from age 3 found that most of the negative effects on speech development seen in early years had resolved by age 7, whether or not the children were treated.[32]

The need for treatment in children in whom speech and language development has progressed normally is less compelling. In addition to having less of an effect on the child's future development, otitis media with effusion is more likely to clear spontaneously as children get older. Additionally, those who have unilateral effusions and initially peaked tympanograms have higher spontaneous cure rates. These factors should all be taken into consideration when treatment decisions are made for children with otitis media with effusion.[33]

The treatment options for otitis media with effusion include the use of decongestants, antibiotics, or steroids or surgical clearance of the effusion with the placement of a tympanostomy tube. Since most effusions eventually clear over time, the success of these modalities should be compared to that of watchful waiting.

DECONGESTANTS The use of decongestants for the treatment of otitis media with effusion is based on the hope that a reduction in edema in the nasopharynx will decompress the eustachian tube and promote restoration of proper middle ear pressures. Most studies of decongestants, however, have not shown a major effect on middle ear effusions.[34] In children with chronic rhinosinusitis, the combination of decongestant nose drops and an antibiotic resulted in a greater rate of clearance of otitis media with effusion than placebo, but the overall results were still poor.[35]

ANTIBIOTICS   Because of the finding that bacterial contamination sometimes exists in effusions that are sampled at the time of placement of tympanostomy tubes, it was thought that a subclinical infection could play a role in the perpetuation of the effusion. Based on these observations, a number of studies have examined the effectiveness of antibiotics in treating otitis media with effusion. Two meta-analyses of antibiotic use for otitis media with effusion found a positive effect on the short-term resolution of the effusion.[36,37] Children with persistent effusions appeared to have a 22 to 25 percent improvement in the short-term clearance rate of fluid. However, longer-term clinical outcomes showed no difference.[36] So, while antibiotics may help in otitis media with effusion, it is not clear whether this benefit is long-lasting or has any impact on speech and language development.

STEROIDS   The use of oral and intranasal steroids in patients with otitis media with effusion also has been evaluated. The results with either intranasal or oral steroids have been disappointing. Two studies showed no short-term benefit of prednisone[38] and dexamethasone[39] in clearing effusions or improving hearing. One study did show a short-term benefit of oral prednisone compared to placebo or ibuprofen. However, within 4 weeks of treatment, the differences began to diminish, and by 1 year there was no difference in hearing loss rates between any of the groups.

The only study using nasal steroids employed beclomethasone along with antibiotics in older children (age 3 to 11) with otitis media with effusion.[40] This study reported that children randomized to antibiotics plus the nasal steroid had greater effusion clearance rates over the 12 weeks

of the study. The benefit was seen in both atopic and nonallergic children. However, no long-term evaluation of the children was performed, so it is unclear whether this effect was transient or sustained.

SURGERY   The role of surgical placement of tympanostomy tubes remains controversial. It is clear that placement of a ventilation tube results in restoration of middle ear pressure and reduction in middle ear fluid. However, the indications for this procedure remain unclear and are open to debate even among the otolaryngologists who perform it.[41] In addition, the benefit of tympanostomy tube placement for speech and language development is open to question.[32,42] One study showed a benefit with tympanostomy tube insertion, but found that watchful waiting for up to 9 months was not detrimental; children who received tubes after a prolonged period of watchful waiting quickly caught up to those who had undergone surgery early.[43] Many of these studies have been performed in children 3 years of age or older, when speech and language development are already well established. However, a recent study also showed no difference in language comprehension or speech development in younger children (between the ages of 1 and 2) who were randomized into ventilation tube surgery and watchful waiting.[44] The results of these studies suggest that surgery may be useful in reducing some of the symptoms of the effusion and restoring normal ear pressures that may prevent subsequent development of otitis media, but has little long-term impact on speech and hearing development in children.

Other surgical procedures for the treatment of recurrent otitis media or for otitis media with effusion have also been advocated. Adenoidectomy has been shown to reduce recurrences of otitis media and reduce effusions, but appears to produce results no better than those achieved with tympanostomy tubes.[45] Other studies have shown a marginal benefit of tonsilloadenoidectomy on recurrences of acute otitis media (1.4 cases per year versus 2.1), but the investigators believed that this small degree of improvement was not worth the increased cost, morbidity, and risk of the procedure.[46]

Taken together, these studies suggest that symptomatic serous otitis media may be successfully treated with antibiotics, but that the effusion is very likely to return. For symptomatic patients who experience recurrent otitis media and who fail antibiotic prophylaxis, placement of tympanostomy tubes may be useful and preferable to tonsillectomy or adenoidectomy. However, no current treatment appears to improve speech and hearing development. But, as indicated earlier, families of children with otitis media with effusion can be reassured that any delays appear to be resolved by the time children reach the age of 7.

Complications

Over the past several decades, the treatment of acute otitis media has greatly reduced the rate of complications from this disease. However, there are still sporadic reports of serious complications. Complications from otitis media are divided into two categories, intratemporal and intracranial. Intracranial complications occur when the disease extends beyond the temporal bone.

INTRATEMPORAL COMPLICATIONS

Hearing loss is the most common complication from otitis media.[47] It is usually temporary and self-limited. However, with recurrent or persistent cases of otitis media, the hearing loss can affect a child's ability to develop language skills and may lead to speech disorders.[48,49] To prevent long-term hearing sequelae from otitis media, it is recommended that patients follow up with their physician 2 to 3 weeks after diagnosis and treatment of the infection if the parents do not see resolution of the infection based on other observations. This is especially important during the period in which children are forming their language skills (age 2 years and under). However, as previously discussed, insertion of tubes early in the course of the effusion has no effect on long-term speech and language attainment.

Perforation of the tympanic membrane is the second most common complication of otitis media. In fact, prior to the availability of antibiotic therapy, perforation was encountered so often that it was considered a normal part of the clinical course of otitis media. The majority of perforations heal spontaneously, but some episodes of perforation do not heal and become chronic perforations or lead to the development of chronic suppurative otitis media. In these latter cases, tympanostomy tube placement or tympanoplasty may be required.[50]

Another complication of acute otitis media is mastoiditis, a natural extension of an acute middle ear infection into the periosteum covering the mastoid process. More severe infections can involve the bony trabeculae that separate the mastoid cells and thus develop into an osteitis.[51] The use of computed tomographic (CT) scanning to make the diagnosis of mastoiditis is recommended. CT findings indicative of mastoiditis include bone destruction, loss of intercellular septae, or air-fluid levels in the mastoid cells. Parenteral antibiotics are needed to treat this infection, and surgery may be required if it does not begin to resolve within 48 h.[47]

Finally, labyrinthitis can occur when the acute otitis media infection moves from the middle ear to the inner ear space. This diagnosis is typically made clinically by the presence of decreased or absent cochlear or vestibular function.[47]

INTRACRANIAL COMPLICATIONS

Intracranial complications occur when the infection spreads beyond the temporal bone. Before the introduction of antibiotics, 2.5 percent of all patients with otitis media suffered an intracranial complication, and many of these complications were fatal.[47,50]

Meningitis, or infection of the cerebrospinal fluid, is the most common intracranial complication of otitis media. The infection can spread to the meninges through venous channels, bone erosion, or bacteremia.[47] The diagnosis is made based upon examination of the cerebrospinal fluid, and treatment is parenteral antibiotics.

Another potential intracranial problem that can develop is an extradural abscess. The most common place for an extradural abscess to form is in the tegmen tympani and perisinus cells. An extradural abscess can also be associated with other complications, including lateral sinus thrombosis.[47,48] Both CT scanning and angiography may be useful in making the diagnosis. Parenteral antibiotics and diagnostic mastoidectomy are used in treating these complications.

Subdural abscess is a rare complication of otitis media that is defined by a collection of pus between the dura mater and the arachnoid membrane. It can occur via direct extension or as the result of a venoembolism. CT scanning is diagnostic, and treatment consists of neurosurgical drainage.

Prevention

The easiest way to prevent otitis media is to reduce the environmental factors that lead to its development. This includes educating parents and other caregivers to stop their tobacco use and encouraging all mothers to breast-feed for at least 3 to 6 months. These two steps alone could greatly reduce the incidence of otitis media in the United States.

There is also hope that the introduction of the conjugated pneumococcal vaccine (Prevnar) in 2000 may reduce the incidence of acute otitis media in young children.[52] Initial testing of the vaccine on over 37,000 children in California showed a 94 percent reduction in invasive *S. pneumoniae* disease as well as a 67 percent reduction in the incidence of acute otitis media caused by serotypes included in the vaccine.[53]

Current recommendations are to administer this vaccine to all infants and to higher-risk children under the age of 5.[54] Because of the effectiveness of the vaccine in stimulating an immunologic response in children who have had several episodes of otitis media,[55] older children who are "otitis-prone" are also prime candidates for vaccination.

Side effects from the vaccine are self-limiting and include a fever less than 102°F, erythema and tenderness at the injection site, and febrile seizures. The vaccine should not be given to anyone with a hypersensitivity to any component of the vaccine or to individuals who have already received a 23-valent pneumococcal vaccine.[54]

Otitis Externa

Definition

Also known as "swimmer's ear," otitis externa is an inflammation and/or infection of the external auditory canal and auricle.[56]

Epidemiology

There are several risk factors for the development of otitis externa. These include the absence of cerumen in the ear canal, local irritants, foreign bodies that cause trauma to the canal, and anatomic deviations in the canal. Anatomic features that increase the risk of otitis externa include narrow ear canals, excessive ear hair, or sharp angles in the curve of the ear canal.[57]

Cerumen acts as an antimicrobial by creating a low pH in the ear canal, which is a poor environment for pathogens. Removing the cerumen can disrupt this pH and allow pathogens to infect the area. Cerumen removal itself can be traumatic to the thin skin in the external auditory canal and can allow bacteria to enter through the damaged skin.[56]

Any irritant that alters the pH of the ear canal can also predispose one to developing otitis externa. The most common irritants include water (especially from pools or other swimming areas), hairsprays, and dyes.[57]

Foreign bodies that can cause trauma to the canal include hearing aids, insects, cotton swabs, bobby pins, or just about any other object that a small child can fit into the ear. Inflammation can occur as a result of trauma caused by the foreign body or through contact sensitivity, especially from the plastic or silastic components of hearing aids.[57]

Pathophysiology

Otitis externa can be caused by either bacteria or fungi. The most common bacteria associated with otitis externa are *Pseudomonas aeruginosa* and *Staphylococcus aureus*. Fungi cause otitis externa in about 10 percent of all patients with this diagnosis. The most common fungi that cause otitis externa are *Aspergillus* (80 to 90 percent of all cases) and *Candida* species.[58]

There are also some noninfectious causes of otitis externa. Most of these are dermatologic conditions, such as psoriasis, atopic dermatitis, acne, and contact dermatitis.[58]

Diagnosis

HISTORY

As with otitis media, a thorough history can help to make the diagnosis of otitis externa. Useful information includes a previous history of otitis externa or otitis media, duration of symptoms, and type of symptoms present. In addition, one should inquire about the various risk factors, including recent swimming history, use of foreign objects to clean ears, use of hearing aids, and allergic reactions to any products that may be used in this area, such as hair care products.

PHYSICAL EXAMINATION

The separate innervation of the middle and external ears can be useful in differentiating the source of pain. In cases of otitis externa or trauma to the external auditory canal, retraction of the pinna will cause pain because of local inflammation of the seventh nerve. However, since the middle ear receives different neural innervation, stimulation of the external ear should not produce pain with an acute otitis media.

Inspection of the ear canal in cases of acute otitis externa will usually reveal erythema, swelling of the canal wall, and debris clogging the canal opening. The material in the canal is usually white or opaque, but may be purulent-appearing. Manipulation of the canal through irrigation or insertion of a cotton-tipped applicator can produce severe pain.

Treatment

The most common organism cultured from the auditory canal in otitis externa is *Pseudomonas*, which can be found in association with other bacteria such as *Staphylococcus* and *Proteus*.[58] Infection causes edema of the ear canal and disrupts the normal squamous cell shedding that occurs on a regular basis. This leads to the accumulation of a keratin layer in the canal, along with exudate and necrotic debris. Treatment includes debridement of necrotic tissue through gentle rinsing followed by the application of a broad-spectrum antibiotic solution that will cover the most common organisms in what is usually a polymicrobial infection. For patients whose canal is obliterated by edema, the insertion of a gauze wick to draw antibiotics into the infected canal may be necessary.

The choice of an antibiotic for otitis externa has not been studied extensively. Neomycin/polymyxin B ear drops and ofloxacin ear drops are both popular because of their ability to eradicate *Pseudomonas* (Table 7-5). Because of

Table 7-5

Antibiotic Therapy for Otitis Externa

DRUG	CONTRAINDICATIONS/ CAUTIONS	DOSAGE	ADVERSE EFFECTS
Neomycin solutions	Rupture of tympanic membrane	3–4 drops q.i.d. for 7 days	Potential ototoxicity with rupture of tympanic membrane
Ofloxacin solutions	Fluoroquinolone allergy	5 drops t.i.d. for 10 days	None

ototoxicity associated with aminoglycosides, neomycin should be avoided when the tympanic membrane is ruptured or cannot be visualized well. The addition of corticosteroids to ear drops is popular, although there is little evidence that this speeds healing or prevents recurrences.

Fungal otitis externa is best treated by a thorough cleansing of the ear canal followed by the use of acidifying drops for 5 to 7 days. Individuals with suspected fungal infections should be rechecked in 1 week to ensure that the treatment has cured the infection. If signs and symptoms of otitis externa persist, patients can be treated with topical solutions of 1% clotrimazole (Lotrimin), thimerosal (Merthiolate), or M-cresyl acetate (Cresylate). If the tympanic membrane is perforated, 1% tolnaftate (Tinactin) should be used.[57]

Complications

Complications from otitis externa tend to occur when the disease presents in its late stages. This is fairly uncommon, as the condition is so painful and disturbing that most of those afflicted seek medical advice early. People who are more likely to have complications are those who are immunocompromised, including diabetic patients and those with cancer.

Patients with diabetes and other immunocompromised states are at highest risk for invasive otitis externa, called malignant otitis externa. Malignant otitis externa is usually caused by invasion of *Pseudomonas aeruginosa* into tissue surrounding the ear canal. One physical finding that indicates invasion of the otitis externa is a seventh nerve palsy associated with otitis externa. Treatment of malignant otitis media must include aggressive use of anti-*Pseudomonas* antibiotics such as an aminoglycoside plus a semisynthetic penicillin. Despite appropriate therapy, mortality rates are high.

Local complications, such as ear canal stenosis and tympanic membrane perforation, are most likely to occur. One can also see regional complications such as auricular cellulitis and chondritis.[56] There have also been reports of necrotizing otitis externa and cases of skull base osteomyelitis that result from otitis externa, but these are much less common.[59]

Prevention

Prevention of recurrent otitis externa includes maneuvers to reduce the intrusion of fluids or other materials into the ear. Cleaning of the ear by sticking instruments into the ear canal should be avoided. Finally, some suggest rinsing the ear with alcohol following bathing or swimming to flush out water that may pool in the canal. While probably harmless, this technique has not been evaluated to determine if it reduces recurrences.

References

1. American Academy of Family Physicians: Facts about family practice, http:www.aafp.org/facts. table17.html.
2. Daly KA, Gebnick GS: Clinical epidemiology of otitis media. *Pediatr Infect Dis J* 19:S31–S36, 2000.
3. Haddad J Jr, Saiman L, San Gabriel P, et al: Non-susceptible *Streptococcus pneumoniae* in children with chronic otitis media with effusion and recurrent otitis media undergoing ventilating tube placement. *Pediatr Infect Dis J* 19:432–437, 2000.
4. Luz JG, Maragno IC, Martin MC: Characteristics of chief complaints of patients with temporomandibular disorders in a Brazilian population. *J Oral Rehabil* 24:240–243, 1997.
5. Kuttila S, Kuttila M, Le Bell Y, et al: Aural symptoms and signs of temporomandibular disorder in association with treatment need and visits to a physician. *Laryngoscope* 109:1669–1673, 1999.
6. Daly KA: Epidemiology of otitis media. *Otolaryngol Clin North Am* 24:775–786, 1991.
7. Shurin PA, Pelton SI, Donner A, et al: Persistence of middle ear effusion after acute otitis media in children. *N Engl J Med* 330:1121–1123, 1997.
8. Paradise JL, Rockette HE, Colborn K, et al: Otitis media in 2253 Pittsburgh-area infants: prevalence and risk factors during the first two years of life. *Pediatrics* 99:318–333, 1997.
9. Casselbrant ML, Mandel EM, Kurs-Lasky M, et al: Otitis media in a population of black American and white American infants, 0–2 years of age. *Int J Pediatr Otorhinolaryngol* 33:2–16, 1995.
10. Uhari M, Mantysaari K, Niemela M: A meta-analytic review of the risk factors for acute otitis media. *Clin Infect Dis* 22:1079–1083, 1996.
11. Difranza JR, Lew RA: Morbidity and mortality in children associated with the use of tobacco products by other people. *Pediatrics* 97:560–568, 1996.
12. Dowell SF, Butler JC, Giebink GS, et al: Acute otitis media: management and surveillance in an era of pneumococcal resistance—a report from the Drug-resistant *Streptococcus pneumoniae* Therapeutic Working Group. *Pediatr Infect Dis J* 18:1–9, 1999.
13. Faden H, Duffy L, Boeve M: Otitis media: back to basics. *Pediatr Infect Dis J* 17:1105–1113, 1998.
14. Kontiokari T, Koivunen P, Miemela M, et al: Symptoms of acute otitis media. *Pediatr Infect Dis J* 17:676–679, 1998.
15. Stewart MH, Siff JE, Cydulka RK: Evaluation of the patient with sore throat, earache, and sinusitis: an evidence based approach. *Emerg Med Clin North Am* 17:153–187, 1999.
16. Froom J, Culpepper L, Grob P, et al: Diagnosis and antibiotic treatment of acute otitis media: report from International Primary Care Network. *Br Med J* 300:528–586, 1990.
17. Nozza RJ, Bluestone CD, Krdatzke D, et al: Towards the validation of aural acoustic immittance measure for the diagnosis of middle ear effusion in children. *Ear Hear* 13:442–453, 1992.
18. Sassen ML, Van Aarem A, Gote JJ: Validity of tympanometry in the diagnosis of middle ear effusion. *Clin Otol* 19:185–189, 1994.
19. Karma PH, Penttila MA, Sipila MM, et al: Otoscopic diagnosis of middle ear effusion in acute and non-acute OM. *Int J Pediatr Otorhinolaryngol* 17:37–49, 1989.
20. Koivunen P, Albo O, Ubari M, et al: Minitympanometry in detecting middle ear fluid. *J Pediatr* 131:419–422, 1997.
21. Kemaloglu YK, Sener T, Beder L, et al: Predictive value of acoustic reflectometry (angle and reflectivity) and tympanometry. *Int J Pediatr Otorhinolaryngol* 48:137–142, 1999.
22. Agency for Healthcare Research and Quality: Management of acute otitis media. Evidence Report/Technology Assessment Number 15, AHRQ publication no. 00-E009, www.ahrq. gov/clinic/otitisum.htm.
23. Rosenfeld RM, Vertrees JE, Carr J, et al: Clinical efficacy of antimicrobial drugs for acute otitis media: metanalysis of 5400 children from thirty-three randomized trials. *J Pediatr* 124:355–367, 1994.
24. Koryrskyj AL, Hildes-Ripstein GE, Longstaffe SEA, et al: Treatment of acute otitis media with a shortened course of antibiotics: a meta-analysis. *JAMA* 279:1736–1742, 1998.
25. Dagan R: Clinical significance of organisms in otitis media. *Pediatr Infect Dis J* 19:378–382, 2000.
26. Hueston WJ, Ornstein S, Jenkins RG, et al: Treatment of recurrent otitis media after a previous treatment failure: which antibiotics work best? *J Fam Pract* 48:43–46, 1999.
27. Pizzuto MP, Volk MS, Hingston LM: Common topics in pediatric otolaryngology. *Pediatr Clin North Am* 45:973–991, 1998.

28. Bernard PA, Stenstrom RJ, Feldman W, et al: Randomized, controlled trial comparing long-term sulfonamide therapy to ventilation tubes for otitis media with effusion. *Pediatrics* 88:215–222, 1991.

29. Hathaway TJ, Karz HP, Dershewitz RA, et al: Acute otitis media: who needs posttreatment follow-up. *Pediatrics* 94:143–147, 1994.

30. Teele DW, Klein JO, Rosner BA: Otitis media with effusion during the first three years of life and development of speech and language. *Pediatrics* 74:282–287, 1984.

31. Van Cauwenberge P, Van Cauwenberge K, Klukskens P: The influence of otitis media with effusion on speech and language development and psycho-intellectual behaviour of the preschool child—results of a cross-sectional study in 1,512 children. *Auris Nasus Larynx* 12(suppl 1): S228–S230, 1985.

32. Grievink EH, Peters SA, von Bon WH, et al: The effects of early bilateral otitis media with effusion on language ability: a prospective cohort study. *J Speech Hear Res* 36:1004–1012, 1993.

33. Gates GA, Wachtendorf C, Holt GR, et al: Medical treatment of chronic otitis media with effusion (secretory otitis media). *Otolaryngol Head Neck Surg* 94:350–354, 1986.

34. Burke P: Otitis media with effusion: is medical management an option? *J R Coll Gen Pract* 39:377–382, 1989.

35. Otten FW, Grote JJ: Otitis media with effusion and chronic upper respiratory tract infection in children: a randomized, placebo-controlled study. *Laryngoscope* 100:627–633, 1990.

36. Williams RL, Chalmers TC, Stange KC, et al: Use of antibiotics in preventing recurrent acute otitis media and in treating otitis media with effusion. *JAMA* 270:1344–1351, 1993.

37. Rosenfeld RM, Post JC: Meta-analysis of antibiotic for the treatment of otitis media with effusion. *Otolaryngol Head Neck Surg* 106:378–386, 1992.

38. Lambert P: Oral steroid therapy for chronic middle ear perfusion: a double-blind crossover study. *Otolaryngol Head Neck Surg* 95:193–199, 1986.

39. Macknin ML, Jones PK: Oral dexamethasone for treatment of persistent middle ear effusion. *Pediatrics* 75:329–335, 1985.

40. Tracy JM, Demain JG, Hoffman KM, et al: Intranasal beclomethasone as an adjunct to treatment of chronic middle ear effusion. *Ann Allergy Asthma Immunol* 80:198–206, 1998.

41. McIsaac WJ, Coyte PC, Corxford R, et al: Otolaryngologists' perceptions of the indications for tympanostomy tube insertion in children. *Can Med Assoc J* 162:1285–1288, 2000.

42. Rach GH, Zielhuis GA, van Baarle PW, et al: The effect of treatment with ventilating tubes on language development in preschool children with otitis media with effusion. *Clin Otolaryngol Allied Sci* 16:128–132, 1991.

43. Maw R, Wilks J, Harvey I, et al: Early surgery compared with watchful waiting for glue ear and effect on language development in preschool children: a randomised study. *Lancet* 353:960–963, 1999.

44. Rovers MM, Staatman H, Ingels K, et al: The effect of ventilation tubes on language development in infants. *Pediatrics* 106:E4, 2000.

45. Dempster JH, Browning GG, Gatehouse SG: A randomized study of the surgical management of children with persistent otitis media with effusion associated with a hearing impairment. *J Laryngol Otol* 107:284–289, 1993.

46. Paradise JL, Bluestone CD, Colborn DK, et al: Adenoidectomy and adenotonsillectomy for recurrent acute otitis media: parallel randomized clinical trials in children not previously treated with tympanostomy tubes. *JAMA* 282:945–953, 1999.

47. Fliss DM, Leiberman A, Dagan R: Medical sequelae and complications of acute otitis media. *Pediatr Infect Dis J* 13:S34–S40, 1994.

48. Shriberg LD, Flipsen P, Thielke H, et al: Risk for speech disorder associated with early recurrent otitis media with effusion: two retrospective studies: *J Speech Language Hear Res* 43:79–99, 2000.

49. Gravel JS, Wallace IF: Language, speech and educational outcomes of otitis media. *J Otolaryngol* 27(suppl 2):17–25, 1998.

50. Bluestone CD: Clinical course, complications and sequelae of acute otitis media. *Pediatr Infect Dis J* 19:S37–S46, 2000.

51. Garcia DJ, Baker AS, Cunningham MJ, et al: Lateral sinus thrombosis associated with otitis media and mastoiditis in children. *Pediatr Infect Dis J* 14:617–623, 1995.

52. Hausdorff WP, Bryant J, Kloek C, et al: The contribution of specific pneumococcal serogroups to different disease manifestations: implications for conjugate vaccine formulation and use, part II. *Clin Infect Dis* 30:122–140, 2000.

53. Black S, Shinefield H, Fireman B, et al: Efficacy, safety and immunogenicity of heptavalent pneumococcal conjugate vaccine in children. Northern California Kaiser Permanente Vaccine Study Center Group. *Pediatr Infect Dis J* 19:187–195, 2000.

54. Advisory Committee on Immunization Practices (ACIP): Preventing pneumococcal disease among infants and young children. *MMWR* 49(Rro9):1–38, 2000.

55. Barnett ED, Pelton SI, Cabral HJ, et al: Immune response to pneumococcal conjugate and polysaccharide vaccines in otitis-prone and otitis-free children. *Clin Infect Dis* 29:191–192, 1999.

56. Bojrab DI, Bruderly T, Abdulrazzak Y: Otitis externa. *Otolaryngol Clin North Am* 20(5):761–782, 1996.

57. Carlson, L (ed): *Sound Advice: Otitis Externa*. London, Daiichi Pharmaceuticals, 2001.

58. Sander R: Otitis externa: a practical guide to treatment and prevention. *Am Fam Physician* 63:927–936, 2001.

59. Slattery WH, Brackmann DE: Skull base osteomyelitis: malignant external otitis. *Otolaryngol Clin North Am* 20(5):795–806, 1996.

Lori M. Dickerson
Peter J. Carek

Chapter

8

Prevention and Treatment of Influenza

Influenza is an acute viral infection of the respiratory tract, with symptoms that include fever, myalgia, headache, malaise, cough, sore throat, rhinitis, and other common coldlike symptoms. Complications of influenza infection include primary influenza pneumonia and secondary bacterial pneumonia. Fortunately, influenza can be prevented with immunization or chemoprophylaxis. The advent of antivirals directed against influenza A and B have made treatment possible, although therapy must be initiated early in the course of illness to have any benefit.

tions, and deaths from influenza occurs in older persons, very young children and persons of any age with certain underlying health conditions have higher complication rates than healthy older children and younger adults (Table 8-1).[1,2,5] Options for controlling influenza in high-risk populations include vaccination, antiviral drugs for prophylaxis of people exposed to active influenza infection, and early initiation of antiviral drugs to treat influenza in those with active infection.

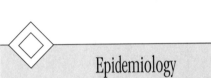

Epidemiology

Pathophysiology

Influenza causes an epidemic during the winter months in the United States; school-age children and young adults have the highest rates of influenza infection and illness.[1,2] Influenza can also cause pandemics, in which rates of illness and death can increase dramatically.[1]

Influenza can lead to considerable morbidity among healthy adults, with associated health care provider visits, lost work days, and antibiotic use. Mortality rates are highest among persons aged 65 years and older and those with preexisting pulmonary and cardiac conditions.[1,3] Death can be the result of influenza pneumonia, but is more commonly the result of secondary bacterial infections that lead to pneumonia. Pneumonia and influenza are listed as one of the ten leading causes of death in the United States.[4] Influenza is associated with 20,000 to 40,000 deaths per year in the United States and is the fifth leading cause of death among persons aged 65 years and older.[1] Influenza also results in nearly 150,000 hospitalizations per year in the United States.[1,5]

Despite the high risk of death and complications among older patients, the rates of influenza infection are highest among children.[6–8] While the highest risk of complications, hospitaliza-

Influenza viruses are spread primarily by small-particle aerosols of virus-containing respiratory secretions that are expelled into the air by an infected person during coughing, sneezing, or talking.[9–11] Spread of the virus through direct contact may also occur. The incubation period for influenza is 1 to 4 days, with an average of 2 days.[12] Persons can be infectious from the day before symptoms begin through approximately 5 days after the onset of illness; children can be infectious for a longer period.

There are two types of influenza virus, A and B, that cause human disease. Type A has historically been the principal cause of influenza and is further subdivided according to surface proteins: hemagglutinin (H) and neuraminidase (N).[1,12] Although many subtypes have been identified, three H subtypes (H1, H2, and H3) and two N subtypes (N1 and N2) of influenza A are known to cause illness in humans. Type B virus is an increasing cause of influenza in humans but is not categorized into subtypes.

The influenza virus attacks the epithelial cells of the respiratory tract and produces abrupt symptoms. The virus replicates rapidly (in 4 to 6 h) and is spread by respiratory secretions through coughing and sneezing.

Table 8-1

Rates of Influenza-Associated Hospitalizations by Age Group

AGE GROUP	HIGH-RISK (I.E., UNDERLYING CARDIAC OR PULMONARY DISEASE*)	WITHOUT HIGH RISK*
0–4	500	100
5–14	200	20–40
15–44	40–60	20–30
45–64	80–400	20–40
>65	>1000	200

*Hospitalization rate per 100,000 population.

The surface proteins of influenza A and B can mutate and cause antigenic variation, also known as antigenic "drift."[1,12] Larger antigenic variations can occur in influenza A and cause an antigenic "shift"; such shifts have been responsible for past pandemics. IgA and IgG antibodies, specific to the surface hemagglutinin and neuraminidase proteins, mediate influenza immunity.

In the 2000–2001 flu season, activity increased in December and peaked at the end of January (with 24 percent of specimens positive for influenza). The most frequently isolated viruses were influenza A (58 percent, primarily H1N1) and influenza B (42 percent). Overall, influenza activity and the rates of death from pneumonia and influenza were lower than in the previous three seasons.[13]

A person's immunity to the surface antigens, especially hemagglutinin, reduces the likelihood of infection and the severity of disease if infection occurs.[14] Antibodies against one influenza virus type or subtype confer little or no protection against another virus type or subtype. Furthermore, antibodies to one antigenic variant of influenza virus may not protect against a new antigenic variant of the same type or subtype. The frequent development of antigenic variants through antigenic drift is the virologic basis for seasonal epidemics and the reason for the incorporation of one or more new strains in each year's vaccine.

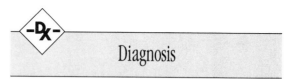

Diagnosis

Clinical Presentation

Uncomplicated influenza illness is characterized by the abrupt onset of constitutional and respiratory signs and symptoms (i.e., fever, myalgia, headache, severe malaise, nonproductive cough, sore throat, and rhinorrhea). Although influenza is often confused with the common cold, patients with an influenza-like illness during the flu season who have both cough and fever within 48 h of symptom onset are likely to have influenza (Table 8-2).[15] Some clinical signs and symptoms may be reported in one age group but not in others (Table 8-3).[12]

Illness typically resolves after several days in most individuals, although cough and malaise may persist for 2 weeks or longer. A fever of 38 to 40°C usually peaks within 24 h and, while typically lasting 2 to 3 days, may persist for 7 days. The myalgias often involve the back, arms, and legs. Other symptoms that occur less frequently include substernal soreness, photophobia and other ocular symptoms, nausea, abdominal pain, and diarrhea.

Children experience symptoms similar to those of adults, but they are more likely to have gastrointestinal problems such as nausea, vomit-

Table 8-2

Common Symptoms of Influenza and the Common Cold

SYMPTOM	INFLUENZA	COMMON COLD
Onset	Abrupt	More gradual
Fever	Characteristic, high, lasting 3–4 days (102 to 104°F)	Rare, or a minimal increase of about 1°F
Myalgia, arthralgia	Severe, common	Rare
Anorexia	Common	Rare
Headache	Prominent	Rare
Malaise	Severe and early	Mild
Fatigue, weakness	Common, lasting 2 to 3 weeks	Very mild, short in duration
Chest discomfort	Common, can be severe	Mild to moderate
Cough (dry)	Severe, common	Mild to moderate
Stuffy nose	Sometimes	Common
Sneezing	Sometimes	Common
Sore throat	Sometimes	Common

Table 8-3

Signs and Symptoms of Influenza in Specific Age Groups

AGE GROUP	SIGN OR SYMPTOM
Children	Otitis media
	Seizures
	Croup
	Conjunctivitis
Children and adults	Pharyngitis
	Dizziness
	Hoarseness
	Abdominal pain
Adults	Arthralgia
	Chest pain
	Insomnia
	Cervical lymphadenopathy
Adults and elderly	Sputum production
Elderly	Dyspnea

ing, abdominal pain, and diarrhea. Maximum temperatures tend to be higher in children, and febrile seizures may occur. Infants and children can present with a nonspecific febrile illness or with a respiratory illness such as croup, bronchi-

olitis, or bronchitis. The clinical presentation of influenza in infants can mimic bacterial sepsis.[16]

In some persons, influenza can exacerbate underlying medical conditions (e.g., pulmonary or cardiac disease) or lead to secondary bacterial pneumonia and primary influenza viral pneumonia. Upper respiratory tract complications include bacterial sinusitis and otitis media. Other cardiac and lower respiratory tract complications include exacerbation of chronic obstructive pulmonary disease and chronic congestive heart failure, croup, bronchitis, and exacerbation of asthma.[9,17]

Complications

Secondary bacterial pneumonias typically occur 5 to 10 days after the initial onset of influenza symptoms.[11] Productive cough, pleuritic chest pain, and chills are commonly present. *Streptococcus pneumoniae*, *Staphylococcus aureus*, and *Haemophilus influenzae* are the most commonly involved organisms.

Reye's syndrome, an acute encephalopathy with cerebral edema and fatty degeneration of the liver, has been reported in patients using aspirin after influenza infection.[12] Other complications involving the central nervous system (CNS) include impaired reaction time, postinfluenza encephalitis, encephalopathy, transverse myelitis, and Guillain-Barré syndrome.[18]

Other complications of an influenza infection may occur, although less commonly. Toxic shock syndrome caused by an underlying *S. aureus* infection has been reported.[19] Myositis may present in early convalescence with an acute onset of pain and tenderness in the gastrocnemius and soleus muscles.[12] This complication is more common in children than in adults and is usually associated with influenza B rather than influenza A virus infections.

Physical Examination

Despite severe subjective complaints by the patient, the physical findings during an uncomplicated influenza infection are usually minimal. The skin may feel hot and dry, with the face demonstrating a flushed appearance. Upper respiratory tract findings may include erythema of mucous membranes, postnasal discharge, and mild cervical adenopathy. In addition, rhonchi, wheezes, and an occasional rale may be detected during lung examination.

Laboratory Findings

Laboratory studies (i.e., electrolytes, complete blood count, etc.) rarely aid in the acute evaluation of an influenza infection. On a complete blood count, the leukocyte count is usually normal. Occasionally, leukopenia with relative lymphocytosis is present.

Specific diagnostic tests for influenza are available. Currently, these tests involve either virus isolation, detection of viral proteins, detection of viral nucleic acid, or serologic diagnosis.[12] The best clinical sample for isolation or detection of influenza is a combination of nasopharyngeal and throat swabs. Serologic diagnosis involves the acquisition of at least two serum samples over a period of 10 to 14 days,

which limits its usefulness in the acute evaluation and treatment of this infection.

Viral isolation is the gold standard for laboratory diagnosis of influenza.[12] The collection of clinical specimens for viral culture is important, as only culture isolates provide information on circulating influenza subtypes and strains. Antigenic and genetic characterization of virus isolates forms the basis for the selection of virus strains to be included in vaccine formulation. However, culture results are not usually available rapidly enough to be the basis for initiation of antiviral therapy or infection-control measures.

Several commercial rapid diagnostic tests (with results available in less than 1 h) are available for detecting influenza viruses.[1] Some of these tests detect only influenza A viruses; others detect both influenza A and B, but do not differentiate between the two types. The use of rapid diagnostic tests can facilitate decisions regarding treatment for individual patients as well as decisions regarding prophylaxis during outbreaks. The sensitivity of these diagnostic kits for the detection of influenza is high (approximately 90 percent) for acutely ill hospitalized children, but only moderate to low for adults and people with less severe illness.[20,21] A reverse transcriptase–polymerase chain reaction assay with a sensitivity similar to that of viral culture is under development but is not yet available commercially.[20,22] The hope is that with the development of accurate rapid testing methods, physicians can monitor the influenza type in their area, diagnose influenza more accurately, and consider treatment options more carefully.

Vaccination

In the United States, the primary mechanism for reducing the burden of influenza illness is through immunoprophylaxis with the inactivated vaccine. The Advisory Committee on Immunization Practices (ACIP) recommends that the vaccine be given to persons aged 50 years and older, plus many populations with chronic underlying medical conditions.[1] Vaccines should be given to patients during routine health care visits or during hospitalizations in order to maximize the vaccine delivery. Many health care providers and persons in close contact with high-risk patients should also be vaccinated to reduce transmission rates and subsequent influenza infection.[22]

Types of Vaccines

The current vaccine for prevention of influenza is the inactivated (i.e., killed-virus, noninfectious) vaccine.[22] In the near future, an attenuated vaccine will also be available for use. In both cases, the hemagglutinin and neuraminidase proteins of the influenza virus are the primary targets of the protective antibody response. The antibodies induced against the hemagglutinin proteins neutralize the virus infectivity, and the neuraminidase antibodies attenuate the severity of disease.[12]

INACTIVATED VACCINES

The inactivated influenza vaccine is prepared from virus grown in chick embryos. Its contents are determined by the Food and Drug Administration (FDA) and the World Health Organization (WHO) each year based on the viruses likely to circulate in the United States in the upcoming winter.[1,22] To determine which viruses to include, the agencies monitor outbreaks of influenza elsewhere in the world in order to identify the new antigenic drift viruses.[10,12,22] In addition, the antibody protection against the new viruses in people who were vaccinated with the previous year's vaccine is evaluated. Finally, the availability of a high-yield strain of viruses for production of vaccine is necessary.

The vaccine is given as an intramuscular injection and contains 15 μg of hemagglutinin per dose from a combination of two strains of influenza A (H1N1 and H3N2) and one strain of influenza B.[1,22] Products contain either whole or split virus; the split virus has a purified surface antigen (Table 8-4). Both types of product have been found to be highly effective in reducing the risk of influenza in children and adults, but offer less protection to the elderly.

Side effects from the inactivated vaccine are primarily local, including mild soreness at the intramuscular injection site for 24 to 48 h in 25 percent of adults.[22] Systemic symptoms are reported, but they occur at the same frequency in patients receiving placebo. Young children may develop fever, but severe reactions are rare. Fever in children can be minimized by administration of the split-virus vaccine, which is less antigenic.[1,23] In adults, there is no difference in side effects from the whole- versus the split-virus vaccine. Earlier concerns about a potential association between vaccination and Guillain-Barré syndrome have been refuted and should not deter patients from receiving the inactivated vaccine.[1,12,22]

The inactivated influenza vaccine is contraindicated for people with a documented egg allergy, although the risk of hypersensitivity reactions appears to be very low. For those with an egg allergy who are likely to derive great benefit from vaccination, the vaccine can be administered safely using a two-dose protocol and preparations that contain no more than 1.2 mg/mL of egg protein.[24] In addition, hypersensitivity reactions may also occur in response to thimerosal or antibiotic preservatives in some vaccine preparations.[1,22]

ATTENUATED VACCINES

A live attenuated influenza vaccine is currently under investigation in the United States. This vaccine will also contain strains of influenza A (H2N2) and B and will be administered intranasally by spray.[12,22] It is hoped that the live attenuated vaccine will better mimic natural infection and provide a greater mucosal and systemic response. The live attenuated vaccine has been found to be as safe and efficacious as

Table 8-4

Available Influenza Vaccines

PRODUCT	MANUFACTURER	PREPARATION	PRESERVATIVES	AWP* PER DOSE
Fluogen	Monarch	Split-virus	0.01% thimerosal	$5.87
Flushield	Wyeth-Ayerst	Purified split-virus	0.01% thimerosal	$5.32
Fluvirin	Medeva	Purified surface antigen	0.01% thimerosal	$4.70
Fluzone	Aventis Pasteur	Whole-virus	0.01% thimerosal	$5.18
		Split-virus	0.01% thimerosal	$5.18

*ABBREVIATION: AWP, average wholesale price.

the inactivated influenza vaccine when given to healthy working adults, young adults, and children.[22,25,26] In the elderly, immunologic response is lower as a result of preexisting antibodies acquired through years of exposure to influenza virus infections. However, antibody responses have been significantly improved in elderly persons who receive a combination of the new live attenuated vaccine and the currently available inactivated vaccine.[27] Advantages to the intranasal vaccine will include increased ease of use and acceptability, and potentially a longer-lasting or broader immune response than that provided by the inactivated vaccine.[12]

Several adverse effects have been reported with the use of the live attenuated vaccine. As a result of its delivery mechanism, the attenuated vaccine can induce mild upper respiratory tract symptoms in 10 to 15 percent of patients.[22] Like the inactivated virus vaccine, the attenuated virus vaccine is also derived from chick-embryo cells, and so the risk of hypersensitivity reactions to eggs may be present.

Clinical Efficacy of the Inactivated Influenza Vaccine

HEALTHY ADULTS AND CHILDREN

The influenza vaccine effectively prevents influenza illness in 70 to 90 percent of healthy adults less than 65 years of age when the vaccine

and the epidemic viruses match antigenically.[1,22] In the presence of a good antigenic match, vaccination has resulted in a 30 to 50 percent decrease in upper respiratory tract illnesses, work absenteeism, and use of health care resources in adults.[22,28–30] It has also been shown to be effective in preventing infection in health care professionals, reducing work absenteeism and febrile respiratory illnesses.[31] When vaccine was given to staff of long-term care facilities, mortality rates among residents decreased, regardless of the vaccination status of the residents.[22,32] In children, the influenza vaccine has resulted in decreased episodes of otitis media and reduced influenza-related morbidity in household contacts of children attending day care.[33–35]

OLDER AND HIGH-RISK ADULTS

Vaccine efficacy is reduced by 30 to 60 percent when there is a poor antigenic match, such as in persons whose immune system responses are weaker (i.e., the elderly and individuals with high-risk chronic medical conditions).[1,22,36,37] Even if the antibody titer is less than optimal, however, vaccination can still be effective in preventing secondary complications of influenza and reducing the risk of hospitalization and death.[38] For example, the influenza vaccine is effective in preventing influenza illness in only 30 to 40 percent of residents of long-term care facilities. However, it is 50 to 60 percent effective in preventing hospitalizations and 80 percent effective in preventing death in the same group. In elderly persons living at home, the vaccine is 30 to 70 percent effective in preventing hospitalization.[1,22] Attempts to increase the efficacy of the live attenuated vaccine in the elderly by using booster doses have not been effective.[39]

Indications for Vaccination

The influenza vaccine is strongly recommended for any person older than 6 months of age who is at increased risk for complications as a result of underlying chronic medical conditions. In 2000, the Centers for Disease Control and the ACIP modified their previous recommendation and lowered the age for routine influenza vaccination to include all persons 50 years of age and older.[1] Other target populations for vaccination include health care workers and persons in close contact with high-risk groups. A detailed list of the indications for vaccination is found in Table 8-5.[1]

The vaccine should be given to members of high-risk groups in October and November, as the influenza season typically peaks between late December and early March. Vaccination prior to October should be avoided, as antibody levels decline within a few months after vaccination and adequate immunity may not be maintained during the peak influenza season.[1] During the 2000–2001 influenza season, a delay in the supply of influenza vaccine resulted in a restriction of vaccination to the elderly and those with chronic diseases, their household contacts, and health care personnel.[40]

The dosage recommendations for the influenza vaccine vary according to age group (see Table 8-6).[1] In general, adults should receive a single dose of the vaccine. Children less than 9 years of age should receive two doses of the vaccine at least 1 month apart (the second dose should be given before December). The intramuscular route of administration is recommended, using the deltoid muscle for adults and the anterolateral aspect of the thigh for children.[1]

The influenza vaccine can be administered in conjunction with other vaccines, such as the pneumococcal vaccine in adults and routine immunizations in children.

Antiviral Agents

Antiviral drugs are an important adjunct in the management of influenza illness, but they should not be considered a substitute for vaccination. Currently, four antiviral agents are available in the United States: amantadine, rimantadine, oseltamivir, and zanamivir. The decision to prescribe an antiviral agent for the prevention of influenza should be based on evidence or a high probability of exposure to an infected individual, the laboratory diagnosis, or a high clinical suspicion of influenza virus infection based on signs and symptoms.[22]

Amantadine and Rimantadine

PHARMACOLOGY

Amantadine and rimantadine are effective in the prevention and treatment of influenza A virus, but do not have activity against influenza B. Amantadine is FDA-approved for the prevention and treatment of influenza A in adults and children 1 year of age and older. Rimantadine is FDA-approved for the prevention and treatment of influenza A in adults. Although in children rimantadine is FDA-approved only for the prevention of infection, many experts consider it to be appropriate also for treatment of children 1 year of age and older.[1]

These drugs interfere with viral penetration into host cells and inhibit the uncoating of the virus through action on a specific protein called M_2.[41] Since influenza B viruses lack the M_2 protein, these viruses are not sensitive to amantadine and rimantadine.

Table 8-5

Indications for Influenza Vaccination

Groups at High Risk for Complications of Influenza:
Persons aged > 50 years
Residents of long-term care facilities
Adults and children with chronic pulmonary (including asthma) and cardiac disease
Adults and children requiring care for chronic metabolic diseases (e.g., diabetes), renal dysfunction, hemoglobinopathies, or immunosuppression (e.g., induced by medication or due to human immunodeficiency virus)
Children (6 months to 18 years) receiving long-term aspirin therapy who might be at risk of Reye's syndrome after influenza infection
Women who will be in the second or third trimester of pregnancy during the influenza season (usually December through March)
Persons Who Can Transmit Influenza to Those at Risk:
Health care personnel in hospital and outpatient facilities, including emergency response workers
Employees of long-term care facilities or residences for persons in high-risk groups
Providers of home care to persons in high-risk groups
Household members (including children) of persons in high-risk groups
Groups to Consider for Vaccination:
Persons at high risk traveling to locations where influenza may be in season, e.g., Southern Hemisphere in July
Persons providing essential community services
Students and others in institutional settings
Any person who wishes to reduce the risk of influenza infection

---

Table 8-6

Dosage of Influenza Vaccine

AGE	PRODUCT	DOSE	NUMBER OF DOSES
6–35 months	Split-virus	0.25 mL	1–2*
3–8 years	Split-virus	0.50 mL	1–2*
9–12 years	Split-virus	0.50 mL	1
> 12 years	Whole- or split-virus	0.50 mL	1

*Two doses of vaccine are recommended for children less than 9 years of age who are receiving the vaccine for the first time.

Both agents are well absorbed after oral administration. They have half-lives of approximately 15 and 30 h, respectively.[22,41] Amantadine is not metabolized in the liver, and is cleared by the kidney. Patients with renal dysfunction (creatinine clearance < 50 mL/min) have a two- to threefold increase in the elimination half-life of amantadine. Rimantadine is extensively hepatically metabolized (but does not interfere with the cytochrome P-450 system) and is renally eliminated. Patients with severe hepatic or renal dysfunction exhibit a twofold increase in the elimination half-life of rimantadine.[22,41]

In more than 25 percent of patients given amantadine or rimantadine for the treatment of influenza, viral resistance to both agents develops quickly (i.e., within days).[22] However, this resistance has not been related to a prolonged illness or illness rebound. Although resistant strains can be transmitted to other persons, the clinical implications of resistant viral infections are unknown.[12] Resistance does not appear to occur when these agents are used for the prevention of influenza.[22]

SAFETY AND TOLERABILITY

The tolerability of these antiviral agents is good. Nausea and vomiting are the primary adverse effects, occurring in approximately 5 to 10 percent of patients receiving amantadine and rimantadine.[42] Insomnia occurs in about 5 percent of patients receiving either drug. Other CNS effects (i.e., depression, anxiety, irritability, hallucinations, confusion) have been reported in approximately 10 percent of patients receiving amantadine and 5 percent of patients receiving rimantadine. This risk is greater in elderly patients and is due to the drug's ability to stimulate the release of catecholamines, particularly dopamine.[22,41] When serum concentrations increase significantly, hallucinations and seizures can occur. In a nursing home population, 19 percent of patients experienced adverse effects and required drug discontinuation with amantadine, whereas only 2 percent had problems with rimantadine.[43] All side effects are dose-related and resolve rapidly with discontinuation. Amantadine can interact with anticholinergic drugs, causing additive CNS side effects. Rimantadine has no significant drug interactions. Both agents are in FDA pregnancy risk category C and are not recommended for use in breast-feeding mothers.[40,44]

EFFICACY

When given within 48 h of the onset of symptoms, amantadine and rimantadine are effective in reducing the severity and duration of illness caused by influenza A viruses. Overall, amantadine reduces the duration of uncomplicated influenza A fever and illness by 1 day.[1,42] The efficacy appears to be similar for rimantadine, although there have been fewer clinical trials. Despite their ability to reduce the duration of influenza illness, these agents have not been shown to prevent serious complications (i.e., viral or bacterial pneumonia) or death from influenza.[1] Studies have primarily included low-risk patients, so the benefit in patients with a greater risk for complications is unknown.

Both drugs are about 50 percent effective in preventing overall influenza A infection and 70 to 90 percent effective in preventing influenza illness after a known exposure.[1,22,42] More specifically, the average effectiveness of amantadine and rimantadine for the prevention of confirmed influenza illness was 61 and 72 percent, respectively.[42,45] Both agents prevent illness while permitting subclinical infection and the production of a protective antibody response to circulating influenza viruses. The use of antiviral agents does not interfere with the protective effect of vaccination. Both drugs have been found to be an effective component of influenza outbreak control programs in long-term care facilities.[46,47]

DOSING REGIMENS

Amantadine and rimantadine are available as tablets or suspensions for oral administration once or twice a day (see Table 8-7) and should be started within 48 h of the onset of symptoms. There does not appear to be any significant clinical benefit associated with initiating treatment after 48 h from the onset of symptoms. Both agents should be given with food to decrease gastrointestinal side effects. The dosage of both agents should be reduced in patients with renal dysfunction.

To reduce the emergence of drug-resistant viruses, the duration of treatment during acute infection should be limited to 3 to 5 days, or 24

Table 8-7

Comparison of Dosing Regimens for Antiviral Agents

Antiviral Agent	Route of Administration	Daily Dosage—Treatment		Duration of Treatment	Daily Dosage—Prophylaxis		Duration of Prophylaxis
		Children	**Adults**		**Children**	**Adults**	
M2 Inhibitors							
Amantadine[a] (Symmetrel)	Oral	<1 year: not recommended; 1–9 years: 5 mg/kg/day divided b.i.d. (up to 150 mg/day); >10 years[b]: 100 mg b.i.d. — 100 mg b.i.d. × 5 days = $6.79[c]	<65 years: 100 mg b.i.d; >65 years: 100 mg q.d.	Continue for 3–5 days or 24–48 h after symptoms disappear	<1 year: not recommended; 1–9 years: 5 mg/kg/day divided b.i.d. (up to 150 mg/day); >10 years[b]: 100 mg b.i.d. — 100 mg BID × 10 days = $13.58	<65 years: 100 mg b.i.d.; >65 years: 100 mg q.d.	Continue for at least 2 weeks or until approximately 1 week after the outbreak. When vaccine is contraindicated, continue throughout influenza season (i.e., up to 90 days).
Rimantadine[d] (Flumadine)	Oral	NA — 100 mg b.i.d. × 5 days = $21.85	≤65 years: 100 mg b.i.d; >65 years: 100 mg q.d.		<1 year: not recommended; 1–9 years: 5 mg/kg/day q.d. or divided b.i.d. (up to 150 mg/day); >10 years[b]: 100 mg b.i.d. — 100 mg b.i.d. × 10 days = $43.70	<65 years: 100 mg b.i.d.; >65 years: 100 mg q.d.	
Neuraminidase Inhibitors							
Oseltamivir[e] (Tamiflu)	Oral	1–13 years: ≤15 kg = 30 mg b.i.d.; >15–23 kg = 45 mg b.i.d.; 23–40 kg = 60 mg b.i.d.; >40 kg = 75 mg b.i.d. — 75 mg b.i.d. × 5 days = $55.67	>13 years: 75 mg b.i.d.	5 days	NA	>13 years: 75 mg q.d. — 75 mg q.d. × 7 days = $77.94	Continue for at least 7 days following a known exposure. Safety and efficacy have been documented for up to 6 weeks.
Zanamivir (Relenza)	Inhaled (oral)	>7 years: 2 inhalations (5 mg/puff, 10 mg/dose) b.i.d. — 2 puffs b.i.d. × 5 days = $47.70		5 days	NA	NA	NA

ABBREVIATIONS: NA, not applicable—not FDA approved for this indication; b.i.d., twice daily; q.d., once daily.

[a] Consult the package insert for amantadine dosing recommendations in patients with impaired renal function (creatinine clearance < 50 mL/min).

[b] Children weighing < 40 kg should be prescribed amantadine or rimantadine 5 mg/kg/day, regardless of age.

[c] Average wholesale prices provided by www.drugstore.com.

[d] Consult the package insert for rimantadine dosing recommendations in patients with impaired renal function (creatinine clearance < 10 mL/min) or severe hepatic dysfunction.

[e] Consult the package insert for oseltamivir dosing recommendations in patients with impaired renal function (creatinine clearance < 30 mL/min).

to 48 h after the disappearance of signs and symptoms. The duration of prophylactic therapy is controversial, but for those exposed to a known case, it is generally recommended that the drug be given for 10 days after the exposure.[1] To be maximally effective, the drug must be taken daily for the duration of influenza activity in the household, long-term care facility, or other community.

Oseltamivir and Zanamivir

PHARMACOLOGY

Oseltamivir and zanamivir are neuraminidase inhibitors with activity against influenza A and B. Activity against influenza A has been extensively documented in vivo, but the majority of data demonstrating the effectiveness of neuraminidase inhibitors against influenza B have been in vitro. Oseltamivir is FDA-approved for prevention of influenza in adults and children older than 13 years, and for the treatment of influenza in adults and children 1 year and older.[41,48,49] Zanamivir is FDA-approved for the treatment of influenza in adults and children older than 7 years.[41,48,49]

Oseltamivir and zanamivir inhibit the neuraminidase protein on the surface of the virus, preventing illness in patients exposed to influenza and reducing the severity of illness in those with active infection.[22,48] Oseltamivir is given orally, and absorption is not affected by food. It is hepatically metabolized but does not interfere with the cytochrome P-450 system. Metabolites are renally eliminated and have a half-life of 6 to 10 h. Patients with renal dysfunction may require a dosage adjustment. Zanamivir, a dry powder formulated for oral inhalation, is less than 15 percent systemically absorbed. It is excreted unchanged in the urine and has an elimination half-life of 3 to 5 h. Influenza A and B viruses with reduced susceptibility to zanamivir have been isolated in vitro and found in 2 percent of adults with influenza

who have been treated with oseltamivir.[41,48] The clinical significance of these resistant strains is unknown, but influenza A viruses that are resistant to neuraminidase inhibitors appear to be sensitive to amantadine and rimantadine.[50]

SAFETY AND TOLERABILITY

Neuraminidase inhibitors are much better tolerated than the older antiviral agents, amantadine and rimantadine. The primary adverse effects with oseltamivir (i.e., nausea, vomiting, and headache) have been reported in about 10 percent of patients.[41,48,51] Nausea and vomiting can be reduced by administering oseltamivir with food. Compared to rimantadine, oseltamivir is better tolerated when used for prevention of influenza.[51] In general, side effects with zanamivir are rare. However, patients with asthma or chronic obstructive pulmonary disease may experience bronchospasm and a decline in forced expiratory volume and peak flow rates.[22,48,49] Therefore, zanamivir is generally not recommended for use in patients with any chronic airway disease. Drug interactions are not present with either agent. Both agents are in FDA pregnancy risk category C and are not recommended for use in breast-feeding mothers.[41,44]

EFFICACY

When given within 48 h of the onset of symptoms, oseltamivir and zanamivir are both effective in reducing the duration of influenza symptoms by 1 to 1.5 days, and in reducing the duration and quantity of virus in respiratory secretions.[22,48] An even greater improvement has been documented in high-risk patients and in those who started treatment on the first day of illness.[52–55] In some studies, treatment has also reduced associated complications such as sinusitis, bronchitis, otitis media, and other infections requiring antibiotic treatment.[48,56–59] In general, treated patients returned to normal activities a half-day sooner and had less sleep disturbance.[51,53,58] However, neither drug has shown significant impact on major complications such as pneumonia. In addition, only a small proportion of patients in these clinical trials had documented influenza B infection, so it is still not certain how effective the neuraminidase inhibitors will be in unselected patients with influenza B.

Both drugs have been shown to be effective in preventing influenza if given before exposure to illness. However, only oseltamivir is FDA-approved for prevention of influenza. In general, oseltamivir and zanamivir prevent infection in 30 to 50 percent of patients and prevent illness in 70 to 90 percent of patients.[48,51,60–62] Both drugs offer protection (80 to 90 percent) against influenza in exposed family members.[62,63] Oseltamivir has also shown significant benefit in the prevention of influenza in vaccinated residents of long-term care facilities. The use of oseltamivir does not interfere with the protective effects of vaccination.

DOSING REGIMENS

Oseltamivir is available as a tablet or as a suspension for oral administration once or twice a day (Table 8-7). It should be given with food in order to minimize the gastrointestinal side effects.

Zanamivir is a dry powder inhaler; two puffs are taken twice a day. For the drug to be effective, patients must have good coordination, and significant respiratory effort is required to deliver the drug to the lungs. Since the drug was approved by the FDA, a warning has been added to the package insert recommending against the use of zanamivir for the treatment of influenza in patients with underlying pulmonary disease (e.g., asthma or chronic obstructive pulmonary disease). This information was added because of the risk of bronchospasm in this population and because there are insufficient data to support the efficacy of zanamivir in this popula-

tion. If a patient develops shortness of breath or bronchospasm while using zanamivir, the drug should be stopped immediately. If zanamivir is given to a patient with respiratory disease, the patient should also have a fast-acting bronchodilator (e.g., albuterol) available for use.[41]

Both drugs should be started within 48 h of the onset of influenza symptoms. Benefits are minimal for patients treated after 48 h from the onset of symptoms. To reduce the emergence of drug-resistant viruses, duration of treatment during acute infection should be limited to 5 days. The duration of prophylactic therapy with oseltamivir is at least 7 days following a known exposure.

Indications for Antiviral Agents

As previously stated, antiviral agents are not a substitute for vaccination. Indications for antiviral agents are found in Table 8-8. Patients with the highest priority for receiving antiviral agents are unvaccinated individuals who are at a high risk for complications.[1] These individuals should receive treatment in the case of an acute infection and prophylaxis if exposed to someone with the flu. High-risk patients, even if vaccinated, should receive treatment if they develop clinical influenza. In addition, these drugs offer a benefit to vaccinated patients in years in which there is a poor antigenic match between the circulating influenza virus and the vaccine virus. Household contacts of high-risk patients should be considered for treatment. Antiviral agents have been shown to be effective if started within 48 h of the onset of symptoms, but treatment initiated earlier offers even greater benefit.[1]

Choice of Antiviral Agent

In seasons in which there is predicted to be substantial influenza B illness, oseltamivir and zanamivir are the preferred antiviral agents for treatment, as they are effective against influenza

Table 8-8

Recommendations for Use of Antiviral Drugs

Treatment

All persons at high risk for complications who develop influenza

Persons with severe influenza

Persons presenting within 48 h of symptom onset who wish to shorten the duration of influenza illness

Prophylaxis

Unvaccinated persons (e.g., those with egg allergies) at high risk

Persons at high risk vaccinated after the onset of an epidemic:

For children, 4 weeks after the first dose of vaccine and 2 weeks after the second dose

For adults, 2 weeks after vaccination

Vaccinated persons at high risk when the vaccine virus and epidemic virus are a poor antigenic match

Persons with immunodeficiencies (e.g., human immunodeficiency virus)

Unvaccinated persons caring for high-risk patients

Unvaccinated persons living with high-risk patients

All unvaccinated residents and staff of long-term care facilities during an outbreak

Consider:

Vaccinated persons at high risk to ensure optimal prophylaxis

All vaccinated staff and residents of long-term care facilities during an institutional outbreak when the vaccine virus and epidemic virus are a poor antigenic match

All unvaccinated persons exposed in the household

A and, in contrast to amantadine and rimantadine, may offer some protection against influenza B viruses. Oseltamivir would be preferred over zanamivir in patients with compromised respiratory function or those lacking the inspiratory effort or coordination required to deliver the drug. Other advantages to the newer antiviral agents include increased tolerability, potentially a decreased risk for resistance, and a decrease in some influenza complications.

In seasons in which influenza A is the primary virus, amantadine and rimantadine would be appropriate choices. Rimantadine is preferred over amantadine because of its increased tolerability, particularly in the elderly or in those with compromised renal function. Amantadine is significantly less expensive than any of the other agents and would be appropriate to use for the treatment of influenza A in otherwise healthy adults.

When considering prophylaxis, however, the choice is more difficult. The cost of neuraminidase inhibitors prohibits their use in the prevention of influenza, particularly if prophylactic therapy is given during a prolonged period of exposure. However, during prolonged therapy, an agent with greater tolerability would offer an advantage. Oseltamivir is the only neuraminidase inhibitor currently approved for prevention of influenza A and B. Amantadine and rimantadine are as effective as oseltamivir in the prevention of influenza A and are much less expensive.

Use in Long-Term Care Facilities

Outbreaks of influenza in long-term care facilities can involve up to 60 percent of residents, and many of these patients develop complications and die from influenza and bacterial pneumonia.[39] Most severe outbreaks have involved influenza A, although influenza B has the potential to reemerge as a significant cause of illness. The ACIP recommends that prophylaxis be started immediately when confirmed or suspected outbreaks of influenza occur in long-term care facilities and other institutions.[1] Early prophylaxis should reduce the spread of the virus and minimize the impact of an outbreak. Antiviral agents should be given to all residents, even those who have received the inactivated vaccine during the current influenza season. Prophylaxis should continue for at least 2 weeks or until approximately 1 week after the outbreak. Prophylaxis should be offered to all unvaccinated staff providing care to high-risk patients, and to all staff if the circulating virus is a poor antigenic match with the vaccine virus. In addition to antiviral therapy, infection control policies such as droplet precautions, restricting contact between residents and visitors, isolating residents with confirmed infection, restriction of movement of staff between cohorts with and without infection, and vaccination of unvaccinated staff and patients should be instituted.[1,64] If the outbreak is due to influenza A infection, rimantadine is the antiviral agent of choice. If influenza B is suspected or if rimantadine is poorly tolerated in this elderly population, oseltamivir can be used.

Conclusion

An influenza epidemic occurs annually in the United States and is associated with significant morbidity and mortality. An inactivated vaccine is currently available for the prevention of influenza and is produced annually based on the FDA and WHO recommendations concerning predicted viral circulation. A live attenuated vaccine is currently under investigation and may offer greater protection against influenza illness and infection, particularly among the elderly and other high-risk populations. Older antiviral agents, amantadine and rimantadine, are effective in the prevention and treatment of influenza A, but are associated with significant side effects. The neuraminidase inhibitors, oseltamivir and zanamivir, offer protection against influenza A and B but are much more expensive than the older agents. Oseltamivir is approved for the prevention and treatment of influenza, whereas zanamivir is approved only for treatment. All

agents must be initiated within 48 h of the onset of symptoms if they are to be effective in the treatment of infection. Efforts should be focused on increasing vaccination rates among those eligible, in order to decrease the impact of an epidemic. In addition, health care providers and the public need to be aware of the symptoms of influenza in order to quickly initiate therapy in appropriate situations. Optimal application of prevention and treatment methods could substantially reduce the impact of influenza in the United States.

References

1. Centers for Disease Control and Prevention: Prevention and control of influenza. Recommendations of the advisory committee on immunization practices. *MMWR* 49(RR03):1–38, 2000.
2. Izurieta HS, Thompson WW, Kramarz P, et al: Influenza and the rates of hospitalization for respiratory disease among infants and young children. *N Engl J Med* 342:232–239, 2000.
3. Glezen WP, Greenberg SB, Atmar RL, et al: Impact of respiratory virus infections on persons with chronic underlying conditions. *JAMA* 283:499–505, 2000.
4. Guyer B, Freedman MA, Strobino DM, Sondik EJ: Annual summary of vital statistics: trends in the health of Americans during the 20th century. *Pediatrics* 106:1307–1317, 2000.
5. Simonsen L, Fukuda K, Schonberger LB, Cox NJ: The impact of influenza epidemics on hospitalizations. *J Infect Dis* 181(3):831–837, 2000.
6. Glezen WP: Serious morbidity and mortality associated with influenza epidemics. *Epidemiol Rev* 4:25–44, 1982.
7. Barker WH, Mullooly JP: Impact of epidemic type A influenza in a defined adult population. *Am J Epidemiol* 112:798–811, 1980.
8. Barker WH: Excess pneumonia and influenza associated hospitalization during influenza epidemics in the United States, 1970–78. *Am J Public Health* 76:761–765, 1986.
9. Betts RF: Influenza virus, in Mandell GL, Bennett JE, Dolin R (eds): *Mandell, Gouglas, and Bennett's Principles and Practice of Infectious Diseases,* 4th ed. New York, Churchill Livingstone, 1995; p. 1546.

10. Ottolini MG, Cheng TL: Influenza update. *Pediatr Rev* 20:33–34, 1999.

11. Cox NJ, Fukuda K: Influenza. *Infect Dis Clin North Am* 12(1):27–38, 1998.

12. Cox NJ, Subbarao K: Influenza. *Lancet* 354:1277–1282, 1999.

13. Centers for Disease Control and Prevention: Influenza activity—United States, 2000–2001 season. *MMWR* 50(11):207–209, 2001.

14. Clements ML, Betts RF, Tierney EL, Murphy BR: Serum and nasal wash antibodies associated with resistance to experimental challenge with influenza A wild-type virus. *J Clin Microbiol* 24:157–160, 1986.

15. Monto AS, Gravenstein S, Elliott M, et al: Clinical signs and symptoms predicting influenza infection. *Arch Intern Med* 160:3243–3247, 2000.

16. Dagan R, Hall CB: Influenza A virus infection imitating bacterial sepsis in early infancy. *Pediatr Infect Dis J* 3:218–221, 1984.

17. Nicholson KD: Clinical features of influenza. *Semin Respir Infect* 7:26–37, 1992.

18. Nicholson KD: Human influenza, in Nicholson KD, Hay AJ, Webster RD (eds): *Textbook of Influenza*. Boston, Blackwell Science, 1998; p. 222.

19. MacDonald KL, Osterholm MT, Hedgerg CW, et al: Toxic shock syndrome. A newly recognized complication of influenza and influenzalike illness. *JAMA* 257(8):1053–1058, 1987.

20. Atmar RL, Baxter BD, Dominguez EA, Taber LH: Comparison of reverse transcription-PCR with tissue culture and other rapid diagnostic assays for detection of type A influenza virus. *J Clin Microbiol* 38:2604–2606, 2000.

21. Noyola DE, Clark B, O'Donnell FT, et al: Comparison of a new neuraminidase detection assay with an enzyme immunoassay, immunofluorescence, and culture for a rapid detection of influenza A and B viruses in nasal wash specimens. *J Clin Microbiol* 38:1161–1165, 2000.

22. Couch RB: Prevention and treatment of influenza. *N Engl J Med* 343(24):1778–1787, 2000.

23. Problems with influenza vaccine. *Med Lett* 42 (1086):79–80, 2000.

24. James JM, Zeiger RS, Lester MR, et al: Safe administration of influenza vaccine to patients with egg allergy. *J Pediatr* 133:624–628, 1998.

25. Nichol KL, Mendelman PM, Mallon KP, et al: Effectiveness of live, attenuated, intranasal influenza virus vaccine in healthy, working adults. A randomized controlled trial. *JAMA* 282(2):137–144, 1999.

26. Mendelman PM, Cordova J, Cho I: Safety, efficacy and effectiveness of the influenza virus vaccine, trivalent, types A and B, live, cold-adapted (CAIV-T) in healthy children and adults. *Vaccine* 19:2221–2226, 2001.

27. Gorse GJ, Campabell MJ, Otto EE, et al: Increased anti-influenza A virus cytotoxic T cell activity following vaccination of the chronically ill elderly with live attenuated or inactivated influenza virus vaccine. *J Infect Dis* 172:1–10, 1995.

28. Demichelvi V, Rivetti D, Deeks JJ, Jefferson TO: Vaccines for preventing influenza in healthy adults (Cochrane Review), in *The Cochrane Library*, Issue 1. Oxford, Update Software, 2001.

29. Nichol KL: Cost-benefit analysis of a strategy to vaccinate healthy working adults against influenza. *Arch Intern Med* 161:749–759, 2001.

30. Bridges CB, Thompson WW, Meltzer MI, et al: Effectiveness and cost-benefit of influenza vaccination of healthy working adults. A randomized controlled trial. *JAMA* 284(13):1655–1663, 2000.

31. Wilde JA, McMillan JA, Serwint J, et al: Effectiveness of influenza vaccine in health care professionals. A randomized trial. *JAMA* 281(10):908–913, 1999.

32. Carman WF, Elder AG, Wallace LA, et al: Effects of influenza vaccination of health care workers on mortality of elderly people in long-term care: a randomised controlled trial. *Lancet* 355:93–97, 2000.

33. Heikkinen T, Ruuskanen O, Waris M, et al: Influenza vaccination in the prevention of acute otitis media in children. *Am J Dis Child* 145:445–448, 1991.

34. Hurwitz ES, Haber M, Chang A, et al: Effectiveness of influenza vaccination of day care children in reducing influenza-related morbidity among household contacts. *JAMA* 284(13):1677–1682, 2000.

35. Clements DA, Langdon L, Bland C, Walter E: Influenza A vaccine decreases the incidence of otitis media in 6 to 30 month old children in day care. *Arch Pediatr Adolesc Med* 149:1113–1117, 1995.

36. Ohmit SE, Arden NH, Monto AS: Effectiveness of inactivated influenza vaccine among nursing home residents during an influenza A (H3N2) epidemic. *J Am Geriatr Soc* 47:165–171, 1999.

37. Gross PA, Hermogenes AW, Sacks HS, et al: The efficacy of influenza vaccine in elderly persons: a meta-analysis and review of the literature. *Ann Intern Med* 123:518–527, 1995.

38. Nichol KL, Wuorenma J, vonSternberg T: Benefits of influenza vaccination for low-, intermediate-, and high-risk senior citizens. *Arch Intern Med* 158:1769–1776, 1998.

39. Arden NH: Control of influenza in the long-term care facility: a review of established approaches and newer options. *Infect Control Hosp Epidemiol* 21:59–64, 2000.

40. Centers for Disease Control and Prevention: Updated recommendations from the advisory committee on immunization practices in response to delays in supply of influenza vaccine for the 2000–2001 season. *MMWR* 49:888–892, 2000.

41. Cada DJ (ed): Anti-infectives, systemic, in *Drug Facts and Comparisons*. St. Louis, MO, Facts and Comparisons/Wolters Kluwer, 2001; pp 1416–1423c.

42. Jefferson TO, Demicheli V, Deeks JJ, Rivetti D: Amantadine and rimantadine for preventing and treating influenza A in adults (Cochrane Review), in *The Cochrane Library*, Issue 1. Oxford, Update Software, 2001.

43. Keyser LA, Karl M, Nafziger AN, Bertino JS: Comparison of central nervous system adverse effects of amantadine and rimantadine used as sequential prophylaxis of influenza A in elderly nursing home patients. *Arch Intern Med* 160:1485–1488, 2000.

44. Montalto NJ, Gum KD, Ashley JV: Updated treatment for influenza A and B. *Am Fam Physician* 62:27–38, 2000.

45. Demicheli V, Jefferson T, Rivetti D, Deeks J: Prevention and early treatment of influenza in healthy adults. *Vaccine* 18:957–1030, 2000.

46. Monto AS, Ohmit SE, Hornbuckle K, Pearce CL: Safety and efficacy of long-term use of rimantadine for prophylaxis of type A influenza in nursing homes. *Antimicrob Agents Chemother* 39(10):2224–2228, 1995.

47. Nicholson KG: Use of antivirals in influenza in the elderly: prophylaxis and therapy. *Gerontology* 42:280–289, 1996.

48. Two neuraminidase inhibitors for treatment of influenza. *Med Lett* 41(1063):91–93, 1999.

49. McNicholl IR, McNicholl JJ: Neuraminidase inhibitors: zanamivir and oseltamivir. *Ann Pharmacother* 35:57–70, 2001.

50. Gubareva LV, Kaiser L, Hayden FG: Influenza virus neuraminidase inhibitors. *Lancet* 355:827–835, 2000.

51. Jefferson T, Demicheli V, Deeks J, Rivetti D: Neuraminidase inhibitors for preventing and treating influenza in healthy adults (Cochrane Review), in *The Cochrane Library*, Issue 1. Oxford: Update Software, 2001.

52. Hayden FG, Osterhaus AD, Treanor JJ, et al: Efficacy and safety of the neuraminidase inhibitor zanamivir in the treatment of influenza virus infections. GG167 Influenza Study Group. *N Engl J Med* 337:874–880, 1997.

53. The MIST (Management of Influenza in the Southern Hemisphere Trialists) Study Group: Randomised trial of efficacy and safety of inhaled zanamivir in treatment of influenza A and B virus infections. *Lancet* 352:1877–1881, 1998.

54. Treanor JJ, Hayden RG, Vrooman PS, et al: Efficacy and safety of the oral neuraminidase inhibitor oseltamivir in treating acute influenza: a randomized controlled trial. US Oral Neuraminidase Study Group. *JAMA* 283:1016–1024, 2000.

55. Lalezari J, Campion K, Keene O, Silagy C: Zanamivir for the treatment of influenza A and B infection in high-risk patients. *Arch Intern Med* 161:212–217, 2001.

56. Kaiser L, Keene ON, Hammond JMJ, et al: Impact of zanamivir on antibiotic use for respiratory events following acute influenza in adolescents and adults. *Arch Intern Med* 160:3234–3240, 2000.

57. Hayden FG, Treanor JJ, Fritz RS, et al: Use of the oral neuraminidase inhibitor oseltamivir in experimental human influenza: randomized controlled trials for prevention and treatment. *JAMA* 282:1240–1246, 1999.

58. Nicholson KG, Aoki FY, Osterhaus AD, et al: Efficacy and safety of oseltamivir in treatment of acute influenza: a randomized controlled trial. Neuraminidase Inhibitor Flu Treatment Investigator Group. *Lancet* 355:1845–1850, 2000.

59. Headrick JA, Barzilai A, Behre U, et al: Zanamivir for treatment of symptomatic influenza A and B infection in children five to twelve years of age: a randomized controlled trial. *Pediatr Infect Dis J* 19:410–417, 2000.

60. Hayden FG, Atmar RL, Schilling M, et al: Use of the selective oral neuraminidase inhibitor oseltamivir to prevent influenza. *N Engl J Med* 341:1336–1343, 1999.

61. Monto AS, Robinson DP, Herlocher, et al: Zanamivir in the prevention of influenza among healthy adults: a randomized controlled trial. *JAMA* 282:31–35, 1999.

62. Hayden FG, Guvareva LV, Monto AS, et al: Inhaled zanamivir for the prevention of influenza in families. *N Engl J Med* 343:1282–1289, 2000.

63. Welliver R, Monto AS, Carewicz O, et al: Effectiveness of oseltamivir in preventing influenza in household contacts. A randomized controlled trial. *JAMA* 285:748–754, 2001.

64. Bradley SF and the Long-term Care Committee of the Society of Healthcare Epidemiology of America: Prevention of influenza in long-term care facilities. SHEA Position Paper. *Infect Control Hosp Epidemiol* 20:629–637, 1999.

Part 3

Lower Respiratory Infections

David L. Hahn

Evaluation and Management of Acute Bronchitis

In this chapter, acute bronchitis will be discussed in the context of the otherwise healthy child or adult. Patients with previous asthma, chronic obstructive pulmonary disease (COPD), heart disease, and diabetes are not included in this discussion. Infant lower respiratory tract illnesses, including bronchiolitis, are also beyond the scope of this chapter. Recent evidence-based guidelines have focused on adults but are also broadly applicable to older children and adolescents.

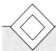

Definition of Bronchitis

A precise, reproducible, and clinically useful definition of acute bronchitis has proven elusive. Some studies have included only patients with a productive cough, but this excludes many patients with an otherwise identical clinical presentation. Current definitions do not include sputum as a necessary criterion for the definition of acute bronchitis.[1,2] Macfarlane et al[2] have proposed a practical and reproducible definition of *acute lower respiratory tract illness* that has practical utility in the primary care setting (Table 9-1). The diagnosis of acute bronchitis requires ruling out the presence of clinically significant pneumonia.

Another term, *wheezy bronchitis*, has been employed to describe the common occurrence of wheezing in children with an acute lower respiratory tract infection. Less well known is the fact that *at least 15 to 30 percent* (some studies have reported 40 to 60 percent) of adults with acute bronchitis also wheeze and/or have objective evidence of reversible airway obstruction.[3] This high prevalence justifies the use of the term *acute asthmatic bronchitis* to describe adults with signs and symptoms of acutely reversible airway obstruction (bronchospasm) in the setting of a nonpneumonic acute lower respiratory tract infection.[3] Such symptoms include complaints of

Table 9-1

Definition of Acute Bronchitis

- Previously well patients not under supervision or management for an underlying disease—for example, patients with asthma, chronic obstructive pulmonary disease, heart disease, and diabetes are excluded.
- Diagnosis of acute lower respiratory tract infection requires all of the following:
  (a) An acute illness present for 21 days or less
  (b) Cough as the cardinal symptom
  (c) At least one other lower respiratory tract symptom (sputum production, dyspnea, wheeze, chest discomfort/pain)
  (d) No alternative explanation—for example, not sinusitis, pharyngitis, or a new presentation of asthma

SOURCE: Reproduced from Macfarlane,[2] with permission from the BMJ Publishing Group.

wheezing, chest tightness, and shortness of breath, particularly with a nocturnal component. In many cases, troublesome nocturnal symptoms are often the main reason that patients visit the doctor in search of relief.

Acute Bronchitis in the Age of Antibiotic Resistance

As currently implemented, the management of acute bronchitis is misguided and probably does more harm than good, mainly because antibiotics are prescribed routinely despite evidence that they are not beneficial to most patients with this condition. In the past this antibiotic misuse could be shrugged off as a small price to pay for giving the impression that "everything possible" was being done. Now, however, the emergence of antibiotic-resistant bacterial pathogens as a direct result of antibiotic overuse requires radical reassessment of current management by both patients and physicians.

New guidelines have recently been developed that have the potential to improve the process of care for acute bronchitis.[1,4,5] These guidelines emphasize that antibiotics should not be prescribed routinely for uncomplicated acute bronchitis because the results of most randomized, controlled trials do not support the benefit of antibiotics for this condition.

An exciting but still speculative future prospect, suggested by an emerging body of research, is the determination that a subset of acute bronchitis will develop into chronic bronchitis and asthma. This research also implicates specific bacterial pathogens as potentially responsible for chronic respiratory sequelae of acute bronchitis. Although the therapeutic applications of this research are as yet unknown, primary care physicians are in an ideal position to observe, document, and research the earliest manifestations of chronic respiratory diseases that later become severe, debilitating, or fatal. Thus, in the future, the evaluation and management of acute bronchitis may become important to the early recognition, management, and perhaps even prevention of severe chronic respiratory conditions such as COPD and asthma.

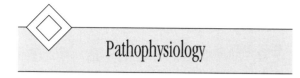

Pathophysiology

Gonzales and coworkers have suggested that the clinical features of uncomplicated acute bronchitis develop in sequential phases.[1] The acute phase results from direct inoculation of the tracheobronchial epithelium by an infectious agent, followed by cytokine release and acute inflammation that produces variable constitutional symptoms, such as fever, myalgias, and malaise. These symptoms may last 1 to 5 days, depending on the infectious agent. Infection with rhinovirus, for example, may be associated with few constitutional symptoms, whereas infection with the influenza virus may cause severe constitutional symptoms lasting 3 to 5 days. A distinguishing clinical feature of acute bronchitis due to *Chlamydia pneumoniae* is the presence of several weeks of low-grade symptoms prior to seeking care.[6]

The pathogenesis of the protracted phase of uncomplicated acute bronchitis has not been formally studied. However, extensive knowledge from the study of the virus-mediated pathogenesis of asthmatic inflammation serves as a basis for extrapolation.[7] According to Gonzales,[1] the protracted phase of uncomplicated acute bronchitis results from hypersensitivity of the tracheobronchial epithelium and airway receptors, leading to bronchial hyperresponsiveness and cough, often in association with phlegm and/or wheeze. Bronchial hypersensitivity does not appear to be related to any specific pathogen. Instead, it is probably a result of a combination of host factors that may include respiratory epithelial dysfunction, adrenergic-cholinergic tone imbalance, and IgE-mediated histamine release. Several studies document that uncomplicated acute bronchitis is often (but not invariably) associated with abnormalities of pulmonary function that are usually transient but may last several months. While there is no hard and fast rule on how long one should observe a patient with persisting symptoms after an episode of acute bronchitis before concluding that the symptoms have become chronic, a reasonable approach is to wait a minimum of a month after an acute episode of bronchitis illness before progressing to evaluation for other conditions.[8]

Microbiology of Acute Bronchitis

Most episodes of uncomplicated acute bronchitis are triggered by respiratory viral infections.[1] The viruses that are most often isolated include influenza A and B, parainfluenza, and respiratory syncytial virus, which target the lower respiratory tract, and rhinovirus, adenovirus, and coronavirus, which also target the upper respiratory tract. *Bordetella pertussis* and *B. parapertussis* can also cause acute bronchitis, even in previously immunized adults. Their recognition usually depends on an enhanced awareness during an epidemic and use of appropriate cultures, as recommended by local public health laboratories.

Mycoplasma pneumoniae can cause acute bronchitis, although it has been thought to contribute to 5 percent or less of cases. Likewise, acute *C. pneumoniae* infection has been shown to cause, in general, approximately 5 percent of acute bronchitis.[6,9] A recent prospective study of the incidence, etiology, and outcome of adult lower respiratory tract infections reported a higher proportion of cases associated with evidence for *M. pneumoniae* (7.3 percent) and *C. pneumoniae* (17 percent) infection.[2] In this study, whether antibiotic treatment was prescribed or withheld in cases of bronchitis associated with atypical pathogens did not seem to affect the outcome as measured by the need to revisit a clinician.

A high prevalence of serologic evidence for possible chronic *C. pneumoniae* infection has been reported in acute bronchitis. Falck et al[10] found evidence for *C. pneumoniae*–specific IgA antibodies in a quarter of patients with acute bronchitis. IgA antibodies may be found in recent secondary infection, and persistent detection of IgA suggests chronic infection, since the half-life of IgA is short (less than 1 week). In a larger study from the same group, IgA antibodies were associated with a "naso-pharyngeal-bronchial syndrome," defined as a constellation of persisting upper and lower respiratory tract illness symptoms.[11] In a case control study using asymptomatic adults as controls, Huittinen et al[12] reported that *C. pneumoniae*–specific IgA antibodies were associated with both acute bronchitis and asthma, but that only asthma was associated with antibodies directed against

chlamydial heat-shock protein 60 (hsp60). Since antibodies against chlamydial hsp60 are associated with the chronic inflammatory sequelae of other chlamydial diseases such as trachoma, pelvic inflammatory disease, and tubal infertility, these data suggest (but do not prove) that chronic inflammation in some cases of asthma also may be related to chlamydial infection. These preliminary findings should not, however, be used as justification for antibiotic use in uncomplicated acute bronchitis. The association between atypical infections and asthma is now an active area of research, and more information should be forthcoming.

Epidemiology

The epidemiology of uncomplicated acute bronchitis has not received as much attention as the epidemiology of other respiratory illnesses.[13] Large surveys of morbidity in general practice carried out in England and Wales between 1970 and 1999 found that the age-specific incidence of acute bronchitis assumed a U-shaped distribution, with the highest incidence in infants, a nadir in the 15- to 25-year age group, and then a progressive increase in incidence throughout adulthood.[14,15] In early childhood, acute bronchitis tends to cluster with pneumonia and asthma, whereas a different group of children are diagnosed with acute upper respiratory illnesses (tonsillitis, otitis media, and the common cold).[16] Studies in adults indicate that women are more likely than men to be diagnosed with acute bronchitis and that most diagnoses occur during the winter months.[2,15] In a stable suburban English population presenting over 1 year with acute lower respiratory tract infections, the incidence in otherwise healthy adults was 64 per 1000 for women compared to 44 per 1000 for men.[2] It is interesting that these age- and sex-specific incidence patterns for the epidemiology of acute bronchitis are the same as those for asthma.[17]

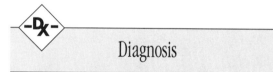

Diagnosis

Differential Diagnosis

Acute asthmatic bronchitis must be distinguished from chronic asthmatic bronchitis. This is a term applied to patients in whom the diagnoses of chronic bronchitis and asthma coexist or are difficult to distinguish. The textbook definition of chronic bronchitis also includes chronic sputum production for at least 3 months of the year for 2 consecutive years. The possibility that these chronic conditions arise following acute bronchitis will be addressed later in this chapter.

In addition to chronic bronchitis and asthma, other acute problems can mimic acute bronchitis. The most important of these to distinguish is pneumonia. Uncomplicated acute bronchitis is a self-limited illness, whereas pneumonia can be more severe and even fatal. The standard for diagnosing pneumonia is chest radiography,[18] but this test is not universally available in primary care settings and is expensive. Thus, many primary care providers do not routinely obtain a chest radiograph to evaluate a patient with a cough. When the diagnosis of pneumonia is suspected, however, clinicians need to be aware that while no individual clinical finding or combination of findings can rule out the possibility of pneumonia,[18] further diagnostic testing is usually not necessary unless the patient's vital signs are abnormal (i.e., heart rate > 100 beats/minute, respiratory rate > 24 breaths/minute, and oral body temperature > 38°C) or findings other than wheezing are present on chest examination (focal consolidation, such as rales, egophony, or fremitus).[1] In making the decision about further diagnostic testing to rule out

pneumonia, the clinician must also consider the possibility of an atypical presentation of pneumonia (without the cardinal vital sign abnormalities) in the elderly and the possible presence of influenza bronchitis (with vital sign abnormalities), depending on the epidemic milieu.

Another possibility that should not be overlooked is that of a lung cancer with localized obstruction of a proximal bronchus. Patients with lung cancer may present with a wheezy cough but often have other systemic symptoms such as weight loss, appetite changes, or night sweats. For high-risk patients, such as smokers or those exposed to occupational agents associated with increased rates of cancer, a new cough associated with systemic signs of malignancy should prompt an evaluation for a bronchial tumor. Similarly, patients who are at risk for lung cancer or who have hemoptysis should be considered for further evaluation.

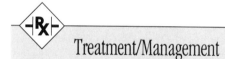

Treatment/Management

Recent evidence-based guidelines for the management of uncomplicated acute bronchitis emphasize the importance of ruling out more severe disease (mainly pneumonia), limiting the use of antibiotics, and focusing on communication, patient education, and symptomatic relief of this usually self-limited condition.

Role for Antibiotics

Antibiotics should not be considered routine treatment for patients with uncomplicated acute bronchitis. Several evidence-based reviews (summarized in reference 5) of existing randomized, controlled trials of antibiotic versus placebo in uncomplicated acute bronchitis have concluded that there is little or no consistent benefit from antibiotics. In particular, giving antibiotics with the aim of reducing the risk of later pneumonia is unwarranted. Regarding the improvement in acute symptoms such as cough, malaise, or time to return to work, conclusions are hampered by the paucity and poor quality of data and by the lack of uniformity in entry and outcome criteria.

The one uncommon circumstance in which antibiotics are indicated is the suspicion of pertussis, which requires a high probability of exposure and a supportive local public health laboratory to aid in diagnosis.[5] Regardless of the limitations of current studies, it is clear that the benefit, if any, of antibiotics in relieving symptoms of acute bronchitis is minimal and that antibiotics should not be regarded as first-line therapy.

The majority of physicians prescribe antibiotics as their first choice for treatment of patients with uncomplicated acute bronchitis.[19] In the United States and the United Kingdom, the probabilities are between two-thirds and three-quarters that an adult primary care outpatient presenting with acute bronchitis will receive a prescription for an antibiotic.[20,21] The antibiotic prescribing rate for acute bronchitis in children is equally high.[22] How this state of affairs evolved is obscure, but it probably resulted from a complex interaction among other factors: a "do everything possible" philosophy on the part of physicians associated with a training effect on patients to equate antibiotics with relief of symptoms. Fortunately, quality improvement initiatives can be successful in stemming the tide of inappropriate prescribing of antibiotics.[23]

Although inappropriate prescribing of antibiotics has been documented for a long time, the recent increase in the prevalence of antibiotic-resistant bacteria has made the lowering of inappropriate antibiotic use an urgent priority.[24] It is hoped that decreased prescribing of antibiotics will result in a generalized lower prevalence of bacterial antibiotic resistance, as demonstrated for group A streptococci after decreased consumption of macrolide antibiotics.[25] Unfortunately, depending on the underlying molecular

mechanisms, restriction of antibiotic use does not always result in decreased resistance.[26]

In addition to antibiotic resistance, other phenomena are also thought to be linked to excessive antibiotic use. Some suspect that injudicious antibiotic use can result in alterations of microbial flora, causing infectious diseases such as antibiotic-associated diarrhea (*Clostridium difficile*) and uncomplicated cystitis in young women.[27] Another note of concern in using antibiotics unnecessarily comes from a recent finding that antibiotics administered to infants during the first 6 months of life may increase the risk for subsequent asthma, possibly by disrupting the development of immune responses against gut flora that protect against asthma.[28,29]

Additional reasons to avoid unnecessary prescribing of antibiotics are listed in Table 9-2. Among these are adverse reactions to and financial costs of antibiotics. Focusing on the prescribing of antibiotics as the primary treatment for acute bronchitis may also have the unintended adverse consequence of diverting attention from more useful symptomatic treatments.

One caveat to this discussion on antibiotics is that few studies have been done to evaluate effective treatment strategies for acute bronchitis. One expert in the field has commented that uncomplicated acute bronchitis is a "homely" disease that is not deemed worthy of significant

Table 9-2

Reasons to Avoid Antibiotic Prescribing in Acute Bronchitis

- Development of antibiotic resistance in the community
- Increased risk for subsequent infections and (possibly) asthma
- Side effects
- Allergic reactions
- Financial cost to the patient
- Financial cost to the health care system
- Training patients to expect antibiotics
- Diverting attention from useful symptomatic treatments

attention.[30] All told, fewer than 1000 patients worldwide with uncomplicated acute bronchitis have been randomized to antibiotic/placebo trials. The largest study of antibiotic therapy in acute bronchitis had a total of only 207 participants and was conducted more than a quarter-century ago. The small number of study participants makes it difficult to identify subgroups for whom antibiotics may be beneficial. In fact, the only study in the last 25 years to have enrolled more than 100 patients found that a subgroup of patients 55 years of age or older taking doxycycline had a significantly shortened illness duration compared to those taking placebo.[31] Consequently, the available data supporting current recommendations against the routine use of antibiotics in acute bronchitis do not exclude the possibility that some patients might benefit from antibiotic treatment. However, at this time it is impossible to identify this potential subgroup on clinical grounds alone, except to note that patients age 55 years or older who feel ill might benefit from doxycycline.[31]

Furthermore, none of the randomized trials performed to date address the question of whether chronic sequelae of acute bronchitis are influenced by treatment.[3] While these studies do not deal with patients with acute bronchitis, it is interesting to note that tetracycline antibiotic treatment of acute exacerbations of chronic bronchitis has been shown to be associated with fewer subsequent relapses when compared to cephalosporins and beta-lactam antibiotic therapy.[32] Whether this finding also applies to relapses or other sequelae of uncomplicated acute bronchitis has not been studied systematically.

Symptomatic/Supportive Care

The most important insight into the successful management of acute bronchitis in recent decades is the observation that a significant proportion of patients with this condition have evidence of reversible airway obstruction[33,34] and that treatment with inhaled bronchodilators,[35–37] but not with oral bronchodilators,[38,39] is beneficial to relieve symptoms. The effectiveness of bronchodilators in relieving the symptoms of acute bronchitis is not surprising, since the protracted phase of uncomplicated acute bronchitis, at least in a subgroup of patients, involves airway hyperresponsiveness and cough.

It is unclear whether all patients with uncomplicated acute bronchitis will benefit from inhaled bronchodilators or whether only the subgroup with signs and/or symptoms of hyperreactive airways will derive symptomatic benefit. The preponderance of evidence favors the latter possibility. Melbye and colleagues found that only a subgroup of patients showed improvement when treated with fenoterol. Patients who came to their physician with either over 7 days of symptoms, wheezes found on auscultation, evidence of reversible airway obstruction after bronchodilator treatment, or a forced expiratory volume in 1 s (FEV_1) less than 80 percent of predicted showed improvement in their symptoms at day 2 with inhaled fenoterol; no effect was observed in patients with normal lung findings.[35] On the other hand, Hueston found that wheezing was not predictive of response to inhaled bronchodilators, but his study did not report on pulmonary function.[36] The evidence favors the use of inhaled bronchodilators in the subgroup of patients with signs or symptoms of bronchial hyperreactivity, although more studies are needed to confirm this possibility.

Antitussives such as dextromethorphan or codeine probably have some benefit in reducing cough severity during the protracted phase of acute bronchitis.

Communication with Patients

Many patients with acute bronchitis come to their physician to rule out the possibility of pneumonia, to be reassured that they will get better, and to seek relief from disturbed sleep or to address other, less predictable concerns that need to be identified.[40] Instead of routine prescribing of an antibiotic, a clinical examination, some reassuring words (if appropriate), and information on the etiology and natural history of acute bronchitis (for example, a quarter of patients are still coughing after 3 weeks[41]), along with a statement that symptomatic treatments are more beneficial than antibiotics, are all that the patient needs. Patients also can be informed that there is only about a 1 in 20 chance that their bronchitis is due to bacteria that are susceptible to antibiotics. Therefore, while an antibiotic might help, the probability is low. Reconsultations for acute lower respiratory tract illness can be reduced by strategies that include information.[42] Furthermore, patient satisfaction with a visit for acute bronchitis depends more on patient education and adequate physician-patient communication than on antibiotic prescribing, even for patients who expect to receive an antibiotic.[43]

Other Approaches

Avoidance of known triggers (cold air, dust, or allergens) and environmental humidification are reasonable options. *Consumer Reports* has published a useful guide for patients ("What to Do about a Cold or Flu," January 1999, pp. 14–15) that includes a table of symptoms linked to a list of over-the-counter remedies.

A proposed algorithm for the evaluation and management of acute cough illness is presented in Figure 9-1.

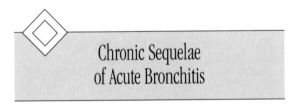

Chronic Sequelae of Acute Bronchitis

Uncomplicated acute bronchitis may be associated with chronic sequelae. Table 9-3 illustrates the typical clinical presentations of acute bron-

chitis (*A*), chronic asthma (*B*), and COPD (chronic asthmatic bronchitis) (*C*). These clinical diagnoses are usually regarded as three separate clinical entities. However, it would probably be more appropriate to regard each of them as a particular clinical manifestation of the same disease process at a different stage of development. In the particular example described in Table 9-3, the clinical scenarios involve the same patient, who was encountered over a 17-year time period.

Chronic Asthma

Often, patients with adult-onset asthma report that it began after an acute lower respiratory tract illness, usually described as acute bronchitis, pneumonia, or an influenza-like illness. This presentation for adult-onset asthma is common enough that it has been formally studied and given the descriptive term *infectious asthma*.[44] Prospective, population-based epidemiologic studies consistently report that asthma in all age groups is significantly associated with a history of preceding lower respiratory tract illnesses.[44] In most of these epidemiologic studies, a history of previous lower respiratory tract illness is more significant than atopy as an associated factor. In fact, a recent comprehensive review of all population-based asthma studies has concluded that less than half of asthma cases, whether of childhood or adult onset, can be attributed to atopy and that other mechanisms for the development of asthma need to be investigated.[45]

A role for acute respiratory viral infection (particularly respiratory syncytial virus) as a precipitating cause for childhood asthma is being actively investigated,[46] and emerging evidence supports the possibility that acute *C. pneumoniae* infection, and to a lesser extent *M. pneumoniae* infection, may initiate chronic asthma in adults.[47] What quantitative contribution these infections may make to the incidence of asthma is unknown. It is also unknown whether specially designed antibiotic treatments will have

Figure 9-1

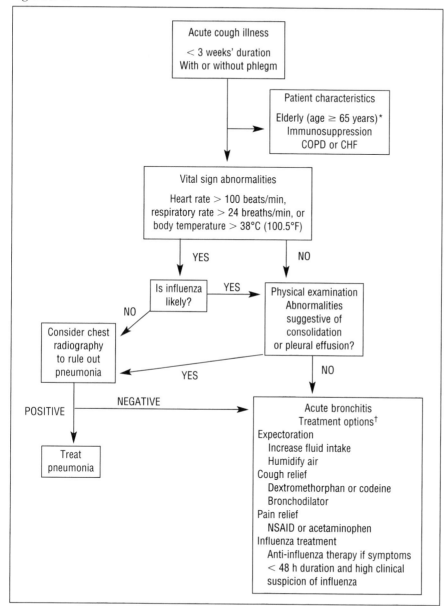

*Pneumonia in elderly persons, those with immunosuppression, and those with chronic obstructive pulmonary disease (COPD) or congestive heart failure (CHF) often presents atypically. A high index of suspicion is warranted when evaluating cough illness in these patients, even when vital signs and chest examination appear normal.

† Consider pertussis treatment if the patient has known exposure to pertussis. Follow local health department testing guidelines; pending results, treat with erythromycin for 14 days.

NSAID = nonsteroidal anti-inflammatory drug.

From Gonzales and Sande,[1] with permission.

Table 9-3

Typical Presentations for Acute Bronchitis and Other Similar Conditions

---

A. Acute bronchitis
- 55-year-old male developed rhinorrhea, nasal congestion, sore throat, cough, and low-grade fever (100°F)
- Diagnosed with acute bronchitis after chest x-ray showed no infiltrate
- Treated with an antihistamine-decongestant combination and erythromycin 250 mg q.i.d. for 1 week

B. Chronic asthma
- 55-year-old pipe-smoking male with no previous history of chronic respiratory complaints or clinical allergies
- Presented with a 2-month history of cough, wheeze, and shortness of breath following a "cold"
- History that erythromycin treatment for "bronchitis" resulted in some improvement, but then symptoms relapsed and persisted
- Symptoms were improved by oral theophylline, an injection of epinephrine, and inhaled albuterol
- FEV_1 was 87 percent predicted without a bronchodilator response (FEV_1/FVC = 72 percent)
- His symptoms worsened, and 3 weeks later his FEV_1 was 27 percent predicted; after steroid bursts and hospitalization, his FEV_1 improved to 119 percent predicted

C. COPD
- 71-year-old ex-smoking male with a diagnosis of "COPD with asthma"
- Current medications:
  Theophylline CR 300 mg t.i.d.
  Albuterol 2 puffs q.i.d.
  Brethine 5 mg t.i.d.
  Prednisone 10 mg/day alternating with 5 mg/day
- Fairly well-controlled symptoms, but having occasional exacerbations
- Stable pulmonary function (FEV_1/FVC = 40–48 percent)
- Comorbidities:
  Chronic sinusitis
  Osteopenia
  Atraumatic lumbar compression fractures
  Posttraumatic glaucoma
- Died suddenly in ventricular fibrillation; no postmortem performed

---

ABBREVIATIONS: FEV_1, forced expiratory volume in 1 s; FVC, forced vital capacity; COPD, chronic obstructive pulmonary disease.

any potential to favorably alter the natural history of infectious asthma. It is known, however, that the standard courses of antibiotics currently used for the treatment of uncomplicated acute bronchitis do not have any benefit in chronic asthma.[47]

Chronic Bronchitis

Recently, evidence for chronic *C. pneumoniae* infection has been found in lung tissue from patients with COPD[48] and emphysema.[49] Nearly half of the young adults sampled were also found to contain *C. pneumoniae* in lung specimens,[48] which raises the possibility that lung carriage of *C. pneumoniae* is common in adults and increases with age. This could contribute to the pathogenesis of obstructive lung diseases such as asthma and COPD. Since many people are infected, yet only some develop disease, genetic or other susceptibility factors must also be operating. As with chronic asthma, therapeutic interventions require further research.

Summary

The diagnosis and management of uncomplicated acute bronchitis should be simple and straightforward. Treatment for uncomplicated acute bronchitis should emphasize communication and provision of information and symptomatic remedies. Antibiotics should be reserved for the rare instances of complications or persistence of illness. Major challenges to implementation appear to involve behavioral factors, mainly resistance on the part of physicians to change current practices and on the part of patients to accept the recommended changes. An important emerging aspect of the management of uncomplicated acute bronchitis relates to evidence that this condition can lead to chronic sequelae, such as asthma and COPD. Current medical practice does not include guidelines for dealing with the chronic sequelae of acute bronchitis.

References

1. Gonzales R, Sande M: Uncomplicated acute bronchitis. *Ann Intern Med* 133:981–991, 2000.
2. Macfarlane J, Holmes W, Gard P, et al: Prospective study of the incidence, aetiology and outcome of adult lower respiratory tract illness in the community. *Thorax* 56:109–114, 2001.
3. Hahn DL: Acute asthmatic bronchitis: a new twist to an old problem. *J Fam Pract* 39:431–435, 1994.
4. Snow V, Mottur-Pilson C, Gonzales R: Principles of appropriate antibiotic use for treatment of acute bronchitis in adults. *Ann Intern Med* 134:518–520, 2001.
5. Gonzales R, Bartlett JG, Besser RE, et al: Principles of appropriate antibiotic use for treatment of acute bronchitis in adults: background. *Ann Intern Med* 134:521–529.
6. Hahn DL, Dodge R, Golubjatnikov R: Association of *Chlamydia pneumoniae* (strain TWAR) infection with wheezing, asthmatic bronchitis and adult-onset asthma. *JAMA* 266:225–230, 1991.
7. Gern JE, Busse WW: The role of viral infections in the natural history of asthma. *J Allergy Clin Immunol* 106:201–212, 2000.
8. Hahn DL: Treatment of *Chlamydia pneumoniae* infection in adult asthma: a before-after trial. *J Fam Pract* 41:345–351, 1995.
9. Grayston JT, Kuo C-C, Wang S-P, Altman J: A new *Chlamydia psittaci* strain, TWAR, isolated in acute respiratory tract infections. *N Engl J Med* 315:161–168, 1986.
10. Falck G, Heyman L, Gnarpe J, Gnarpe H: *Chlamydia pneumoniae* (TWAR): a common agent in acute bronchitis. *Scand J Infect Dis* 26:179–187, 1994.
11. Falck G, Gnarpe J, Gnarpe H: Comparison of individuals with and without specific IgA antibodies to *Chlamydia pneumoniae* with regard to morbidity and the metabolic syndrome. Proceedings, Fourth Meeting of the European Society for Chlamydia Research, Helsinki, Finland, 2000; p. 256.
12. Huittinen T, Hahn D, Anttila T, et al: Host immune response to *Chlamydia pneumoniae* heat shock protein 60 is associated with asthma. *Eur Respir J* 17:1078–1082, 2001.
13. File TM Jr: The epidemiology of respiratory tract infections. *Semin Respir Infect* 15:184–194, 2000.
14. Fleming DM, Crombie DL: Prevalence of asthma and hayfever in England and Wales. *Br Med J* 294:279–283, 1987.
15. Fleming DM, Ross AM, Cross KW, Cobb WA: *Annual Report of the Weekly Returns Service for 1999.* Birmingham, UK, Birmingham Research Unit of the Royal College of General Practitioners, 1999.
16. Kolnaar BGM, van den Bosch WJHM, van den Hoogen HJM, van Weel C: The clustering of respiratory diseases in early childhood. *Fam Med* 26:106–110, 1994.

17. Pedersen P, Weeke ER: Epidemiology of asthma in Denmark. *Chest* 91:107S–114S, 1987.

18. Metlay JP, Kapoor WN, Fine MJ: Does this patient have community-acquired pneumonia? *JAMA* 278:1440–1445, 1997.

19. Oeffinger K, Snell LM, Foster BM, et al: Treatment of acute bronchitis in adults. A national survey of family physicians. *J Fam Pract* 46:469–475, 1998.

20. Gonzales R, Steiner JF, Sande M: Antibiotic prescribing for adults with colds, upper respiratory tract infections, and bronchitis by ambulatory care physicians. *JAMA* 278:901–904, 1997.

21. Macfarlane J, Lewis SA, Macfarlane R, Holmes W: Contemporary use of antibiotics in 1089 adults presenting with acute lower respiratory tract illness in general practice in the U.K.: implications for developing management guidelines. *Respir Med* 91:427–434, 1997.

22. Nyquist A-C, Gonzales R, Steiner JF, Sande M: Antibiotic prescribing for children with colds, upper respiratory tract infections, and bronchitis. *JAMA* 279:875–877, 1998.

23. Gonzales R, Steiner JF, Lum A, Barrett PH Jr: Decreasing antibiotic use in ambulatory practice. Impact of a multidimensional intervention on the treatment of uncomplicated acute bronchitis in adults. *JAMA* 281:1512–1519, 1999.

24. Spach DH, Black D: Antibiotic resistance in community-acquired respiratory tract infections: current issues. *Ann Allergy Asthma Immunol* 81:293–303, 1998.

25. Seppälä H, Klaukka T, Vuopio-Varkila J, et al: The effect of changes in the consumption of macrolide antibiotics on erythromycin resistance of group A streptococci in Finland. *N Engl J Med* 337:441–446, 1997.

26. Enne VI, Livermore D, Stephens P, Hall LMC: Persistence of sulphonamide resistance in *Escherichia coli* in the UK despite national prescribing restriction. *Lancet* 357:1325–1328, 2001.

27. Smith H, Hughes JP, Hooton TM, et al: Antecedent antimicrobial use increases the risk of uncomplicated cystitis in young women. *Clin Infect Dis* 25:63–68, 1997.

28. Patel BP, Johnson CC, Carter PM, et al: Early antibiotic use and asthma and bronchial hyperreactivity at age 6–7. *Am J Respir Crit Care Med* 163(Part 2 of 2):A970, 2001.

29. McKeever TM, Lewis SA, Smith C, et al: Antibiotics and incidence of allergic disease: a birth cohort study using the UK general practice research database. *Am J Respir Crit Care Med* 163(Part 2 of 2):A971, 2001.

30. Williamson H: Acute bronchitis: a homely prototype for primary care research. *J Fam Pract* 23:103–104, 1986.

31. Verheij T, Zermansky A, Hahn DL: Antibiotics in acute bronchitis. *Lancet* 345:1244–1245, 1995.

32. Chodosh S, Tuck J, Pizzuto D: Comparative trials of doxycycline versus amoxicillin, cephalexin and enoxacin in bacterial infections in chronic bronchitis and asthma. *Scand J Infect Dis* 53(suppl):22–28, 1988.

33. Williamson HA: Pulmonary function tests in acute bronchitis: evidence for reversible airway obstruction. *J Fam Pract* 25:251–256, 1987.

34. Melbye H, Kongerud J, Vorland L: Reversible airflow limitation in adults with respiratory infection. *Eur Resp J* 7:1239–1245, 1994.

35. Melbye H, Aasebø U, Straume B: Symptomatic effect of inhaled fenoterol in acute bronchitis: a placebo-controlled double-blind study. *Fam Pract* 8:216–222, 1991.

36. Hueston WJ: Albuterol delivered by metered-dose inhaler to treat acute bronchitis. *J Fam Pract* 39:437–440, 1994.

37. Huhti E, Mokka T, Nikoskelainen J: Association of viral and mycoplasma infections with exacerbations of asthma. *Ann Allergy* 33:145–149, 1974.

38. Tukiainen H, Karttunen P, Silvasti M, et al: The treatment of acute transient cough: a placebo-controlled comparison of dextromethorphan and dextromethorphan-beta$_2$-sympathomimetic combination. *Eur J Respir Dis* 69:95–99, 1986.

39. Littenberg B, Wheeler M, Smith DS: A randomized, controlled trial of oral albuterol in acute cough. *J Fam Pract* 42:49–53, 1996.

40. Bergh KD: The patient's differential diagnosis. Unpredictable concerns in visits for acute cough. *J Fam Pract* 46:153–158, 1998.

41. Williamson H: A randomized, controlled trial of doxycycline in the treatment of acute bronchitis. *J Fam Pract* 19:481–486, 1984.

42. Macfarlane JT, Holmes W, Macfarlane RM: Reducing reconsultations for acute lower respiratory tract illness with an information leaflet: a random-

ized, controlled study of patients in primary care. *Brit J Gen Pract* 47:719–722, 1997.

43. Hamm RM, Hicks RJ, Bemben DA: Antibiotics and respiratory infections: are patients more satisfied when expectations are met? *J Fam Pract* 43:56–62, 1996.

44. Hahn DL: Infectious asthma: a reemerging clinical entity? *J Fam Pract* 41:153–157, 1995.

45. Pearce N, Pekkanen J, Beasley R: How much asthma is really attributable to atopy? *Thorax* 54:268–272, 1999.

46. Douglass JA, O'Heheir RE: What determines asthma phenotype? *Am J Respir Crit Care Med* 161:S211–S214, 2000.

47. Hahn DL: Is there a role for antibiotics in the treatment of asthma? Involvement of atypical organisms. *Biodrugs* 14:349–354, 2000.

48. Wu L, Skinner SJM, Lambie N, et al: Immunohistochemical staining for *Chlamydia pneumoniae* is increased in lung tissue from subjects with chronic obstructive pulmonary disease. *Am J Respir Crit Care Med* 162:1148–1151, 2000.

49. Theegarten D, Mogilevski G, Anhenn O, et al: The role of chlamydia in the pathogenesis of pulmonary emphysema. Electron microscopy and immunofluorescence reveal corresponding findings as in atherosclerosis. *Virchows Arch* 437:190–193, 2000.

Mark A. Knox

Croup, Epiglottitis, Bronchiolitis, and Pertussis

Causes of cough in children are numerous and range from the trivial to the life-threatening. This chapter will first introduce a framework for evaluating children who present with cough, and then discuss in detail some of the most common and serious causes of cough.

General Evaluation

History

In evaluating a child with a cough, the history usually provides important clues to the nature of the underlying disease (Table 10-1). For example, the duration of the symptoms is an important clue. A mild cough of more than 2 weeks' duration in a child who does not appear ill is less likely to be due to infection than to allergies or reactive airway disease. The timing of the cough also may be important, with a nocturnal cough suggesting asthma rather than infection. The parents should be asked about other signs of infection, such as fever, irritability, lethargy, or poor feeding, although these symptoms must be interpreted in light of the age of the child.

A cough that is productive is more likely to indicate the presence of an infectious process than is a dry cough, although sputum that is green or yellow in color does not necessarily indicate the presence of a bacterial infection.[1] Bloody or rust-colored sputum may, however, be associated with pneumonia. Wheezing may be an important symptom, although parents do not understand what this symptom truly is and will often report a croupy cough or harsh breathing as wheezing.

Dyspnea, tachypnea, and stridor are other important symptoms. The parents should be asked whether these are present, and if so, whether they are present only with agitation or exertion or are present at rest as well.

The season of the year may offer some important clues as to the nature of the symptoms. Croup, for example, is most common in the autumn, and bronchiolitis is more common between November and April, when respiratory syncytial virus (RSV) is more prevalent.[2] Exposure to other ill children or adults at day care or at school may be a useful historical item.

Exposure to certain irritants and a family history of respiratory problems are other important aspects of the history. Passive exposure to cigarette smoke is associated with an increased incidence of respiratory infections.[3] A wood-burning stove may trigger asthma in susceptible children, and nearby industrial discharges may also be associated with reactive airway disease. A family history of atopic disorders may suggest

Table 10-1

Helpful Symptoms in Evaluating Respiratory Infections in Children

Cough duration	Less than 2 weeks more likely to be infectious
	Over 2 weeks suggestive of asthma or allergy
Timing of cough	Nighttime worsening suggestive of asthma
	or bronchiolitis
Productive cough	Indicative of infection rather than asthma or allergy
Sputum character	Bloody or rusty sputum associated with pneumonia
Stridor	Indicative of laryngeal or tracheal inflammation
Wheezing	Indicative of lower respiratory infection or asthma
	(may be difficult for some parents to distinguish
	from congested upper airways)

asthma or allergic rhinitis as a cause for the cough.

Physical Examination

The physical examination provides most of the remaining information necessary to make a diagnosis in a child with a cough. The most important vital signs are temperature and respiratory rate. The presence of cyanosis, its severity, and whether it is only peripheral or also central can provide a clue to the severity of hypoxia. The degree of respiratory distress can be ascertained by observing for the presence of alar flaring, subcostal retractions, and use of accessory muscles of respiration. Stridor is an important finding, with stridor at rest being of slightly more concern than stridor that is present only with agitation. The lungs should be carefully auscultated for the presence of wheezes, rales, rhonchi, and areas of decreased breath sounds. Purulent nasal drainage and sinus tenderness in an older child may indicate the presence of sinusitis. Finally, the clinician should be alert for signs of cardiac dysfunction, since congestive heart failure in children may present as a cough.

Bronchitis

Although acute bronchitis is a diagnosis that is commonly made in primary care, it probably does not exist as a distinct clinical entity, but may represent a viral respiratory infection in which cough is the most prominent symptom.[1] Even though these are viral infections, numerous prescriptions for antibiotics are written each year to treat them.[1] While sputum cultures may show *Streptococcus pneumoniae, Haemophilus influenzae, Staphylococcus aureus,* or various other species of *Streptococcus,* it has not been shown that these are causative agents, and antibiotics

have not been shown to be effective treatments.[4] Further discussion of acute bronchitis can be found in Chap. 9.

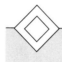

Croup (Acute Laryngotracheobronchitis)

Croup is a relatively common infection in children, causing between 27,000 and 62,000 hospitalizations each year.[5] Most cases occur in the autumn and early winter, with a higher incidence in alternate years associated with epidemics of parainfluenza virus 1.[5] Hospitalizations peak in October and February, coincident with peaks in parainfluenza virus 1 activity.[5] The peak age incidence of croup is 3 months to 5 years of age,[5] with 91 percent of hospitalizations occurring in children less than 5 years of age.[5]

As its name would suggest, croup is caused by an infection of the upper airways—the larynx, trachea, and upper levels of the bronchial tree—and obstruction of these airways caused by edema produces most of the symptoms of the disease. As noted, nearly all cases of croup are caused by viruses. Parainfluenza viruses, types 1, 2, and 3, cause 75 percent of cases, with type 1 the most common cause.[5] Adenovirus and RSV cause most of the remaining cases. Bacteria, predominantly *Mycoplasma pneumoniae,* account for only a small percentage (3 to 4 percent) of cases.[5]

Diagnosis of Croup

HISTORY

The symptoms of croup are usually typical, and diagnosis usually is not difficult. Most children present with several days of prodromal upper respiratory tract infection (URI) symptoms, followed by the gradual onset of a barking, "seallike" cough. Stridor is generally mild and intermittent at first, primarily with inspiration and worse when the child is agitated. Typically, respiratory distress is only mild to moderate. In most children, this is the maximum extent of the disease. The symptoms are usually more severe at night than during the day and are worse on the first or second day, with gradual resolution over several days. However, some children have a more severe infection that includes respiratory distress, more pronounced and continuous stridor, and cyanosis.

PHYSICAL EXAMINATION

The physical findings of croup vary depending on the severity of the illness. In most patients with mild illness, the lungs are clear. The degree of subcostal and intercostal retractions, the degree of stridor, and the presence of cyanosis are important clues to the severity of the illness. If the child is cyanotic and in respiratory distress, manipulation of the pharynx, such as when trying to examine the pharynx using a tongue depressor, may trigger respiratory arrest. This maneuver should therefore be avoided until the clinician is in a position to manage the child's airway by endotracheal intubation.

LABORATORY AND IMAGING

Laboratory findings in this disease are generally minimal. The white blood cell count is usually normal or slightly elevated, with counts greater than 15,000 occurring in about 20 percent of cases.[7] The blood oxygen saturation may be normal or decreased, depending on the severity of the disease. The chest x-ray is normal. In 40 to 50 percent of cases, anteroposterior soft-tissue x-rays of the neck will show subglottic narrowing, causing the classic "steeple" sign of croup.[8]

Treatment

Perhaps the most critical decision to make when evaluating a child with croup is determining whether the patient needs to be treated in the hospital or will do well at home. Between 1.5 and 15 percent of children with croup are hospitalized for treatment, and of these, 1 to 5 percent will require endotracheal intubation and mechanical ventilation.[8] While there are no commonly accepted scoring systems for croup severity, there are several signs and symptoms that indicate more serious illness. High fever, toxic appearance, worsening stridor, respiratory distress, cyanosis or pallor, hypoxia, and restlessness or lethargy are all symptoms of more severe disease and should prompt the physician to admit the child for inpatient treatment.[6] A summary of treatment options is shown in Table 10-2.

Most children with croup can be treated safely at home. The mainstay of treatment has long been held to be cool, moist air, although re-

Table 10-2
Treatment for Croup

OUTPATIENT MANAGEMENT
Cool, humidified air
Dexamethasone single dose of 0.6 mg/kg
Racemic epinephrine (useful before discharge from emergency department because dexamethasone may take 6 h to be effective)

INPATIENT MANAGEMENT
Cool, humidified air with oxygen supplementation
Racemic epinephrine
Steroids
Dexamethasone 0.6 mg/kg (single dose)
Nebulized budesonide (optional)
Close observation for respiratory compromise

search has not confirmed the effectiveness of this treatment.[9,10] While corticosteroids have long been an accepted part of inpatient treatment, their role in outpatient management of this disease has not been studied until recently. At least one placebo-controlled trial has demonstrated the effectiveness of a single intramuscular dose of dexamethasone, 0.6 mg/kg, in reducing the severity of moderately severe croup in patients discharged from the emergency department to be treated at home.[11] Since dexamethasone requires about 6 h for onset of action, a single dose of racemic epinephrine may be given before the child is sent home.[12] Racemic epinephrine is commonly used in hospitalized patients, but beta$_2$ agonist bronchodilators have not been shown to be effective.[6]

Inpatient treatment of croup has changed little in recent years. As with home treatment, the mainstay of therapy is cool, humidified air, using a croup tent. Although there are no controlled studies documenting the effectiveness of oxygen,[13] supplemental oxygen is generally used even if the patient is not hypoxemic; if the patient's oxygen saturation is low, the level of supplemental oxygen should be adjusted to correct hypoxemia. Racemic epinephrine has long been the mainstay of treatment for patients who do not respond to cool, moist air or who have respiratory distress. Numerous studies have confirmed its effectiveness. The drug is usually given in a dose of 0.25 to 0.5 mL of a 2.25% solution mixed with 2 mL of normal saline and administered via nebulizer and face mask. It has a duration of action of 1 to 2 h. Why racemic epinephrine has come to be used is unclear. Although it was long suspected that L-epinephrine should be equally effective, this was not proven until 1992, when a study showed that 5 mL of 1:1000 L-epinephrine diluted with saline was equally as effective as racemic epinephrine.[14]

Systemic corticosteroids have for many years been an important part of inpatient treatment of croup. Dexamethasone is the most widely studied drug, and numerous studies have shown it to be effective in reducing both the severity and duration of the disease and the need for intubation.[15] Because of its long action, it can be given as a single dose, which remains effective for the remainder of the course of the disease. The dose is 0.6 mg/kg intramuscularly, and it should be given as early as possible in the course of the disease. It has not been associated with any deleterious effects.[6] Numerous studies have been done examining the effectiveness of different steroids, primarily nebulized budesonide, relative to that of dexamethasone. Nebulized budesonide is superior to placebo and equally as effective as oral dexamethasone.[16] While both are superior to placebo, intramuscular dexamethasone is more effective than nebulized budesonide.[17]

Children hospitalized for treatment of croup should be observed carefully for any signs of respiratory distress. Intubation and mechanical ventilation are necessary in a small percentage of children with this disease.

Prognosis

The natural history of croup is that recurrences are common. However, as the child grows, his or her airways grow larger and are less affected by edema, and symptoms tend to be less severe over time.

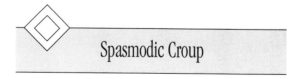

Spasmodic Croup

Spasmodic croup is a disorder that is clinically similar to infectious croup, but with some important differences. It primarily affects children between 1 and 3 years of age. Unlike infectious croup, spasmodic croup has no viral prodrome, and the disease presents with the sudden onset of a nocturnal croupy cough with variable degrees of stridor and respiratory distress. These symptoms gradually decrease over several hours, only to recur each night for one to two more nights, decreasing in severity each night.

Like those of infectious croup, the symptoms of spasmodic croup respond to cool air and racemic epinephrine.[18] The cause of this disorder is unclear. It may be caused by a viral infection or an allergic response to viral antigens, but no good evidence exists to support the concept that spasmodic croup is an entity distinct from infectious croup. These two diseases may simply be different manifestations of the same disease.[13]

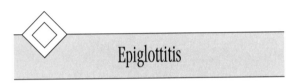

Epiglottitis

Epiglottitis is a life-threatening bacterial infection of the epiglottis. The infection causes edema of the epiglottis, which has the potential to cause fatal airway obstruction. Untreated, the disease has a high mortality rate, but appropriate treatment can reduce the mortality rate to less than 1 percent.[6] Fortunately, as a result of widespread use of vaccines against *H. influenzae* type B, the disease frequency has been reduced by approximately 80 percent.[18] Estimates of annual incidence range from a low of 0.63 per 100,000 children[18] to a high of 14 per 100,000 children.[19]

Since epiglottitis has become so uncommon, retropharyngeal abscess is now a more common cause of acute respiratory distress than epiglottitis.[20] This disease is caused primarily by *H. influenzae* type B, and the majority of cases occur in children who either have not been immunized or have incomplete immunizations.[21] Occasionally, cases of retropharyngeal abscess may be caused by *Streptococcus pyogenes.*[22] The disease affects children between the ages of 2 and

7 years of age, with a peak incidence at 3 to 4 years of age.[6]

Diagnosis

HISTORY

The initial presentation of epiglottitis is dramatic and usually suggests the diagnosis. However, milder cases of epiglottitis may be confused with croup. The symptoms of epiglottitis include a high fever, hoarseness, croupy cough, stridor, and respiratory distress, typically with an abrupt onset. Symptoms may worsen and may progress to death from airway obstruction within hours.[6]

PHYSICAL EXAMINATION

The physical examination is likewise dramatic and distinctive. The child usually has a high fever and looks toxic. The child will typically be sitting, leaning forward, and often drooling because of dysphagia. The child often is unable to speak, but if he or she is able to talk, the voice is notably hoarse because of inflammation of the vocal cords and surrounding tissue. Respiratory distress can be moderate to severe. Visualization of the epiglottis is diagnostic, with the epiglottis erythematous and markedly enlarged. However, attempts to visualize the epiglottis have the potential to precipitate complete and fatal airway obstruction and should be attempted only by a physician who has the skill to manage acute airway obstruction, including performing an emergency tracheostomy. While one well-done study in 1988 suggests that visualization of the epiglottis may not be as dangerous as has long been believed, the authors still take the conservative position that this not be done unless a specialist who can manage the child's airway is present.[23] Visualization of the epiglottis is usually done with direct laryngoscopy, but flexible endoscopy can be a useful tool for diagnosis when direct laryngoscopy could be difficult.

LABORATORY AND IMAGING

Laboratory tests are not generally of much value in the patient with epiglottitis. The white blood cell count is usually elevated at greater than 10,000/mm^3.[19] Blood cultures will be positive in the majority of cases but are not useful acutely. X-rays of the chest are normal. If epiglottitis is suspected, soft-tissue lateral x-rays of the neck may be helpful. The classical finding is an enlarged, thumb-shaped epiglottis, but these films are positive in only about 50 percent of cases. All x-rays should be done as portable films in the emergency department. Because of the risk for acute airway obstruction, children with suspected epiglottitis should not be sent to a radiology department where they could sit unobserved for a period of time.

Treatment

The treatment of epiglottitis depends on rapid diagnosis, airway management, and institution of appropriate antibiotic therapy. The clinical picture is suggestive of the disease, but definitive diagnosis depends on visualization of the epiglottis. All children with confirmed epiglottitis require endotracheal intubation. The mortality rate in unintubated children is as high as 6 percent, compared to less than 1 percent in intubated children.[6] This procedure should be done only in the operating room, with the capacity to perform an emergency tracheostomy if a failed attempt at intubation triggers airway obstruction. Intubation should be attempted only by an otolaryngologist, an anesthesiologist, or another physician with similar airway and surgical skills.

In addition to airway management, antibiotics directed at the primary causative organisms are essential. Because of the high proportion of beta-lactamase-producing organisms, second- and third-generation cephalosporins are considered the drugs of first choice.[19] Antibiotic therapy should be continued for 7 to 10 days.[6] Unlike with croup, steroids and racemic epi-

nephrine are of no value in this disease.[6] The child will generally remain intubated for 2 to 3 days, until the epiglottal edema has subsided enough that the child is no longer in danger of airway obstruction. Serial flexible endoscopy can be used to follow the course of the disease and decide when extubation is safe.[19]

Bacterial Tracheitis

Bacterial tracheitis, also known as pseudomembranous croup or membranous laryngotracheitis, is another cause of crouplike coughing in children; it is much less common than infectious croup and generally less severe than epiglottitis. This is a bacterial infection of the trachea that usually follows infectious croup or other viral respiratory infections and may represent a complication of these viral infections.[19] *S. aureus* is the most common cause, with group A streptococci, *Moraxella catarrhalis*, *H. influenzae*, and *S. pneumoniae* being less common causes.[19]

Diagnosis

HISTORY

The typical picture of bacterial tracheitis is that of a child with apparent croup or other upper respiratory symptoms who starts to get worse after several days, when the usual course would be gradual improvement. Fever is usually moderate to high, and respiratory distress is variably moderate to severe.

PHYSICAL EXAMINATION

Physical examination will reflect the severity of respiratory distress but will be otherwise normal. The diagnosis is based on clinical suspicion. Endoscopy below the vocal cords often will show purulent secretions or a pseudomembrane in the trachea.

LABORATORY AND IMAGING

Chest x-rays will show pulmonary infiltrates in about 50 percent of cases, especially if the symptoms have been present for more than 24 h.[19] Soft-tissue films of the neck may be normal or may show a membrane in the trachea. Culture of a transtracheal or bronchoscopic aspirate is usually required to identify the causative organism.

Treatment

Treatment is with antibiotics effective against *S. aureus* and the other possible causative organisms. If a large membrane is present, its removal during bronchoscopy may provide immediate and significant improvement. Intubation is not necessary in all cases; the decision to intubate is based on the degree of respiratory distress.

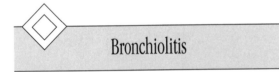

Bronchiolitis

Bronchiolitis is a common disease of infants. In one prospective study, 7 percent of infants were diagnosed with bronchiolitis during the first 2 years of life, and 1 percent were admitted to the hospital for treatment of bronchiolitis.[25] In 1996, the hospitalization rate in the United States for bronchiolitis in children under 1 year of age was 31.2 per 1000.[26] Bronchiolitis is seen most commonly in the first 2 years of life, with a peak at an age of about 6 months.[27]

Bronchiolitis is an infection that causes edema and obstruction of the small airways. Older children and adults contract the same infection, but because they have larger airways, they do not experience the same degree of airway obstruc-

tion. In fact, an older sibling or a parent is often the source of the infant's infection.

Bronchiolitis is almost always viral in etiology. RSV causes more than half of cases, causing approximately 90,000 hospitalizations and 4500 deaths each year.[2] RSV is a common human pathogen, with most children having been infected by the age of 2.[26] Bronchiolitis also can be caused by parainfluenza and other viruses, with a few cases being caused by *M. pneumoniae*.[27] Adenoviruses can cause a severe necrotizing infection called bronchiolitis obliterans.

Pathologically, edema and accumulated cellular debris cause obstruction of small airways. Because air flow in a tube is proportional to the fourth power of the radius of the tube, a small reduction in airway diameter leads to a large reduction in air flow. This obstruction causes a ventilation-perfusion mismatch, with wasted perfusion, a right-to-left shunt, and hypoxemia early in the course of the disease.[27]

An important item in the differential diagnosis of bronchiolitis is acute asthma, as there may be many similarities in history and physical examination between these two conditions. Asthma is unusual in the first year of life, whereas the incidence of bronchiolitis peaks at 6 months of age. The presence of one or more of the following favors the diagnosis of asthma: family history of asthma, sudden onset without a preceding URI, repeated attacks, a markedly prolonged expiratory phase of respiration, eosinophilia, and response to one dose of epinephrine.[27]

Diagnosis

HISTORY

The typical course of bronchiolitis begins with the exposure of the infant to another person with an URI. The infant will generally have URI symptoms for several days, with or without fever. The child then experiences the gradual onset of respiratory distress, with a paroxysmal wheezy cough and dyspnea. The child may be irritable and feed poorly, but there are usually no other systemic symptoms. The temperature is often in the range of 38.5 to -39°C (101 to -102°F), although it may be subnormal to greatly elevated.[27]

PHYSICAL EXAMINATION

Physical examination shows the child to be tachypneic, with a respiratory rate as high as 60 to 80 breaths per minute, and often in severe respiratory distress. Alar flaring, retractions, and use of accessory muscles of respiration may be evident. Examination of the lungs often shows a prolonged expiratory phase with diffuse wheezes. Diffuse fine rales at the end of expiration and the beginning of inspiration are typical findings. The lungs are often hyperinflated with shallow respirations, and breath sounds may be nearly inaudible if the obstruction is severe.

LABORATORY AND IMAGING

The laboratory finding that is of most utility is the oxygen saturation level, since children with hypoxia should be admitted to the hospital. A nasopharyngeal swab should be performed and sent for RSV culture. X-rays usually show signs of hyperinflation. In about one-third of cases, x-rays will show scattered areas of consolidation. These may represent postobstructive atelectasis or inflammation of alveoli. It may not be possible to exclude early bacterial pneumonia solely on the basis of x-ray findings.[27]

Treatment

Treatment of bronchiolitis is primarily supportive. The decision to hospitalize the child is usually based on the degree of respiratory distress. Placing the child in a tent with cool humidified oxygen both relieves hypoxemia and reduces water loss from tachypnea. Intravenous fluid administration may be necessary if the child

is not taking sufficient oral fluids because of the tachypnea.

The most critical phase of bronchiolitis is the first 2 to 3 days of the illness. Most cases will resolve in 1 to 3 days without much difficulty. However, in severe cases, symptoms may develop within hours and may be protracted.[27]

ANTIBIOTICS AND STEROIDS

Antibiotics are of no value in bronchiolitis but may be given if the x-ray picture suggests pneumonia. Steroids have been shown to be of no benefit in this disease.[28]

BRONCHODILATORS

The use of inhaled bronchodilators is controversial. Bronchodilators are not helpful in bronchiolitis per se, but some infants with what appears to be bronchiolitis respond to these medications, suggesting a possible link between bronchiolitis and reactive airway disease. One recent meta-analysis showed that bronchodilators may provide short-term benefit in children with mild to moderate disease.[29] Another recent study showed that inhaled epinephrine was somewhat more effective than albuterol in improving oxygen saturation and reducing the need for hospital admission.[30] Given this information, many physicians elect to use bronchodilators for children in whom wheezing is a prominent feature of the disease.

ANTIVIRAL AGENTS

In the early 1980s, studies showed that the mortality from RSV infection in children with underlying cardiac or pulmonary disease or immune deficiency was 35 to 40 percent.[31,32] For this reason, there was great interest in a drug that could reduce morbidity and mortality rates in these children. Based on initial favorable results in water-placebo controlled trials,[33,34] ribavirin was approved in 1985 for use in high-risk children with RSV infection. In 1993, the

Committee on Infectious Diseases (COID) of the American Academy of Pediatrics recommended the use of ribavirin for certain high-risk infants.[35] In more recent years, the mortality rate has been shown to be 1 to 2 percent for all infants and 3 to 4 percent in children with underlying cardiac or pulmonary disease.[36] Much higher mortality rates, in the range of 20 to 67 percent, are reported in immunocompromised children.[33]

Recent studies have not shown a beneficial effect of ribavirin in clinical practice,[37,38] and in 1996, the COID reassessed its earlier recommendation for the use of ribavirin, changing the wording "should be used"[35] to "may be considered."[37] Because ribavirin is also expensive,[40] its use has become much more limited. The COID has not recommended discontinuance of this drug, however, and physicians treating certain high-risk or critically ill children may opt to use it.[37]

Complications

There appears to be a relationship between bronchiolitis and reactive airway disease, although the exact connection is unclear. Children who develop bronchiolitis do not appear to have family histories of asthma or atopy or histories of exposure to cigarette smoke that are different from those of children who do not develop the disease.[25] Some studies have shown an increased incidence of airway hyperreactivity in children who have had bronchiolitis that may persist for years.[39,40] However, a similar, although somewhat lesser, phenomenon can be seen in children who have been diagnosed with pneumonia in early childhood.[39] Treatment with anti-inflammatory medications such as nebulized budesonide or cromolyn sodium after an episode of bronchiolitis can reduce wheezing episodes and hospital admissions for bronchospasm.[41] Whether such treatment is useful for all children or should be reserved for those children with clinically apparent wheezing after bronchiolitis has not been established.

Prevention

In 1999, palivizumab (Synagis), a monoclonal antibody targeted to an RSV protein, became available in the United States for prevention of RSV disease in high-risk infants. The drug has been shown to decrease hospitalization rates among high-risk infants with and without chronic lung disease, although the death rates in the initial studies were not significantly different between the treatment and placebo groups.[42] The decision to use this drug is based on the age of the child at the onset of RSV season and the child's medical history.

The American Academy of Pediatrics recommends prophylaxis with palivizumab for a number of populations (Table 10-3).[43] Palivizumab is given in a dose of 15 mg/kg intramuscularly once a month beginning with the onset of the local RSV season and continuing for 4 to 5 months.[44] Protective antibody levels are achieved in 66 percent of infants after one injection and in 86 percent after a second injection.[45]

Table 10-3

Indications for Use of Palivizumab for Prevention of RSV Bronchiolitis

- Child less than age 2 with chronic lung disease who has required medical treatment in the previous 6 months
- Infant less than 1 year of age who was born at 28 weeks gestation or earlier
- Infant less than 6 months of age who was born at 29 to 32 weeks gestation
- Infant less than 6 months of age who was born at between 32 and 35 weeks gestation who has another risk factor for RSV infection, such as day-care attendance or three or more siblings

ABBREVIATION: RSV, respiratory syncytial virus.

Pertussis

Pertussis is a bacterial infection that affects airways lined with ciliated epithelium. The most common cause of pertussis is *Bordetella pertussis*, but *B. parapertussis* occasionally causes the disease, as do adenoviruses. Pertussis is endemic in the general population, with epidemics occurring every 3 to 4 years.[46] It is most common in unimmunized infants and in adults, as immunity wanes 5 to 10 years after the last immunization.

Since 1995, 95 percent of children between the ages of 19 and 35 months have received at least three doses of pertussis-containing vaccine.[47] However, immunization does not confer complete protection,[46] and immunized children may be asymptomatic reservoirs for infection.[48] Of the 7288 cases reported in 1999, 27 percent occurred in children less than 7 months of age, i.e., in children too young to have received the full initial course of three doses of pertussis vaccine. Some 11 percent of cases occurred in children between the ages of 1 and 4 years, and 28 percent were in children between the ages of 10 and 19 years.[49]

Pertussis causes serious disease in children and mild or asymptomatic disease in adults. Infants less than 6 months of age have greater morbidity than older children, and those under 2 months have the highest rates of pertussis-related hospitalization, pneumonia, seizures, encephalopathy, and death.[46] Pertussis is highly contagious, with attack rates as high as 100 percent in susceptible individuals exposed at close range.[46]

Pathologically, the bacteria attack ciliated epithelium in the respiratory tree, where they produce toxins and other active factors. These cause inflammation and necrosis of the walls of small airways, which lead in turn to plugging of airways, bronchopneumonia, and hypoxemia.

Diagnosis

HISTORY

In China, pertussis is called the "cough of one hundred days," reflecting the long duration of symptoms. Fever of greater than 38.4°C is unusual in all ages. Children under the age of 2 show the most typical symptoms of the disease. In these children, 100 percent will have paroxysms of coughing, with 60 to 70 percent manifesting the "whoops" that give this disease its nickname of "whooping cough." Some 60 to 80 percent will have vomiting induced by coughing, 70 to 80 percent will have dyspnea lasting more than 1 month, and 20 to 25 percent will have seizures. Children over the age of 2 have lower incidences of all these symptoms and a shorter duration of disease, while adults often have atypical symptoms.[46]

Pertussis has an incubation period lasting 3 to 12 days. After that, the disease progresses through three stages, each lasting approximately 2 weeks.[46]

The first stage is the catarrhal stage. This stage lasts from 1 to 2 weeks and is characterized by symptoms typical of an URI. The child may have especially thick nasal discharge during this stage, but the symptoms are nonspecific, and the diagnosis of pertussis is usually not considered.

The second stage, called the paroxysmal stage, lasts 2 to 4 weeks, but can occasionally be longer. During this stage, episodes of coughing increase in severity and number. The typical paroxysm is five to ten hard coughs in a single expiration, followed by the classic "whoop" as the patient inspires. Facial redness or cyanosis, bulging eyes, lacrimation, and salivation are common. The paroxysms recur until the mucus plugs causing the cough are dislodged. Coughing to the point of vomiting is common, and the diagnosis of pertussis should be considered in any patient with this symptom. The paroxysms are exhausting, and the child may appear apathetic and may lose weight because he or she is too weak to eat or drink. The paroxysms may be frequent enough to cause hypoxemia, which may be severe enough to cause anoxic encephalopathy. Between the paroxysms, however, the patient may not appear otherwise especially sick.

The final convalescent stage lasts from 1 to 2 weeks. During this stage, the paroxysms gradually decrease in frequency and number. The patient may experience a cough for several months after the disease has otherwise resolved.

The diagnosis of pertussis can usually be made in the paroxysmal stage, but it requires a certain level of suspicion. A cough lasting more than 2 weeks that is associated with posttussive vomiting should prompt the physician to consider the diagnosis.[46] As a diagnostic feature, the finding of an acute cough of presumed infectious etiology that lasts for more than 14 days has a sensitivity of 84 percent and a specificity of 63 percent.[50]

PHYSICAL EXAMINATION

There are no specific physical findings in pertussis.

LABORATORY AND IMAGING

A high white blood cell count (20,000 to 50,000/mm^3) with an absolute lymphocytosis is common but is not specific to the disease.[46] The organism can be obtained for culture or staining by a nasopharyngeal swab. The sensitivity of culture is related to the stage of the disease, with the greatest sensitivity occurring early in the disease, when pertussis is least suspected. Culture is about 80 percent sensitive during the first 2 weeks of infection, 14 percent after the fourth week of infection, and zero after 5 weeks.[51] Direct fluorescent antibody staining can provide a rapid diagnosis, but it has variable sensitivity and specificity, and all suspected cases should be cultured for definitive identification.[51]

Serology is highly sensitive but is accurate only after convalescent serum has been assayed for antibody titers. It is useful for retrospective diagnosis but is not useful in acutely ill patients.

Treatment

The treatment of pertussis is primarily supportive and includes hydration, pulmonary toilet, oxygen, and often antibiotics. The decision to hospitalize the patient depends on the patient's age and general condition. Essentially all children less than 3 months of age are admitted to the hospital, as are children between the ages of 3 and 6 months, unless witnessed paroxysms are not severe. Nearly all children who require ventilation are less than 3 months of age. Older children may be admitted if they experience complications of the disease or if their families are unable to provide care at home. Infants who were born prematurely and those with underlying cardiac, pulmonary, or neuromuscular disorders are also at higher risk for complications.[46]

Patients with pertussis should be placed in respiratory isolation until at least 5 days of antibiotics have been given.[46] Erythromycin given for 14 days will eliminate the bacteria from the respiratory tract within 3 to 4 days. Clarithromycin given for 7 days or azithromycin given for 5 days may be equally effective but are more expensive.[52] Trimethoprim-sulfamethoxazole for 14 days may be as effective as erythromycin in clearing the organism from the nasopharynx,[53] but the clinical effectiveness of this regimen is unknown.

If antibiotics are given within 14 days of the onset of the disease, they may abort or shorten the course of the disease, but the diagnosis of pertussis is rarely made in this stage of the illness. Once the paroxysmal stage begins, erythromycin will not affect the course of the disease, although it will shorten the period of infectivity and reduce communicability.[54] Other appropriate antibiotics should be given if pneumonia or another secondary bacterial infection is suspected.

Bronchodilators and steroids are of no proven benefit.[46] Cough suppressants are likewise not helpful.

Complications

Complications of pertussis are numerous and often severe. Pneumonia is the most frequent complication and is seen in almost all fatal cases.[55] *S. pneumoniae, S. aureus,* and oral flora are the most common organisms involved.[46] A high fever or absolute neutrophilia in a patient with pertussis may be the only clues to a secondary bacterial infection.

Other complications may arise from the severity of the cough in pertussis. Coughing may rupture alveoli and may cause interstitial and subcutaneous emphysema or pneumothorax. The cough may also cause epistaxis, melena, subconjunctival hemorrhage, spinal epidural hematoma, intracranial hemorrhage, rupture of the diaphragm, or umbilical or inguinal hernia. The paroxysms of cough may cause an inability to eat or drink and lead to dehydration, electrolyte imbalances, or nutritional deficiencies, primarily in settings where intravenous fluids are not available. Seizures can be caused by cough-associated anoxia but also are associated with hyponatremia secondary to inappropriate antidiuretic hormone secretion. Tetanic seizures also can occur as a result of electrolyte imbalances. Finally, anoxia may be severe enough to lead to coma.[46]

Prognosis

The prognosis of pertussis depends primarily on the age of the patient. Mortality is rare in adults and children. With proper supportive care, the mortality rate for children under 2 months of age, the group at highest risk, is approximately

1 percent.[46] Most mortality is due to pneumonia and cerebral anoxia. The incidence of long-term pulmonary sequelae is not known, but it appears that infants less than 6 months of age who are hospitalized with severe disease may have minor pulmonary function abnormalities and lower respiratory tract abnormalities, including wheezing, that persist into adulthood.[46]

Prevention

Prevention of pertussis remains the most effective way of reducing morbidity and mortality. Completing a basic series of immunizations provides the best protection from the disease. During a pertussis epidemic, newborns should receive their first immunization at 4 weeks of age, with repeat doses given at 6, 10, and 14 weeks of age.[56] Partially immunized children less than 7 years of age should complete the immunization series at the minimum intervals, and completely immunized children under the age of 7 should receive one booster dose, unless they have received one in the preceding 3 years. Children over the age of 7 do not need further immunizations.[57] Children who have had documented pertussis at any age are exempt from further pertussis immunizations.[46]

All contacts of patients with pertussis should be given erythromycin for 14 days after the date of their last contact with the patient. Continuous contacts of the patient (e.g., parents) should be given erythromycin until the patient's cough has stopped, or until the patient has received 7 days of erythromycin.[46]

References

1. Hueston W, Mainous AG 3d, Dacus EN, Hopper JE: Does acute bronchitis really exist? A reconceptualization of acute viral respiratory infections. *J Fam Pract* 49(5):401–406, 2000.

2. Centers for Disease Control and Prevention: Update: respiratory syncytial virus activity—United States, 1997–98 season. *MMWR* 46(49):1163–1165, 1997.

3. American Academy of Pediatrics Committee on Environmental Health: Environmental tobacco smoke: a hazard to children. *Pediatrics* 99(4):639–642, 1997.

4. Stern R: Bronchitis, in Behrman R, Kliegman R, Arvin A (eds): *Nelson Textbook of Pediatrics*, 15th ed. Philadelphia, WB Saunders, 1996; p. 1210.

5. Marx A, Torok TJ, Holman RC, et al: Pediatric hospitalizations for croup (laryngotracheobronchitis): biennial increases associated with human parainfluenzavirus 1 epidemics. *J Infect Dis* 176(6):1423–1427, 1997.

6. Orenstein D: Acute inflammatory upper airway obstruction, in Behrman R, Kliegman R, Arvin A (eds): *Nelson Textbook of Pediatrics*, 15th ed. Philadelphia, WB Saunders, 1996; pp. 1201–1205.

7. James JA: Dexamethasone in croup. *Am J Dis Child* 117:511–516, 1969.

8. Baugh R, Gilmore BB: Infectious croup: a critical review. *Otolaryryngol Head Neck Surg* 95:40–46, 1986.

9. Bourchier D, Fergusson DM: Humidification in viral croup: a controlled trial. *Aust Paediatr J* 20:289–291, 1984.

10. Henry R: Moist air in the treatment of laryngotracheitis. *Arch Dis Child* 58:577, 1983.

11. Cruz MN, Stewart G, Rosenberg N: Use of dexamethasone in the outpatient management of acute laryngotracheitis. *Pediatrics* 96(2 Pt 1):220–223, 1995.

12. Skolnik N: Croup. *J Fam Pract* 37(2):165–170, 1993.

13. Skolnik N: Treatment of croup: a critical review. *Am J Dis Child* 143:1045–1049, 1989.

14. Waisman Y, Klein BL, Boenning DA, et al: Prospective randomized double-blind study comparing L-epinephrine and racemic epinephrine aerosols in the treatment of laryngotracheitis (croup). *Pediatrics* 89(2):302–306, 1992.

15. Kairys SW, Olmstead EM, O'Connor GT: Steroid treatment of laryngotracheitis: a meta-analysis of the evidence from randomized trials. *Pediatrics* 83(5):683–693, 1989.

16. Klassen TP, Craig WR, Moher D, et al: Nebulized budesonide and oral dexamethasone for treatment of croup: a randomized controlled trial. *JAMA* 279(20):1629–1632, 1998.

17. Johnson DW, Jacobson S, Edney PC, et al: A comparison of nebulized budesonide, intramuscular dexamethasone, and placebo for moderately severe croup. *N Engl J Med* 339(8):498–503, 1998.

18. Frantz TD, Rasgon BM: Acute epiglottitis: changing epidemiologic patterns. *Otolaryngol Head Neck Surg* 109(3 part 1):457–460, 1993.

19. Cunningham M: Acute laryngotracheal infections, in Burg FD, Ingelfinger JR, Wald ER, Polin RA (eds): *Gellis and Kagan's Current Pediatric Therapy*, 15th ed. Philadelphia, WB Saunders, 1996; pp. 134–136.

20. Lee SS, Schwartz RH, Bahadori RS: Retropharyngeal abscess: epiglottitis of the new millennium. *J Pediatr* 138(3):435–437, 2001.

21. Hickerson SL, Kirby RS, Wheeler JG, Schutze GE: Epiglottitis: a 9-year case review. *South Med J* 89(5):487–490, 1996.

22. Lacroix J, Ahronheim G, Arcand P, et al: Group A streptococcal supraglottitis. *J Pediatr* 109(1):20–24, 1986.

23. Mauro RD, Poole SR, Lockhart CH: Differentiation of epiglottitis from laryngeotracheitis in the child with stridor. *Am J Dis Child* 142(6):679–682, 1988.

24. Damm M, Eckel HE, Jungehulsing M, Roth B: Management of acute inflammatory childhood stridor. *Otolaryngol Head Neck Surg* 121(5):633–638, 1999.

25. Young S, O'Keefe PT, Arnott J, Landau LI: Lung function, airway responsiveness, and respiratory symptoms before and after bronchiolitis. *Arch Dis Child* 72(1):16–24, 1995.

26. Centers for Disease Control and Prevention: Respiratory syncytial virus activity—United States, 1999–2000 season. *MMWR* 49(48):1091–1093, 1998.

27. Orenstein D: Bronchiolitis, in Behrman R, Kliegman R, Arvin A (eds): *Nelson Textbook of Pediatrics*, 15th ed. Philadelphia, WB Saunders, 1996; pp. 1211–1213.

28. Roosevelt G, Sheehan K, Grupp-Phelan J, et al: Dexamethasone in bronchiolitis: a randomized controlled trial. *Lancet* 348 (9023):292–295, 1996.

29. Kellner JD, Ohlsson A, Gadomski AM, Wang EE: Efficacy of bronchodilator therapy in bronchiolitis: a meta-analysis. *Arch Pediatr Adolesc Med* 150(11):1166–1172, 1996.

30. Menon K, Sutcliffe T, Klassen TP: A randomized trial comparing the efficacy of epinephrine with salbutamol in the treatment of acute bronchiolitis. *J Pediatr* 126(6):1004–1007, 1995.

31. MacDonald NE, Hall CB, Suffin SC, et al: Respiratory syncytial virus infection in infants with congenital heart disease. *N Engl J Med* 307:397–400, 1982.

32. Hall CB, Powell KR, MacDonald NE, et al: Respiratory syncytial virus infection in children with compromised immune function. *N Engl J Med* 315:77–81, 1986.

33. Hall CB: Aerosolized ribavirin treatment of infants with respiratory syncytial virus infection. *N Engl J Med* 308:1443–1447, 1983.

34. Taber LH, Knight V, Gilbert BE, et al: Ribavirin aerosol treatment of bronchiolitis associated with respiratory syncytial virus infection in infants. *Pediatrics* 72:613–618, 1983.

35. American Academy of Pediatrics, Committee on Infectious Diseases: Use of ribavirin in the treatment of respiratory syncytial virus infection. *Pediatrics* 92:501–504, 1993.

36. Wheeler JG, Wofford J, Turner RB: Historical cohort evaluation of ribavirin efficacy in respiratory syncytial virus infection. *Pediatr Infect Dis J* 12:209–213, 1991.

37. American Academy of Pediatrics, Committee on Infectious Diseases: Reassessment of the indications for ribavirin therapy in respiratory syncytial virus infections. *Pediatrics* 97(1):137–140, 1996.

38. Feldstein TJ, Swegarden JL, Atwood GF, Peterson CD: Ribavirin therapy: implementation of hospital guidelines and effect on usage and cost of therapy. *Pediatrics* 96(1 Part 1):14–17, 1995.

39. Korppi M, Kuikka L, Reijonen T, et al: Bronchial asthma and hyperreactivity after early childhood bronchiolitis or pneumonia: an 8-year follow-up study. *Arch Pediatr Adolesc Med* 148(10):1079–1084, 1994.

40. Kattan M: Epidemiologic evidence of increased airway reactivity in children with a history of bronchiolitis. *J Pediatr* 135(2 Part 2):8–13, 1999.

41. Reijonen T, Korppi M, Kuikka L, Remes K: Anti-inflammatory therapy reduces wheezing after bronchiolitis. *Arch Pediatr Adolesc Med* 150(5):512–517, 1996.

42. The IMpact-RSV Study Group: Palivizumab, a humanized respiratory syncytial virus monoclonal antibody, reduces hospitalization from respiratory syncytial virus infection in high-risk infants. *Pediatrics* 102(3 Part 3):531–537, 1998.

43. American Academy of Pediatrics, Committee on Infectious Diseases and Committee on Fetus and Newborn: Prevention of respiratory syncytial virus infections: indications for the use of palivizumab and update on the use of RSV-IGIV. *Pediatrics* 102(5):1211–1216, 1998.

44. Synagis revisited. *Med Lett* 43(1098):13–16, 2001.

45. Saenz-Lorens X, Castano E, Null D, et al: Safety and pharmacokinetics of an intramuscular humanized monoclonal antibody to respiratory syncytial virus in premature infants and infants with bronchopulmonary dysplasia: the MEDI-493 study group. *Pediatr Infect Dis J* 17(9):787–791, 1998.

46. Long S: Pertussis, in Behrman R, Kliegman R, Arvin A (eds): *Nelson Textbook of Pediatrics*, 15th ed. Philadelphia, WB Saunders, 1996; pp. 779–784.

47. Centers for Disease Control and Prevention: National, state, and urban area vaccination coverage levels among children aged 19–35 months—United States, 1999. *MMWR* 49(26):585–589, 2000.

48. Srugo I, Benilevi D, Madeb R, et al: Pertussis infection in fully-vaccinated children in day-care centers, Israel. *Emerg Infect Dis* 6(5):526–529, 2000.

49. Centers for Disease Control and Prevention: Summary of notifiable diseases, United States—1999. *MMWR* 48(53):1–91, 2001.

50. Patriarca PA, Biellik RJ, Sanden G, et al: Sensitivity and specificity of clinical case definitions for pertussis. *Am J Public Health* 78:833–836, 1988.

51. Onoratio IM, Wassilak SG: Laboratory diagnosis of pertussis: the state of the art. *Pediatr Infect Dis J* 6:145–151, 1987.

52. Aoyama T, Sunakawa K, Iwata S, et al: Efficacy of short-term treatment of pertussis with clarithromycin and azithromycin. *J Pediatr* 129(5):761–764, 1996.

53. Henry RL: Antimicrobial therapy in whooping cough. *Med J Aust* 2(1):27–28, 1981.

54. Statement on management of persons exposed to pertussis and pertussis outbreak control. *Can Commun Dis Rep* 20:193–200, 1994.

55. Wortis N, Strebel PM, Wharton M, et al: Pertussis deaths: report of 23 cases in the United States, 1992 and 1993. *Pediatrics* 97(5):607–612, 1996.

56. Onoratio IM, Wassilak SG, Meade B: Efficacy of whole-cell pertussis vaccine in preschool children in the United States. *JAMA* 267:2745–2749, 1992.

57. Pertussis, in Atkinson W, Wolfe C, Humiston S, Nelson R, et al (eds): *Epidemiology and Prevention of Vaccine-Preventable Diseases*, 2d ed. Atlanta, Centers for Disease Control and Prevention, Department of Health and Human Services, 1995.

William J. Hueston

Pneumonia

Pneumonia refers to infection of the parenchyma of the lung and may occur in tandem with distal bronchial infection. For pneumonia to occur in healthy individuals, the infecting organisms must overcome a number of mechanisms that protect the lung from pathogens. These include the mucociliary transport system, which removes inhaled particles and microbes; the cough reflex, which expels foreign matter; and reflexive closure of the glottis to prevent aspirations. Breakdowns in any of these mechanisms increase the risk that pathogens will be aspirated and deposited in the distal airways, causing infection.

In addition to the physical barriers just noted, immunologic mechanisms in the lung also help prevent the development of infection once microbes are present in the airways. IgA is secreted into the bronchial and alveolar spaces, which helps prompt early identification and removal of foreign substances. Alveolar macrophages are another mechanism for clearing bacterial and other pathogens that are deposited in the lung. Any disruption of the immunologic defenses, such as the congenital absence or impairment of the immune system, administration of immunosuppressing drugs, or infections that disturb normal immunologic function, can increase the risk of pneumonia.

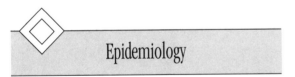

Epidemiology

Pneumonia is one of the most common reasons for hospitalization and the sixth leading cause of death in the United States. It causes over 10 million visits to physicians annually and accounts for 3 percent of all hospitalizations in the United States.[1,2] The total cost of pneumonia in the United States is estimated to be between $20 and $23 billion per year. This includes both direct costs to the health care system and indirect costs due to lost productivity.

Age is a major risk factor for the development of pneumonia. Pneumonia occurs in about 12 per 1000 per year in the population, but the incidence is much higher in the elderly population.[3] In one population-based study in Minnesota, the incidence of pneumonia among the elderly was estimated at about 30 cases per 1000 people per year.[4] In addition to age as a risk factor for pneumonia, institutionalization and debilitation increase the risk for acquiring pneumonia.[5] One study estimates that up to 2 percent of elderly individuals living in extended care facilities have pneumonia at any one time.[5] In addition to a higher incidence of pneumonia in the elderly population, this disease carries a much higher morbidity and mortality with advancing age. The highest mortality for pneumonia is seen in older patients with pneumococcal pneumonia.[6]

Other chronic medical conditions also influence the morbidity and mortality from pneumonia. In particular, chronic pulmonary diseases carry a high risk for the development of pneumonia.[7] This is probably due to impairment of the normal mucociliary clearance mechanism, less effective coughing so that secretions are not cleared as effectively, disruption of the immunologic functioning in the lung, and the creation of larger pools of mucus, which can support the growth of pathogens. Other co-morbidities that are associated with higher incidences of pneumonia and death include congestive heart failure, cerebrovascular diseases, cancer, diabetes mellitus, and poor nutritional status.

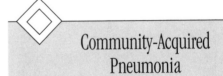

Community-Acquired Pneumonia

Community-acquired pneumonia refers to pneumonia in noninstitutionalized individuals who have not been hospitalized recently. While this definition may also encompass individuals who are immunosuppressed, those with immunodeficiencies generally are at higher risk for atypical infections. For this reason, patients with immunologic disorders should be considered differently from those with other community-acquired pneumonias. The special considerations for patients with immunodeficiencies are discussed in Chapter 12.

Etiology

In the past, over 80 percent of patients who had positive sputum cultures with pneumonia grew *Streptococcus pneumoniae*. *S. pneumoniae* pneumonia not only was common in the past, but also had a high mortality rate—between 20 and 40 percent.[2] In more recent studies, pneumococcal pneumonia still represents the largest single organism isolated from patients with pneumonia, but it no longer constitutes the majority of cases. Starting in the early 1980s, studies suggested that other bacteria were becoming more common in patients hospitalized with pneumonia (Table 11-1). The prevalence of *S. pneumoniae* has fallen from 80 percent to about a third of all cases of pneumonia. Other bacteria are found in about one-third of cases, and unidentified agents cause the remaining third of cases. Among these unidentified agents,

atypical bacteria such as *Legionella* and *Mycoplasma* are probably responsible for about half of all infections, with viruses being responsible for the other half.[2]

However, these data are based on hospitalized patients and may not describe the typical patient seen in ambulatory practices. Patients who are admitted to the hospital with community-acquired pneumonia are likely to have an underlying co-morbidity, such as chronic obstructive pulmonary disease (COPD), or to be more ill than those who can be treated as outpatients. Consequently, the spectrum of infection found in patients who are hospitalized might not reflect the types of agents that cause pneumonia in healthier, ambulatory patients.

The increase in the number of patients who are immunosuppressed from drug therapy or human immunodeficiency virus (HIV) disease may skew the population of individuals hospitalized with pneumonia even further. Data from Johns Hopkins Hospital in 1991 showed that pneumococcus was still the most common cause of pneumonia, but was followed in frequency by *Pneumocystis carinii*, which accounted for 13 percent of all cases.[2] It is unlikely that 13 percent of all people living in Baltimore at that time who got pneumonia had *Pneumocystis* pneumonia!

Table 11-1

Frequency of Organisms Causing Bacterial Pneumonia

Bacteria	Atlanta, GA 1967–68	Milwaukee, WI 1967–70	Hartford, CT 1980–81
Streptococcus pneumoniae	62%	71%	36%
Staphylococcus aureus	10%	10%	8%
Haemophilus influenzae	8%	4%	15%
Enteric gram-negative	19%	13%	16%
Legionella pneumophilia	—	—	14%
Pseudomonas	1%	0%	3%

SOURCE: Based on Garibaldi RA, Epidemiology of community-acquired respiratory tract infections in adults: incidence, etiology, and impact. *Am J Med* 78(suppl 6B):32–37, 1985, with permission.

Another factor that makes it difficult to rely on culture-derived data for determining the prevalence of pneumonia is that suitable sputum specimens can be obtained from only a minority of patients with pneumonia. Even in the hospital setting, only about a third of sputum cultures grow any bacteria at all. In the outpatient setting, where obtaining a suitable specimen for culture is even more difficult, sputum cultures are rarely performed. The true distribution of pathogens in ambulatory practices, especially in young, healthy individuals, has not been determined. For this population, empiric therapy is usually instituted, with no attempt to arrive at a bacteriologic diagnosis.

Based on demographics and co-morbidities, the American Thoracic Society has provided a framework to help clinicians predict the most likely etiologic agent for a patient with community-acquired pneumonia (Table 11-2).[8] These guidelines have been used to suggest treatment protocols that depend upon age, co-morbidity, and the initial severity of illness of the individual with pneumonia. These protocols will be discussed in more detail later in this chapter.

Diagnosis

HISTORY

The most common presenting complaints for patients with pneumonia are fever, dyspnea, pleuritic chest pain, and cough.[2] None of these symptoms, however, is specific for pneumonia. The cough may be either productive or nonproductive and, if productive, can produce hemoptysis. Of the symptoms found in pneumonia, the most common is fever, which in one study was found to be present in 80 percent of patients.

In older patients, symptoms of pneumonia may be vague.[5] Confusion, poor appetite, and falls in the elderly may all be associated with an underlying occult pneumonia.[9] Patients who are older, have preexisting cognitive impairment, or depend on someone else for support of their

Table 11-2

Other Conditions that Can Be Confused with Pneumonia

Other lung infections:
  Acute bronchitis
  Bronchiectasis
Cardiopulmonary diseases:
  Congestive heart failure
  Pulmonary embolism
Other conditions:
  Sarcoidosis
  Wegener's granulomatosis
  Hypersensitivity pneumonitis
  Collagen vascular disease pneumonitis
  Pulmonary alveolar proteinosis

daily activities are at highest risk for not exhibiting typical symptoms of pneumonia.[9]

PHYSICAL EXAMINATION

The most common physical examination findings in pneumonia are fever, tachycardia, and tachypnea. In one study of older patients, tachypnea was often the first abnormality identified in patients subsequently diagnosed with pneumonia. Tachypnea preceded other physical findings of pneumonia by as much as 3 to 4 days.[10] Rales or crackles are often considered the hallmark of pneumonia, but these may be absent in up to 25 percent of patients with pneumonia.[2,5] Other findings on lung examination that are usually believed to be indicative of consolidation, such as dullness to percussion or egophony, are present in less than a third of patients and are not sensitive indicators of pneumonia.[2]

DIFFERENTIAL DIAGNOSIS

Other conditions can cause the common symptoms seen in patients with pneumonia. Some of the conditions that can be confused with pneumonia are shown in Table 11-2. The most common respiratory conditions that produce a productive cough, fever, and some shortness of breath include acute bronchitis, exacerbation of chronic bronchitis, and bronchiectasis. In acute bronchitis and acute exacerbation of chronic bronchitis, the pulmonary infection resides in the bronchial tree and does not extend into the alveolar space. Patients may experience hypoxemia and other findings similar to those of pneumonia, but they generally will have wheezes rather than rales and do not have an infiltrate on chest x-ray. Patients with bronchiectasis tend to have a chronic cough that produces large amounts of putrid-smelling sputum. Because bronchiectasis usually originates from scarring caused by previous bronchopneumonia, an exacerbation of this condition could signal a recurrent pneumonia. However, patients usually have few signs of systemic infection, and the chest x-ray usually shows a fluid-filled dilated bronchus, sometimes with an air-fluid level. If there is a question as to whether this fluid accumulation represents pneumonia or bronchiectasis, confirmation with a spiral computed tomography (CT) scan is useful.[11,12]

Congestive heart failure (CHF) can be confused with pneumonia, since both present with tachycardia, tachypnea, and hypoxia and can be accompanied by altered mental status. The presence of a fever or an elevated white count can help distinguish between pneumonia and CHF, but in elderly patients with pneumonia these signs may be absent. Other signs of CHF such as an S_3, elevated jugular venous distention, and a recent increase in lower extremity edema may be useful in differentiating these two conditions.

Pneumonia also can be confused with an acute pulmonary embolism (PE). The triad of tachypnea, tachycardia, and air hunger that is characteristic of a PE overlaps with common symptoms of pneumonia. Pulmonary infarction from emboli can even produce a localized infiltrate on chest x-ray that can be confused with a pneumonic infiltrate. Because of physiologic shunting of pulmonary blood flow away from areas of pneumonia that have poor aeration, a ventilation-perfusion scan in the patient with pneumonia may not be able to differentiate pneumonia from a PE. If a patient with suspected pneumonia is experiencing profound hypoxia that does not improve with oxygen administration, suspicion for PE should be high. In addition, PE should be considered in patients with other risk factors for a PE, such as previous pulmonary embolism, estrogen use, or a history of cancer or a hereditary condition that results in a hypercoagulable state.

Individuals with sarcoidosis can be misdiagnosed with pneumonia. Patients with sarcoid often have high fevers, systemic symptoms suggestive of infection, cough, and dyspnea. About half of patients with sarcoidosis have an abnormal chest x-ray including infiltrates. However, most patients with sarcoidosis also have hilar adenopathy, which may help distinguish this disease from pneumonia.

Wegener's granulomatosis is a vasculitis that extends through the respiratory tract and the kidneys. It can produce migratory infiltrates as well as hemoptysis. Findings of red cell casts in the urine can help differentiate this condition from pneumonia.

Finally, hypersensitivity pneumonitis can present with fever, malaise, and a cough that can mimic pneumonia. Both pneumonia and hypersensitivity pneumonitis are caused by alveolar inflammation, but in the latter condition the mechanism for the inflammation is immune-mediated rather than infectious. Symptoms of acute hypersensitivity pneumonitis are often transient and related to exposure to the irritant. The lack of response to antibiotics and a history of exposure to common causes of lung hypersensitivity help distinguish this condition from pneumonia.

IMAGING AND LABORATORY EVALUATION

CHEST X-RAY   When pneumonia is suspected on history and physical examination, chest radiography is the most useful tool for confirming the diagnosis. Rarely, the chest x-ray may be falsely negative for pneumonia. Conditions associated with false negative chest x-rays include severe dehydration, early pneumonia (infection within the first 24 h), *P. carinii* infections, and neutropenia.[2] Some conditions other than pneumonia also can produce an infiltrate on chest x-ray that may mimic infections. These conditions include postobstructive pneumonitis, pulmonary infarct from an embolism, radiation pneumonitis, and interstitial edema from congestive heart failure.[1]

Some association between the appearance of the infiltrate on chest radiograph and the etiologic agent has been suggested, but this remains controversial. One study found that an alveolar pattern (which is described as patchy, segmental, or lobar with mixed alveolar/interstitial infiltrate) was associated with a bacterial infection rather than infections due to mycoplasma or viruses,[13] but other studies were unable to confirm any consistent relationship between the pathogen causing the infection and the pattern of the infiltrate on x-ray.[5]

Despite the questionable ability to distinguish bacterial from nonbacterial etiology based on the infiltrate pattern, some individual etiologic agents are associated with atypical infiltrates on a chest x-ray. The presence of a specific pattern can increase the index of suspicion for that particular agent. For example, *Staphylococcus aureus* pneumonia frequently causes bilateral pneumonia with formation of cavities and lung abscesses along with a pleural effusion. *P. carinii* also causes a bilateral pneumonia, but generally with a granular, interstitial appearance that is spread diffusely throughout the lung fields. Acute *Mycobacterium tuberculosis* also causes an interstitial pattern, but the infiltrate occurs predominantly in the lower lung fields.

The presence of a pleural effusion also may be detected on chest x-ray. Between 30 and 50 percent of patients with pneumonia have a parapneumonic effusion.[2] Patients with a significant pleural effusion should have a thoracentesis performed, with the aspirated fluid analyzed for cell count and differential, Gram stain and culture, cytology, lactic dehydrogenase (LDH), and protein, glucose, and pH evaluation. Effusions with very low pH (<7.20) are less likely to clear with antibiotic therapy alone and may require chest tube drainage for definitive treatment. It has been recommended that any effusion greater than 10 mm in width on a lateral decubitus chest x-ray be evaluated through a diagnostic thoracentesis.[14]

Once the diagnosis is made and antibiotic therapy is begun, routine follow-up x-rays are not needed if the patient is improving clinically. Following serial radiographs to determine a clinical response to treatment may not be useful, since radiographic resolution of the infiltrate may lag considerably behind clinical improvement. If patients are not making an adequate recovery, however, additional chest imaging studies may be useful to evaluate for the formation of a lung abscess, empyema, or other complications of the pneumonia. Segmental pneumonias that fail to improve with therapy may be caused by obstruction of a proximal bronchus by either an inflammatory problem or a tumor. Further imaging with CT can be helpful to determine if a proximal bronchial mass is present. For patients who recover uneventfully from their initial pneumonia, a routine follow-up chest radiograph in an otherwise healthy individual is not indicated unless there is suspicion of an underlying malignancy or other pulmonary disease.[3]

SPUTUM EVALUATION In addition to an initial chest x-ray, examination and culture of the sputum is often performed in patients with pneumonia. Sputum Gram stains can be a useful tool when selecting initial drug therapy,[15] but the use of sputum Gram stains and cultures is hampered by the inability of many patients to produce specimens suitable for culture. Between 10 and 30 percent of patients with pneumonia do not have a cough or cannot produce sputum. For these individuals, a sputum specimen sometimes can be induced with hypertonic saline inhalation, but often patients have difficulty producing an adequate specimen even with saline induction techniques. Furthermore, another 30 percent of patients have taken antibiotics on an outpatient basis before the decision to hospitalize them has been made. For these patients, sputum cultures may not be accurate. Even among those who can produce sputum that appears to be free of oropharyngeal contamination, 30 to 65 percent of specimens do not grow out a predominant organism. Some associations between patient populations and the likely pathogens on sputum examination are shown in Table 11-3.

Because of the low diagnostic yield from sputum examination and culture, these tests are rarely performed on outpatients. In hospitalized patients, sputum studies can be useful in guiding initial drug selection. Obtaining a positive sputum culture in hospitalized patients also can provide data on drug resistance. Drug sensitivity studies for individual institutions are useful, as they allow an institution to follow the antibiotic resistance of organisms in that particular hospital and can be helpful in identifying the development of new drug-resistant organisms in communities.

BLOOD CULTURES   As with sputum cultures, routine performance of a blood culture is controversial for patients with pneumonia. In patients who will be treated on an outpatient basis, blood cultures rarely produce clinically useful data. Even in hospitalized patients, the clinical usefulness and cost-effectiveness of blood cultures in otherwise healthy nonimmunosuppressed patients is questionable.[16] Despite reservations about the cost-effectiveness of obtaining a blood culture, however, most experts advocate routine blood cultures, if for no other reason than to identify the occasional drug-resistant strain that may require a change in antibiotic therapy.[3]

OTHER TESTS   When a patient appears moderately to severely ill or when there is a question about whether hospitalization is warranted for a patient with suspected pneumonia, further tests are indicated. In these individuals, serum electrolytes, blood urea nitrogen (BUN)/creatinine, and arterial oxygen saturation should be determined. Patients with significant disturbances in their electrolytes, evidence of renal insufficiency, or hypoxemia are more likely to benefit from hospital care. In patients who were otherwise healthy before their pneumonia, who appear well, and for whom outpatient management is expected, assessment of oxygen saturation with a pulse oximeter may be sufficient. Patients who

Table 11-3

Pathogens Most Likely Responsible for Pneumonia in Certain Age Groups

PATIENT POPULATION	LIKELY PATHOGENS
≤ 60 years old with no co-morbidities	*Streptococcus pneumoniae, Mycoplasma pneumoniae,* viruses, *Chlamydia pneumoniae, Haemophilus influenzae*
> 60 years old and/or co-morbid illness	*S. pneumoniae,* viruses, *H. influenzae,* aerobic gram-negative bacilli, *Staphylococcus aureus*
Patients requiring hospitalization	*S. pneumoniae, H. influenzae,* polymicrobial infections, aerobic gram-negative bacilli, *Legionella, S. aureus, C. pneumoniae,* viruses
Patients requiring ICU care	*S. pneumoniae, Legionella,* aerobic gram-negative bacilli, *M. pneumoniae,* viruses

ABBREVIATION: ICU, intensive care unit.
From Areno et al,[1] with permission.

have underlying pulmonary disease should have further assessment of their blood pH and carbon dioxide content in addition to a determination of oxygenation status.

The Centers for Disease Control and Prevention (CDC) also recommends routine HIV-1 testing in all hospitalized pneumonia patients between the ages of 15 and 54 who live in an area where the prevalence of HIV disease is greater than 1 in 1000 people.[2]

Treatment

Treatment decisions for patients with community-acquired pneumonia center on two issues: (1) Does the patient need to be hospitalized or can she or he be treated safely as an outpatient, and (2) what is the most appropriate drug to use and how does the possibility of the patient's having a drug-resistant organism influence this decision?

HOSPITALIZE OR TREAT AS AN OUTPATIENT?

The decision to hospitalize a patient with pneumonia as opposed to instituting outpatient antibiotic therapy can be difficult. Several studies have helped clarify which patients are at the highest risk for a complication or mortality from pneumonia and might benefit from receiving more intensive care of their disease. However, there are few longitudinal studies that show the outcomes of the decisions based on these protocols. It is useful to recognize underlying co-morbidities or "red flags" that indicate a higher risk of complications in a patient with community-acquired pneumonia. Some of the strongest factors that are associated with higher death rates from pneumonia are tachypnea (respiratory rate $\geq$ 30/min), hypotension (diastolic blood pressure $\leq$ 60 mmHg), and a BUN of more than 7 mmol/L.[17] If these three factors are considered alone, they are accurate in predicting mortality or survival in 82 percent of cases. Unfortunately, these values are based on studies that included only hospitalized patients. Therefore, these data do not help clinicians decide which patients to admit to the hospital, since it is unlikely that clinicians would elect to treat hypotensive, tachypneic patients with renal failure as outpatients. Rather than helping with the decision to hospitalize patients with these findings, the real utility of this study is identifying a group of high-risk hospitalized patients who require intensive management.

A more useful classification that can assist clinicians in deciding which patients might be treated at home identifies four categories of patients who vary in their risk of mortality from pneumonia (Table 11-4).[18] The lowest mortality occurs in patients under age 60 with no co-morbid illnesses. Individuals in this low-risk group have a very low mortality rate (1 percent), suggesting that most of them can be managed on an outpatient basis. Patients who are over 60 and healthy or younger patients with a co-morbid condition have a higher mortality rate, about 3 percent. Depending upon the severity of the co-morbid illness and the patient's physiologic reserve, many of these patients (about 80 percent) can be treated as outpatients.

Moderate-risk patients are those over 60 years old who also have a significant co-morbidity. Mortality in these individuals ranges from 13 to 25 percent. These patients should be cared for in the hospital setting.

The highest risk category includes patients who are extremely ill and present with hypotension, respiratory distress, and other signs of serious compromise. Many of these patients are younger, but are infected with aggressive organisms or have serious co-morbidities that accentuate the effects of pneumonia. Mortality in these individuals is about 50 percent, and they obviously need hospital care, usually in an intensive care unit (ICU).

In addition to these clinical criteria, other factors may enter into the decision to hospitalize a patient with community-acquired pneumonia (Table 11-5). These include factors such as whether the patient has the social support or

Table 11-4

Factors Associated with Mortality from Community-Acquired Pneumonia

CATEGORY	CHARACTERISTICS	MORTALITY	LOCATION OF CARE
Very low risk	Age < 60, no co-morbidities	<1%	Outpatient
Low risk	Age > 60, but healthy	3%	80% can be cared for
	Age < 60, mild co-morbidity		as outpatient (depending on co-morbidity)
Moderate risk	Age > 60 with co-morbidity	13–25%	Hospitalization
High risk	Serious compromise present on presentation (hypotension, respiratory distress, etc.) regardless of age	50%	Intensive care unit

Table 11-5

Other Factors to Consider in Deciding to Hospitalize Patients with Pneumonia

Social/demographic factors
- Home care not available
- Compliance with therapy questionable
- Mental impairment or disability

Host factors
- Coexisting illness such as COPD, diabetes, renal failure, congestive heart failure, chronic liver disease, or previous hospitalization in last year
- Aspiration pneumonia likely
- Alcohol abuse or malnutrition
- Immunosuppression

ABBREVIATION: COPD, chronic obstructive pulmonary disease.
Adapted from Areno et al,[1] with permission.

cognitive ability to successfully manage his or her illness at home as well as other host factors that could complicate the current infection.

ANTIBIOTIC SELECTION FOR COMMUNITY-ACQUIRED PNEUMONIA

Once the decision to either hospitalize a patient with pneumonia or start treatment as an outpatient is made, it is important to select a drug that will provide coverage for the organisms most likely to be causing the disease. Since the most common bacterial cause of pneumonia is *S. pneumoniae*, it is essential that the initial drug regimen provide adequate coverage for this organism. Until the last decade, *S. pneumoniae* was uniformly sensitive to penicillin, other beta-lactam drugs, and several other classes of antibiotics such as macrolides.

Since a wide spectrum of agents provided coverage of *S. pneumoniae*, often the specific antibiotic was selected to provide additional coverage for other common organisms found in community-acquired pneumonia patients, such as *Mycoplasma pneumoniae* or *Haemophilus influenzae*. Initial drug selection in a newly diagnosed patient with pneumonia hinged on whether the patient had COPD (which can increase the likelihood of *H. influenzae*) or whether symptoms were mild and indolent, suggesting *Mycoplasma* or other atypical infections. The introduction of broad-spectrum macrolides that provide adequate coverage for both of these organisms as well as *S. pneumoniae* has reduced the complexity of initial antibiotic selection.

DRUG-RESISTANT *STREPTOCOCCUS PNEUMONIAE* In the last 10 to 15 years, an increase in drug resistance of *S. pneumoniae* has been noted. At first, resistance was found only to penicillin, but increased resistance to multiple drugs has developed recently.[19] Drug-resistant *S. pneumoniae* (DRSP) strains have become commonplace in other countries. In South Africa in the early 1990s, for example, over half of all pneumococcal strains that were isolated were resistant to penicillin and other drugs. In the last decade, drug-resistant strains have become prevalent in the United States as well. The problem with resistance is widespread and is found in both rural and urban sites.[20]

DRSP strains are categorized as either intermediately resistant or highly resistant, depending on the level of drug required to kill the organism. Minimal inhibitory concentrations for intermediately resistant strains can often be achieved with higher doses of the same drug. However, drug concentrations are unlikely to reach levels high enough to be effective against organisms in the highly resistant category. While most resistance was originally intermediate, in recent years a greater percentage of strains have been exhibiting high levels of resistance to multiple drugs.

For organisms that are intermediately resistant, treatment with penicillin or other beta-lactams and many cephalosporins at usual dosing ranges is not effective. Some of this resistance can be overcome using high-dose regimens. For organisms in the highly resistant category, treatment with vancomycin offers the best chance of recovery.

Fluoroquinolones show varied degrees of activity against DRSP. Some quinolones, such as ciprofloxacin, have poor activity against intermediately resistant strains of *S. pneumoniae*, while other members of this class, such as levofloxacin and gatifloxacin, have much better activity. Quinolones with improved activity against intermediately resistant *S. pneumoniae* have been classified as having "enhanced pneumococcal activity."

While DRSP colonization is common and these strains are being isolated increasingly in hospitalized patients, it is unclear how common this phenomenon is in mildly ill patients seen in the ambulatory setting. There are a number of risk factors that have been identified that are linked with a higher probability that a patient harbors DRSP (Table 11-6). When the patient is elderly, is debilitated, has multiple or severe co-morbidities, and/or has recently been hospitalized or treated with beta-lactam agents, DRSP is more likely. For these patients, antibiotics active against intermediately resistant pneumococcus should be started. If the patient is critically ill or appears to be deteriorating despite antibiotic therapy, vancomycin should be added.

TREATMENT GUIDELINES Guidelines from the American Thoracic Society (ATS) and the Infectious Disease Society of America can be useful in selecting specific drugs for either outpatient or initial inpatient management of pneumonia. The ATS guidelines for antimicrobial use in pneumonia were originally published in 1993, before pneumococcal drug resistance was a serious concern. The updated guidelines by the Infectious Disease Society of America were published in 1998 and are summarized in Table 11-7.

For most patients in an ambulatory setting, monotherapy with a fluoroquinolone with enhanced pneumococcal activity, such as levofloxacin, or a macrolide with enhanced *H. influenzae* coverage, such as azithromycin, will provide adequate bacteriologic coverage for intermediately resistant pneumococcus plus atypical organisms.

Table 11-6

Risk Factors for Infection with Drug-Resistant *Streptococcus Pneumoniae*

Risk factors identified for colonization:
- Age under 2 or over 70
- Beta-lactam use in last 3 months
- Children in a day-care center
- Staff member in a day-care center

Risk factors for disease:
- Renal, oncologic, hepatic co-morbidity
- Recent hospitalization
- Age over 70

Table 11-7

Guidelines for Empiric Treatment for Community-Acquired Pneumonia by Infectious Disease Society of America

---

Treatment of Patient Not Requiring Hospitalization:

Preferred (in no special order): Macrolide, fluoroquinolone with enhanced pneumococcal activity,* doxycycline

Alternatives not active against atypical agents: Amoxicillin/clavulinic acid, selected second-generation cephalosporins (cefuroxime, cefpodoxime, or cefprozil)

Treatment of Hospitalized Patients Not Critically Ill:

Preferred (in no special order): Beta-lactam with or without a macrolide or fluoroquinolone with enhanced pneumococcal activity*

Alternatives: Cefuroxime with or without a macrolide or azithromycin alone

Treatment of Critically Ill Hospitalized Patients:

Preferred (in no special order): Erythromycin, azithromycin, or fluoroquinolone with enhanced pneumococcal activity,* *PLUS* cefuroxime, ceftriaxone, or a beta-lactam with beta-lactamase inhibitor

Other situations:

Treatment of patients with penicillin allergy: Fluoroquinolone with enhanced pneumococcal activity*

Suspected aspiration: Fluoroquinolone with enhanced pneumococcal activity* *PLUS* clindamycin or a beta-lactam with beta-lactamase inhibitor

---

*Includes levofloxacin, sparfloxacin, grepafloxacin, trovofloxacin.
From Bartlett JG, Breiman RF, Mandell LA, File TM Jr: Guidelines from the Infectious Diseases Society of America. Community-acquired pneumonia in adults: guidelines for management. *Clin Infect Dis* 26:811–838, 1998, with permission.

Patients who are seriously ill and require hospitalization should receive antimicrobial coverage for *H. influenzae*, pneumococcus, and atypical organisms. In these individuals, providing gram-negative coverage with a second- or third-generation cephalosporin (which also provides staphylococcal coverage) plus an agent for atypical organisms such as a macrolide is an alternative to levofloxacin or another of the fluoroquinolones with enhanced pneumococcal activity.

Critically ill patients are at higher risk for having gram-negative organisms or *S. aureus* and require broader gram-negative coverage in addition to an antimicrobial for atypical organisms. For critically ill patients who are at high risk for drug-resistant pneumococcal disease, empiric treatment with vancomycin also is indicated.

Prevention of Pneumonia

The development of resistance and the rapid spread of resistant strains appear to be linked to excessive use of antibiotics for other respiratory conditions.[21–23] In areas where antibiotics are accessible and are prescribed frequently for equivocal indications, resistance has become more prevalent. Primary care physicians can help limit the development of further resistance by minimizing the injudicious prescribing of antibiotics for conditions such as acute bronchitis or colds where antibiotics are of little benefit.

Pneumococcal pneumonia may be prevented through immunization with multivalent pneumococcal vaccine. The multivalent pneumococcal vaccination is indicated for individuals over age 65; those 2 years of age or older with diabetes mellitus or chronic pulmonary or cardiac disease; and those without a spleen. Additionally, people in certain high-risk populations such as the Native American and Alaskan Native populations and people over age 50 living in chronic care facilities should be vaccinated. Immunosuppressed patients, including those with HIV, alcoholism, cirrhosis, chronic renal failure, sickle cell disease, or multiple myeloma, also should be immunized, but the evidence is less convincing.

Clinicians should also advise patients that the duration of protection is uncertain. For those at particularly high risk of mortality from pneumococcal pneumonia, such as patients over age 75 and those with chronic pulmonary disease or lacking a spleen, revaccination every 5 years is a worthwhile precaution.

The original pneumococcal vaccination was not effective for children under the age of 2. For that reason, a conjugate pneumococcal vaccine was developed and was approved for use in February 2000. The American Academy of Family Physicians recommended routine administration of the conjugate vaccine to all children under the age of 2 and to children under the age of 5 with high-risk conditions such as sickle cell disease, HIV, functional or anatomic asplenia, immunosuppression, and other chronic illnesses that could be complicated by pneumonia. In addition, children under 5 years old in high-risk ethnic groups such as Alaskan Natives and Native Americans were included in those who should receive the immunization.

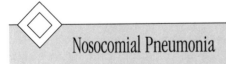

Nosocomial Pneumonia

Nosocomial pneumonia is a pneumonia acquired during a hospitalization. Specifically, it is defined as a pneumonia presenting more than 2 days after hospitalization in a patient who was not admitted with a pneumonia.[24] Because

pneumonia in these settings frequently is caused by atypical organisms and involves a host who is already under physiologic stress, nosocomial pneumonia is associated with a higher mortality rate than community-acquired pneumonia.

Individuals living in institutions such as nursing homes and prisons also are more likely to have atypical pathogens causing pneumonia. Infections acquired in institutions other than the hospital require greater vigilance than community-acquired infections, but generally are not as virulent as hospital-acquired infections.

Epidemiology

Urinary tract infections and pneumonia are the two most common nosocomial infections. Nosocomial pneumonias account for between 13 and 18 percent of all nosocomial infections.[24] A hospital-acquired pneumonia complicates about 0.5 percent of all admissions, with higher percentages occurring in patients hospitalized in an ICU. The rates of hospital-acquired pneumonia vary considerably among institutions, with tertiary-care facilities having higher nosocomial pneumonia rates than community hospitals. Nosocomial pneumonias account for half of all deaths from nosocomial infections.[25] Factors associated with an increased risk of death from hospital-acquired pneumonia are shown in Table 11-8.

There are a number of risk factors that increase the likelihood of a hospital-acquired pneumonia (Table 11-9). Patients with underlying pulmonary disease and other co-morbid conditions are at higher risk for acquiring a nosocomial pneumonia because of breakdown in host defenses. Older individuals are more likely to acquire a nosocomial pneumonia, but when adjusted for other risk factors such as co-morbid conditions, age is not an independent predictor of a patient's getting a hospital-acquired pneumonia.[24]

Table 11-8

Factors Associated with Higher Mortality from Nosocomial Pneumonias

Infection with *Pseudomonas aeruginosa* or another aerobic gram-negative bacillus
Severe underlying disease
Inappropriate antibiotic use during hospital stay
Advanced age
Shock
Bilateral infiltrates
Neoplastic disease
Duration of prior hospitalization
Supine head position in patients on mechanical ventilator

From Weber et al,[29] with permission.

Table 11-9

Risk Factors for Hospital-Acquired Pneumonia

Intrinsic (patient-related) factors
Severity of underlying illness
Malnutrition
Impaired consciousness
Immunosuppression
Prolonged hospitalization
Chronic lung disease
Hospital factors
Poor hand-washing practices by health providers
Inappropriate use of gloves
Contaminated respiratory devices
Contamination of hospital water supply
Treatment-related factors
Intensive care unit admission
Mechanical ventilation
Use of acid-reducing agents
Overuse of antibiotics
Nasogastric tube use
Oversedation
Lengthy surgical procedures

Infection-control practices by hospitals and health providers also have a significant impact on the risk of patients' acquiring a nosocomial pneumonia. Reductions in transmission of organisms from one patient to another through hand washing and changing gloves can reduce the risk of a hospital-acquired pneumonia. Appropriate decontamination and storage of equipment can reduce nosocomial pneumonia rates as well.[26] In addition, nosocomial pneumonia outbreaks caused by *Legionella* have been associated with contamination of hospital water supplies. One study found that 23 percent of all *Legionella* pneumonia was hospital-acquired and could be linked to contamination of the hospital's water supply.[27] Protection of the hospital water supply from contamination is a key step in reducing nosocomial respiratory infections.

Several medical procedures and treatments also expose patients to a higher risk of nosocomial pneumonia. Mechanical ventilation and admission to an ICU are highly associated with developing pneumonia. Suppression of gastric acid with antacids, an H_2-blocker, or a proton-pump inhibitor can increase the overgrowth of gastric bacteria, which can increase the incidence of pneumonia with small amounts of aspiration.

Etiology

Nosocomial pneumonias are believed to develop from the aspiration of small droplets ("microaspirates"), allowing the lower respiratory tract to be colonized with bacteria from the oropharynx and gastric tract.[24] Studies in ventilated patients with depressed neurologic function show that the respiratory tract is often colonized with bacteria within 3 days of intubation. In the presence of impaired defenses, this colonization may progress to a lower respiratory infection.

The specific organisms associated with hospital-acquired pneumonias are often unique to institutions. Even different areas within the same institution may have different microbiologic environments, resulting in different bacteria causing hospital-acquired infections. In addition, there are differences between early-onset nosocomial pneumonias, defined as those that occur within 2 to 3 days after hospitalization, and pneumonias after longer stays or in patients on ventilators (Table 11-10).

For patients with early-onset infections, the spectrum of organisms is similar to that in patients with community-acquired pneumonia. This suggests that early-onset infections probably arise from transmission of organisms from other patients or staff rather than from colonization with hospital-dwelling organisms. Late-onset and ventilator-associated pneumonias are more likely to stem from organisms that have colonized the hospital, the equipment, and, ultimately, the patient. Gram-negative bacilli such as *Pseudomonas, Enterobacter, Acinetobacter*, and *Serratia* have been reported as the most frequent cause of late-acquired nosocomial pneumonia, with many of these being polymicrobial infections.[28,29]

Diagnosis

Rapid recognition of a nosocomial infection results in less morbidity and a higher chance of recovery. The development of a fever, a cough (especially with purulent-appearing sputum), or changes on pulmonary examination should prompt further evaluation for a possible pneumonia as well as other nosocomial sources of infection. Additionally, other potential sources of respiratory deterioration (such as congestive heart failure or myocardial ischemia) should not be overlooked.[25]

When pneumonia is suspected, a chest x-ray, white blood count, Gram stain of sputum, and cultures of sputum, blood, and, if indicated, pleural fluid should be obtained promptly. A sputum specimen obtained by suctioning the endotracheal tube of an intubated patient can provide some insight into possible etiologic agents, but contamination is possible from organisms that have colonized the trachea and endotracheal tube.[30]

Table 11-10

Etiologic Agents in Nosocomial Pneumonias

TYPE OF ORGANISM	PERCENT OF NOSOCOMIAL CASES
Early-onset pneumonia	
Streptococcus pneumoniae	5–20
Haemophilus influenzae	5–15
Late-onset pneumonia/ventilator-associated pneumonia	
Gram-negative aerobes	20–60
Staphylococcus aureus (including methicillin-resistant S. aureus)	20–40
Anaerobes	0–35
Legionella	0–10
Viruses	<1
Pneumocystis carinii	<1
Candida	<1

From Weber et al,[29] with permission.

Blood cultures are important in nosocomial infections. These are positive in between 10 and 20 percent of patients with nosocomial pneumonia; one should keep in mind, however, that additional sites of infection are often present in severely ill patients and may be the source of the bacteremia.[29]

Bronchial alveolar lavage (BAL) for the diagnosis of nosocomial infections can provide reliable culture results. However, BAL does not appear to influence patient outcomes.[30]

Treatment

The treatment of hospital-acquired pneumonias is difficult because of the large number of organisms that may be involved in an infection. To provide treatment for the wide spectrum of potential infectious agents, therapy with broad-spectrum antibiotics (Table 11-11) should be instituted while cultures are pending.[29]

For patients with mild to moderate infections or severe early-onset nosocomial pneumonia,

Table 11-11

Recommended Treatment for Nosocomial Pneumonia

Mild/moderate infection with no risk factors or severe early onset:
Piperacillin-tazobactam 3.375 g IV q4h or 4.5 g IV q6h *OR*
cefotaxime 1–2 g IV q8h *OR*
ceftriaxone 1 g IV q12h
If allergic to penicillin/cephalosporins:
Clindamycin *OR* vancomycin *PLUS*
quinolone *OR* aztreonam
Severe infection or early-onset infection with risk factors:
Aminoglycoside *OR* quinolone *OR* piperacillin-tazobactam *OR* imipenem 500 mg IV q6h *OR* ceftazidime 2 g IV q8h *PLUS*
consider addition of vancomycin

Adapted from Weber et al,[29] with permission.

a broad-spectrum agent is recommended that provides sufficient coverage for gram-positive organisms as well as for gram-negative bacilli excluding *Pseudomonas.* Piperacillin-tazobactam, cefotaxime, or ceftriazone is useful in patients who are not allergic to penicillin or cephalosporins. For penicillin- or cephalosporin-allergic individuals, clindamycin, vancomycin, aztreonam, or a quinolone with enhanced streptococcal activity such as levofloxacin or oflaxin are alternatives.

Additional antibiotic coverage is indicated in patients who have specific risk factors for certain types of infection. For example, clindamycin may be added to piperacillin-tazobactam if an anaerobic infection is likely. When *S. aureus* is more likely, consideration should be given to using vancomycin, since methicillin-resistant *S. aureus* (MRSA) is common in many institutions. Patients in institutions that experience high numbers of nosocomial *Legionella* infections should receive erythromycin or a broad-spectrum macrolide in their initial antibiotic regimen. For patients at high risk for *Pseudomonas* infection or in patients who are severely ill, coverage with an aminoglycoside or other anti-*Pseudomonas* drug, plus addition of vancomycin for methicillin-resistant *S. aureus*, should be considered.

Prevention

Attention to several areas of patient care can help reduce rates of nosocomial infection (Table 11-12). First, selective use of acid suppressants and sedatives can help patients maintain their natural protective mechanisms. Second, avoiding use of the ICU for patients who are not severely ill or in need of intensive nursing services and limiting ICU stays to as short a period as possible can help lower the chance of acquiring a nosocomial infection. Finally, careful hand washing before and after every patient encounter will reduce cross-contamination between patients.

Table 11-12

Strategies for Avoiding Nosocomial Pneumonia

RISK FACTOR	PREVENTIVE STRATEGY
Host factors	
Chronic obstructive pulmonary disease	Incentive spirometry, positive end-expiratory pressure for ventilation
Immunosuppression	Avoid exposure to pathogens such as in ICU
Depressed consciousness	Use CNS depressants cautiously
Abdominal/thoracic surgery	Position patient to avoid aspiration, early ambulation, appropriate pain control
Institutional factors	
Intubation/mechanical ventilation	Gently suction secretions, elevate head of bed, use nonalkylinzing gastric cytoprotectants, do not change ventilation circuits routinely more often than every 48 h, use heat-moisture exchanger
Nasogastric tube placement	Verify proper tube placement, remove NG tube when not needed, elevate head of bed
Antibiotic administration	Use antibiotics prudently, especially in ICU

ABBREVIATIONS: ICU, intensive care unit; CNS, central nervous system; NG, nasogastric.
Adapted from Weber et al,[29] with permission.

Pneumonia in Children

Infants

Pneumonia in the infant is really four different diseases, depending upon when the infant becomes infected. Because of the differences among the infections, pneumonia is categorized as (1) transplacentally acquired or congenital pneumonia; (2) intrauterine infection from ascending infection; (3) early neonatal pneumonia (within first 4 weeks of life); and (4) late neonatal pneumonia.[31] The timing of the infection can give clues to the etiologic agents and guide therapy.

CONGENITAL PNEUMONIA

Congenital and intrauterine pneumonias result in death shortly after birth (usually in less than 24 h) or stillbirth. These pneumonias are associated with birth asphyxia and chorioamnionitis. Neonates with congenital pneumonia demonstrate poor tolerance of labor and are severely depressed at birth. Newborns with congenital pneumonia usually require management in a neonatal ICU and have a low survival rate.

EARLY-ONSET PNEUMONIA IN INFANCY

Pneumonia acquired in the first month of life is usually caused by organisms acquired during transit through the birth canal. Premature infants and those who require ventilatory support or have anomalies such as tracheoesophageal fistulae, choanal atresia, or diaphragmatic hernia are at increased risk for early neonatal lung infections. Prolonged rupture of membranes, prolonged labor, excessive intrauterine manipulations, and foul-smelling amniotic fluid are other risk factors for an early neonatal pneumonia. One study also showed that early neonatal pneumonia was associated with African American ethnicity and was found more often in families of lower socioeconomic status;[32] the mechanism by which race and income influence early neonatal pneumonia is unclear.

Signs of infection in the infant such as lethargy, poor feeding, nasal flaring, grunting, or fever should prompt evaluation for possible pneumonia. In addition to these symptoms, other findings may include hypoxemia, unstable blood glucose, thrombocytopenia, and leukocytosis. Chest x-rays usually demonstrate an infiltrate or streaking that represents early infection. Blood cultures should be done, and a lumbar puncture with cerebrospinal fluid cultures should be performed in children with suspected sepsis. Early administration of antibiotics, oxygen, and fluid to support blood pressure is important to improve survival.

Initial antibiotic therapy is based on the most likely cause of the pneumonia and may be altered once the pathogen is isolated. Organisms causing early neonatal pneumonias include streptococci and gram-negative bacilli, especially *Escherichia coli*. *Chlamydia trachomatis* also may cause an early neonatal pneumonia. Broad-spectrum coverage with ampicillin and an aminoglycoside or a third-generation cephalosporin such as ceftriaxone or cefotaxime provides coverage for most organisms. Dosages are shown in Table 11-13. If a cephalosporin is chosen, coverage with ampicillin is still needed for *Listeria*. If *Chlamydia* infection is suspected, a macrolide should be added to the antibiotic regimen.

Finally, in some newborn nurseries, epidemics of *Staphylococcus* pneumonia have been reported. These instances underscore the importance of good hand washing and isolation of sick infants in nurseries.

LATE-ONSET PNEUMONIA IN INFANCY

After the first few weeks of life, pneumonia is uncommon in infants. Children who contract pneumonia during this period are usually infected with the same organisms that cause infection in adults.

Since infants frequently present with respiratory infections, several criteria that predict the

Table 11-13

Antibiotic Treatment of Pneumonia in Neonates and Infants

Neonates and infants 3 months old:
Ampicillin 200–400 mg/kg/day in 4 doses
  PLUS gentamicin 5 mg/kg/day in 3 doses *OR*
  ceftriaxone 50–100 mg/kg/day in 2 doses
  OR cefotaxime 100–150 mg/kg/day in
  3 doses (200 mg/kg/day if meningitis is
  suspected)

Infants 3 months and older:
Ceftriaxone 50–100 mg/kg/day in 1 or 2 doses
  OR cefotaxime 100–150 mg/kg/day in
  3 doses (200 mg/kg/day if meningitis is
  suspected)

likelihood of pneumonia are useful. In an outpatient study of noninstitutionalized children under 2 months of age, several factors were found that lowered the probability that a child had pneumonia. These included respiratory tract infection in the summer months, absence of cough, a respiratory rate under 60 breaths per minute, presence of normal skin color, the absence of rales or decreased breath sounds, and a white blood count under 19,000/mm^3.[33]

Treatment of infants with pneumonia includes oxygen therapy, fluid support, and ventilatory support if necessary. Antibiotic therapy should be directed at common community-acquired organisms, including *H. influenzae*. Antibiotic coverage with a cephalosporin that provides adequate *H. influenzae* coverage should be given. Because of the risk of sepsis in infants in the first few months of life, most of these children are managed in a hospital setting.

Older Children

Pneumonia in children is similar to that in adults, except that viral infections are more common and the evaluation of sputum is limited because of the inability of many young children to provide adequate sputum specimens. As in adults, most therapy is empiric, and one of the early key decisions is whether to treat the patient in the hospital or as an outpatient.

In older children, as in adults, *S. pneumoniae* and *Mycoplasma* are the most common bacterial causes of pneumonia. With universal administration of *H. influenzae* type B vaccine, cases of *H. influenzae* pneumonia have declined substantially in older children. *S. aureus* should be considered in children with pneumonia associated with influenza.

As noted previously, the evaluation and management of pneumonia in younger children is complicated by the difficulty in obtaining adequate sputum specimens for culture. A recent study of 168 otherwise healthy children between 6 months and 16 years of age showed that in only 43 percent could an etiologic agent be identified despite extensive cultures and serologic testing.[34] In those children in whom a diagnosis could be established, pneumococcal pneumonia (27 percent), *M. pneumoniae* (13 percent), and *C. pneumoniae* (12 percent) were the most common agents. However, it should be noted that the majority of these diagnoses came from matched serologic specimens obtained after convalescence. These investigators did not find that chest x-ray appearance, white blood counts, or blood cultures were useful in predicting the cause.

Unless a blood culture is obtained and is positive, generally treatment should be based on the relative likelihood of the various etiologic agents. In ambulatory children who are only mildly ill, treatment with a broad-spectrum agent that provides coverage for pneumococci and *Mycoplasma*, such as erythromycin or another macrolide, should provide sufficient coverage.

For children who show signs of significant infection such as tachypnea, tachycardia, confusion, or hypoxia, hospitalization may be necessary. Additionally, children at high risk for overwhelming infection or pulmonary compromise, such as those with sickle cell disease, HIV infection, postsplenectomy, leukemia, asthma, cystic fibrosis, or other chronic metabolic diseases, should be carefully managed in a hospital setting. In these children, in addition to a chest x-ray to confirm the diagnosis of pneumonia, blood cultures and possible culture of the cerebrospinal fluid may be advisable to rule out sepsis.

References

1. Areno JP, San Pedro GS, Campbell GD: Diagnosis and prognosis in community-acquired pneumonia: when and where should the patient be treated? *Semin Respir Crit Care Med* 17:231–236, 1997.
2. Bartlett JG, Mundy LM: Community-acquired pneumonia. *N Engl J Med* 333:1618–1624, 1995.
3. Brown PD, Lerner SA: Community-acquired pneumonia. *Lancet* 352:1295–1302, 1998.
4. Houston MS, Silverstein MC, Suman VJ: Community-acquired lower respiratory tract infection in the elderly: a community-based study of incidence and outcome. *J Am Board Fam Pract* 8:247–256, 1995.
5. Sims RV: Bacterial pneumonia in the elderly. *Emerg Med Clin North Am* 8:207–219, 1990.
6. Mufson MA, Oley G, Hughey D: Pneumococcal disease in a medium-sized community in the United States. *JAMA* 248:1486–1489, 1982.
7. LaCroix AZ, Lipson S, Miles TP, White L: Prospective study of pneumonia hospitalizations and mortality of U.S. older people: the role of chronic conditions, health benefits and nutritional status. *Public Health Rep* 104:350–360, 1989.
8. Neiderman MS, Bass JB, Campbell GD Jr, et al: ATS Consensus Committee. Guidelines for the initial management of adults with community-acquired pneumonia: diagnosis, assessment of severity, and initial microbial therapy. *Am Rev Respir Dis* 148:1418–1426, 1993.
9. Harper C, Newton P: Clinical aspects of pneumonia in the elderly veteran. *J Am Geriatr Soc* 37:867–872, 1989.
10. McFadden JP, Price RD, Eastweek HD, et al: Raised respiratory rate in elderly patients: a valuable physical sign. *Br Med J* 1:626–628, 1982.
11. Smith IE, Flower CDR: Review article: imaging in bronchiectasis. *Br J Radiol* 69:589–593, 1996.
12. Hansell DM: Bronchiectasis. *Radiol Clin North Am* 36:107–128, 1998.

13. Levy M, Dromer F, Brion N, et al: Community-acquired pneumonia: importance of initial non-invasive bacteriologic and radiographic investigators. *Chest* 92:43–48, 1988.

14. Sahn SA: Management of complicated parapneumonia effusions. *Am Rev Respir Dis* 148:813–817, 1993.

15. Gleckman R, DeVita J, Hilert D, et al: Sputum gram-stain assessment in community-acquired bacteremic pneumonia. *J Clin Microbiol* 26:846–849, 1988.

16. Chalasani NP, Valdecanas AL, Gopal AK, et al: Clinical utility of blood cultures in adult patients with community-acquired pneumonia without defined underlying risks. *Chest* 108:932–936, 1995.

17. Farr BM, Sloman AJ, Fisch MJ: Predicting death in patients hospitalized for community-acquired pneumonia. *Ann Intern Med* 115:428–436, 1991.

18. Fine MJ, Smith DN, Singer DE: Hospitalization decision in patients with community-acquired pneumonia: a prospective cohort study. *Am J Med* 89:713–721, 1990.

19. Jernigan DB, Cetron MS, Breiman RF: Minimizing the impact of drug-resistant *Streptococcus pneumoniae* (DRSP). *JAMA* 275:206–209, 1996.

20. Mainous AG III, Evans ME, Hueston WJ, et al: Patterns of antibiotic-resistant *Streptococcus pneumoniae* in children in a day-care setting. *J Fam Pract* 46:142–146, 1998.

21. Austin DJ, Kristinsson KG, Anderson RM: The relationship between the volume of antimicrobial consumption in human communities and the frequency of resistance. *Proc Natl Acad Sci U S A* 96:1152–1156, 1999.

22. Deeks SL, Palacio R, Ruvinsky R, et al: Risk factors and course of illness among children with invasive penicillin-resistant *Streptococcus pneumoniae*. The *Streptococcus pneumoniae* Working Group. *Pediatrics* 103:409–413, 1999.

23. Chen DC, McGeer A, de Azavedo JC, et al: Decreased susceptibility of *Streptococcus pneumoniae* to fluoroquinolones in Canada. *N Engl J Med* 341:233–239, 1999.

24. McEachern R, Campbell GD Jr: Hospital-acquired pneumonia: epidemiology, etiology and treatment. *Infect Dis Clin North Am* 12:761–779, 1998.

25. Baughman RP, Tapson V, McIvor A: The diagnosis and treatment challenges in nosocomial pneumonia. *Diagn Microbiol Infect Dis* 33:131–139, 1999.

26. Tablen O, Anderson L, Arden N, et al: Guidelines for the prevention of nosocomial pneumonia. *Am J Infect Control* 22:247–292, 1994.

27. Kloski C, Cage G, Johnson B, et al: Transmission of nosocomial legionnaires' disease. *JAMA* 277:1927–1928, 1997.

28. Kollef MH, Silver P, Murphy DM, Trovillion E: The effect of late-onset ventilator-associated pneumonia in determining patient mortality. *Chest* 108:1655–1662, 1995.

29. Weber DJ, Rutala WA, Mayhall CG: Nosocomial respiratory infections and gram-negative pneumonia, in Elias JA, Fishman JA, Grippi MA, et al (eds): *Fishman's Pulmonary Diseases and Disorders*, 3d ed. New York, McGraw-Hill, 1998; pp. 2213–2233.

30. Niederman MS, Torres A, Summer W: Invasive diagnostic testing is not needed routinely to manage suspected ventilator-associated pneumonia. *Am J Respir Crit Care Med* 150:565–569, 1994.

31. Marks MI, Klein JO: Bacterial infections of the respiratory tract, in Remington JS, Klein JO (eds): *Infectious Diseases of the Fetus and Newborn*. Philadelphia, WB Saunders, 1995; pp. 891–908.

32. Naeye RL, Dellinger WS, Blanc WA: Fetal and maternal features of antenatal bacterial infections. *J Pediatr* 79:733–739, 1971.

33. Losek JD, Kishaba RG, Berens RJ, et al: Indications for chest roentgenogram in the febrile young infant. *Pediatr Emerg Care* 5:149–152, 1989.

34. Wubbel L, Muniz L, Ahmed A, et al: Etiology and treatment of community-acquired pneumonia in ambulatory children. *Pediatr Infect Dis J* 18:98–104, 1999.

Robert Mallin
Edwin A. Brown

Chapter

12

Respiratory Infections in the Immunocompromised Patient

The increasing number of patients with HIV infections, diabetes, and organ transplantation, or who are undergoing treatment for cancer, has made dealing with patients with compromised immune systems an everyday experience in primary care practice. Respiratory infections in immunocompromised patients are more frequent and more severe, and may be caused by organisms that are not usually considered in the care of patients with competent immune defenses. The increased morbidity and mortality from respiratory infections in immunocompromised patients has made it mandatory that primary care physicians understand how to care for these patients. In this chapter we provide a framework for the initial evaluation and treatment of respiratory infections, concentrating on pneumonia, in the patient with an impaired immune system.

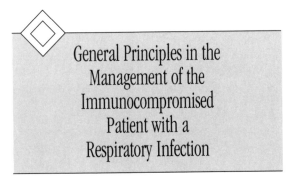

General Principles in the Management of the Immunocompromised Patient with a Respiratory Infection

Although immunocompromised patients can acquire complex infections that are difficult to treat, the initial evaluation and treatment is relatively straightforward. When encountering patients with immunosuppression, clinicians must lower their threshold for considering a lower respiratory infection, requesting invasive diagnostic tests, and initiating broad-spectrum antibiotics. Questions that need to be asked when caring for immunocompromised patients with signs or symptoms of an upper respiratory infection include: (1) How does presentation of

pneumonia differ in the immunocompromised host? (2) What other nonroutine radiographic and laboratory studies should be obtained? (3) What infecting organisms may be involved in addition to the usual community-acquired pathogens? (4) What epidemiologic risk factors need to be considered? (5) What empiric therapy should be initiated, and how does that differ from therapy in a nonimmunocompromised host? and (6) How closely should the patient be followed and what should the clinician watch for?

History

Patients with community-acquired pneumonia and a normal immune system present with complaints of cough, sputum production, fever, rigors, sweats, dyspnea, and chest discomfort that lead the clinician to the diagnosis of a lower respiratory tract infection. Because the presenting symptoms and signs are determined by the host's inflammatory response, the immunocompromised patient is likely to have fewer clinical findings, and those that are present will have diminished intensity (Table 12-1). Therefore, the most important diagnostic tool is awareness—the clinician must consider the diagnosis of pneumonia in the presence of subtle clinical findings. Failure to consider the diagnosis of pneumonia and initiate therapy will lead to the patient's becoming sicker, requiring more intensive medical care, and having a poorer prognosis.

Although the signs and symptoms may be subtle, the rate of their progression may give an important clue to the likely etiology. A rapid onset in hours is more likely in a bacterial infection, while a course of days to weeks is more typical of a mycobacterial or fungal infection. Additionally, less specific symptoms such as malaise, fatigue, and anorexia may provide clinical clues that the patient has a chronic respiratory tract infection.

Table 12-1

Immunocompromising Conditions

Alcoholism—neutrophil dysfunction
Autoimmune disorders—T-cell dysfunction
Cancer chemotherapy—neutropenia, B- and
   T-cell dysfunction
Lymphoproliferative disorders—neutropenia,
   B- and T-cell dysfunction
Diabetes—neutrophil dysfunction
Geriatric—B- and T-cell dysfunction
HIV/AIDS—B- and T-cell dysfunction
Corticosteroids—T-cell dysfunction
Renal failure/hepatic failure—neutrophil
   dysfunction
Solid organ transplants—T-cell dysfunction
Bone marrow transplant—neutropenia, B- and
   T-cell dysfunction

Physical Examination

Physical examination findings may be diminished in the immunocompromised patient as a result of the patient's impaired inflammatory response. Fever is often present, but not always. In neutropenic patients with pneumonia, cough may not be present in up to 30 percent of patients, and sputum production may be absent in over 90 percent of cases.[1] Neurologic deficits may reflect disseminated infection. Skin lesions that may not appear initially to be significant may be due to opportunistic fungal infections, so new dermatologic findings should always be thoroughly investigated. Ecthyma gangrenosum, a skin lesion with a necrotic central ulcer surrounded by a rim of erythema, may be seen with *Pseudomonas aeruginosa* or other gram-negative infections. Necrotic lesions in the oropharynx may be caused by *P. aeruginosa* or filamentous fungi. Mouth and throat ulcers are seen with viral and *Histoplasma capsulatum* infections.[2]

Laboratory and Imaging Evaluations

Once the diagnosis of pneumonia is considered in an immunocompromised patient, the diagnostic studies listed in Table 12-2 should be performed in the initial work-up of pneumonia. An algorithm for evaluating the results from these studies is presented in Fig. 12-1. As for any algorithm, changes in diagnostic studies and patient management are appropriate depending on the clinical presentation, the patient population, and the technical competence of the laboratory.

SPUTUM STUDIES

The evaluation of the immunocompromised patient is often more extensive than that of an immunocompetent patient with a similar infection. For example, community-acquired pneumonia protocols used at many hospitals suggest that sputum Gram stain and culture are not useful in the diagnosis of pneumonia, mostly because of the difficulty of obtaining sputum and the low yield of sputum cultures. This does not hold true for the immunosuppressed patient because atypical organisms can be detected on sputum Gram stain and culture. For this reason, sputum studies may be of great significance in

Table 12-2

Diagnostic Studies for Immunocompromised Patients with Pneumonia

History and physical examination
CBC with differential
PA and lateral chest radiographs
Electrolytes, liver function tests, BUN,
   creatinine, serum glucose
Arterial blood gas
Sputum for Gram stain and culture
Blood cultures X 2

ABBREVIATIONS: CBC, complete blood count; PA, posteroanterior; BUN, blood urea nitrogen.

Figure 12-1

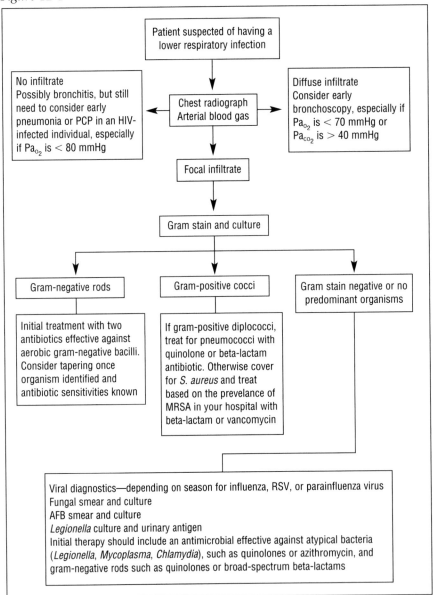

ABBREVIATIONS: PCP, *Pneumocystis carinii* pneumonia; HIV, human immunodeficiency virus; MRSA, medication-resistant *Staphylococcus aureus*; AFB, acid-fast bacillus.

directing therapy and suggesting additional evaluation.

In the immunocompromised patient, the usual rules regarding the adequacy of the specimen [i.e., >10 polymorphonuclear leukocytes per high-power field (PMN/HPF)] may not apply, since neutropenic patients often may not produce sufficient white blood cells (WBCs) to fulfill this criterion. If an organism is identified, the question will arise, "Is it a causative agent or a colonized organism?" This can be difficult to answer, but the following pathogens are always considered indicative of disease: *Mycobacterium tuberculosis, Legionella,* and dimorphic fungi (*H. capsulatum, Blastomyces dermatitidis,* and *Coccidioides immitis*).[2] If uncertainty persists as to the etiology of the pneumonia or if sputum for diagnostic studies cannot be obtained, an invasive procedure such as bronchoscopy or percutaneous lung biopsy may be necessary.

BLOOD GAS

Arterial blood gases are helpful in guiding patient management. If a patient is in minimal distress with an arterial $P_{O_2} > 90$ mmHg and the clinician is certain of the pathogen, outpatient management may be considered. In contrast, a similar patient with a $Pa_{O_2} < 70$ mmHg or an $Pa_{CO_2} > 40$ mmHg should be admitted to the hospital. Since antibiotics, even if appropriate for the infecting organism, may take days to have an effect, the patient's respiratory and functional status will continue to decline. Close in-hospital supervision is necessary to watch for complications of respiratory distress.

IMAGING STUDIES

Chest radiographs, although helpful in making the diagnosis of pneumonia, often underestimate the extent of disease. For example, *Pneumocystis carinii* pneumonia may present with a clear chest radiograph in a severely hypoxic immunocompromised human immunodeficiency virus (HIV)-infected patient with extensive infection. Although the radiographic presentation may be helpful in suggesting a pathogen (Table 12-3), causes of pneumonia cannot be determined reliably based on radiographic presentation. Computed tomography (CT) scans of the chest may demonstrate nodules or cavities or show the full extent of disease and

Table 12-3

Differential Diagnosis Based on Radiographic Appearance

Consolidation
  Bacterial pneumonia
  Streptococcus pneumoniae
  Enterobacteriaceae
  Pseudomonas aeruginosa
  Staphylococcus aureus
  Legionella pneumophila
  Fungal
  Nocardial
  Tuberculous
Peribronchovascular
  Viral
  Pneumocystis carinii
Nodular
  Fungal
  Nocardial
  Tuberculous
Cavitary lesions
  Fungi
  Nocardia
  Gram-negative bacteria—*Klebsiella* and *Pseudomonas*
  S. aureus

should be considered, especially if fungal pathogens are in the differential.

BLOOD CULTURES

Blood cultures often are positive in the immunosuppressed patient. As many as 30 percent of blood cultures are positive in immunocompromised patients with pneumonia, compared to 11 percent in the immunocompetent patient.[3] Positive blood cultures provide clear evidence of the infecting pathogen. Some organisms such as fungi, mycobacteria, *Mycoplasma,* and *Nocardia* are less readily detected in blood cultures, so negative blood cultures are not helpful in diagnosing these pathogens. Pleural aspirates, urine cultures, and stool cultures may add to the ability to find the causative organism.

Role of Risk Profiling in Selecting Initial Treatment

Often, the classic presentations of infectious agents are not seen in immunocompromised patients. Thus, the patient's risk factors and underlying disease process are important in helping make the diagnosis and suggesting the underlying pathogen (Table 12-4). Most important, determining what components of the patient's immune system are not functioning is very helpful in deciding what organisms must be considered in the differential diagnosis. It also should be emphasized that while Table 12-4 provides information on common opportunistic infections, common respiratory pathogens are still common in immunocompromised patients.

The first step in the evaluation of an immunocompromised patient with pneumonia is to assess what epidemiologic risk factors are present and how they alter the likelihood of specific infectious agents in the particular patient. Some risk factors that should be considered are listed in Table 12-5. These include the time of the year; recent hospitalization; geographic location, including previous places the patient has lived; travel to other areas; infectious agents existing in the community; hobbies; contact with others that may be ill; medication changes (including immunosuppressive drugs); and vaccination history. These questions are in addition to the usual

Table 12-4

Infectious Respiratory Agents in Patients with Immunosuppression

Bacteria	Fungi	Viruses	Parasites
A. Patients with Impaired Cell-Mediated Immunity			
Common organisms			
Mycobacterium tuberculosis	Cryptococcus neoformans	Adenovirus	Pneumocystis carinii
Legionella spp.	Histoplasma capsulatum	Respiratory syncytial virus	
Nocardia spp.	Coccidioides immitis	Parainfluenza virus	
	Aspergillus spp.	Influenza	
Uncommon causes			
Mycobacterium avium complex	Candida spp.	Cytomegalovirus	Toxoplasma gondii
		Herpes simplex	Strongyloides stercoralis
		Varicella zoster	
B. Patients with Neutropenia			
Staphylococcus aureus	Aspergillus spp.		
Escherichia coli			
Pseudomonas aeruginosa			
Klebsiella pneumoniae			
Enterobacter spp.			
C. Patients with Impaired Humoral Immunity—Complement Defects or Hypogammaglobulinemia			
Streptococcus pneumoniae			
Haemophilus influenzae			

Table 12-5

Epidemiologic Risk Factors for Lower Respiratory Infections

RISK FACTOR	CONSEQUENCE
Recent hospitalization	Gram-negative bacilli
Intravascular catheters	*Staphylococcus aureus* infection
Community outbreaks	Viral pneumonia, especially influenza and RSV
Splenectomy or functional hyposplenism	Increased severity of infections with encapsulated organisms
Winter to spring	Respiratory syncytial virus and influenza virus epidemics
Spring and fall	Parainfluenza virus outbreaks
Previous exposure to tuberculosis	Reactivation of *Mycobacterium tuberculosis*
Place of residence, travel history	Endemic fungi—histoplasmosis, coccidioidomycosis
Residence in a nursing home or long term care facility	Enteric gram-negative bacilli, *Streptococcus pneumoniae*, tuberculosis
Recent antibiotic therapy	Drug-resistant pneumococci, gram-negative bacilli, *Pseudomonas aeruginosa*
Influenza epidemic	Influenza, *S. pneumoniae*, *S. aureus*, *Haemophilus influenzae*

ABBREVIATION: RSV, respiratory syncytial virus.

social history of smoking, drinking, illicit drug use, occupation, etc.

Treatment

When considering antibiotics options, the clinician should consider the most likely organisms given the patient's underlying immunosuppression and exposure history, how ill the patient is, and the results of the initial diagnostic work-up, if available. As noted previously, the sicker the patient and the greater the uncertainty of the diagnosis, the broader the therapy and the more invasive the diagnostic evaluation should be. Although the antimicrobial therapy suggested in Fig. 12-1 can be used as a guideline, only the physician at the patient's bedside can decide if more or less aggressive therapy is indicated. Antibiotic regimens used in community-acquired pneumonia protocols should be disregarded, as they cannot effectively be applied to immunocompromised patients.

Suggestions for empiric antibiotic treatment are provided in Table 12-6. A critical concept to consider is that therapeutic success is dependent on selection of initial antimicrobial therapy to which the pathogen is sensitive. Modification of therapy days into the illness based on clinical course or diagnostic test may not improve clinical outcome.

Many immunocompetent patients with community-acquired pneumonia can and should be managed as outpatients. Because these patients are healthier, recovery is still possible even if there are errors in diagnosis and initial treatment, assuming that close follow-up is provided. This option often is not available for immunocompromised patients with pneumonia. Initial diagnostic cultures indicating the need for changes in therapy may not return for 2 or more days, at which point the patient may be severely ill. After appropriate therapy is initiated, a clinical response may take days, during which the patient's condition can deteriorate significantly.

Table 12-6

Empiric Antimicrobial Treatment Recommendations in Immunocompromised Hosts When Bacterial Pneumonia Is Suspected but the Etiologic Agent Is Unknown

SETTING/RISK FACTOR	ANTIMICROBIAL THERAPY
Outpatient	Fluoroquinolone*
Inpatient	Fluoroquinolone* or macrolide[†] + extended-spectrum cephalosporin[‡]
Intensive care unit	Fluoroquinolone* + extended-spectrum cephalosporin[‡]
Aspiration	Fluoroquinolone* + clindamycin or metronidazole or piperacillin-tazobactam alone
Increased risk for *Pseudomonas aeruginosa*	Antipseudomonal beta-lactam[§] plus ciprofloxacin (if allergic, replace beta-lactam with aztreonam and aminoglycoside)

*Gatifloxacin, levofloxacin, or moxifloxacin.
[†]Azithromycin or clarithromycin.
[‡]Cefotaxime or ceftriaxone.
[§]Cefepime, imipenem, or meropenem.

The sicker or more immunosuppressed the patient is, the less time the clinician has to make the correct diagnosis and initiate appropriate therapy. Consequently, the sicker the patient, the faster and more extensive the diagnostic work-up and the broader the empiric antimicrobial coverage must be. On the other hand, broad-spectrum coverage using multiple antimicrobial agents increases the chances of drug-related side effects and encourages the proliferation of antimicrobial-resistant organisms. These resistant organisms may cause difficult-to-treat superinfections in the immunocompromised host or be spread by health care workers to other patients, increasing the cost of health care to the patient and society. However, when caring for immunosuppressed patients, erring on the side of caution when making decisions regarding hospital admission, antimicrobial use, and diagnostic testing is appropriate.

If the patient does not improve, the following factors must be considered: Was the diagnosis correct? Instead of pneumonia, does the patient have congestive heart failure, cancer (metastatic or lung primary), or a pulmonary embolism? Are the correct pathogens being treated? Consider drug-resistant organisms, nonbacterial pathogens (viral or fungal), mycobacteria, or *Nocardia*. Has the correct drug and dose been chosen? Are there host factors delaying response to therapy? Look for obstruction, superinfection, or empyema.[4]

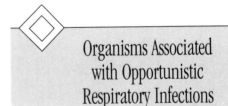

Organisms Associated with Opportunistic Respiratory Infections

Viruses

The presenting symptoms in viral pneumonia are often nonspecific and of little help in determining the etiology of the infection. The physical examination in viral pneumonia is often significant for fever, increased respiratory rate, and, on pulmonary examination, the presence of diffuse rales and wheezes. Chest radiographs in viral pneumonia typically demonstrate bilateral interstitial or patch infiltrates and thus are not useful in differentiating between different viral pathogens. The overall presentation, however, may suggest a viral process.

INFLUENZA

Influenza is a common respiratory virus infection in immunocompromised patients, with outbreaks occurring most often in the winter months. Patients may present with fever, sore throat, headache, dry cough, and myalgias. The symptoms of influenza infection may be blunted by the immunocompromised state, but the morbidity and mortality of infection are increased. Prevention of influenza infection by yearly vaccination should be attempted in all immunocompromised patients, although the protection afforded by vaccination is decreased in such patients. Chemoprophylaxis with antiviral drugs can be initiated during outbreaks to provide some protection against infection.

The diagnosis can be made clinically if influenza is present in the community and patients have a typical presentation, or diagnostic assays such as rapid antigen detection or the slower culture may be used. If patients develop influenza, the use of antiviral agents such as amantadine, rimantadine, or oseltamivir within 48 h of initial symptoms may significantly reduce the consequences of influenza. Patients may need hospitalization depending on respiratory status. All immunocompromised patients must be closely followed for the development of bacterial superinfection.

RESPIRATORY SYNCYTIAL VIRUS

After influenza, respiratory syncytial virus (RSV) is the second most common cause of viral pneumonia in the elderly and is a common although underappreciated cause of pneumonia in other immunocompromised patients. Infection with RSV occurs during the winter months and is associated with outbreaks in health care facilities, especially nursing homes. Symptoms include fever, cough without sputum production, and dyspnea. The diagnosis can be made with antigen detection assays or by enzyme immunoassay (EIA) with respectable sensitivity and specificity.

Treatment is supportive, although there is significant debate as to the merits of ribavirin or anti-RSV immunoglobulin preparations. Treatment with these agents should not be undertaken without consultation with physicians experienced in the treatment of RSV.

PARAINFLUENZA VIRUS

Parainfluenza virus infection in the immunocompetent host is mostly an annoyance, but it can result in life-threatening pneumonia in the immunocompromised host. Symptoms include fever, cough, dyspnea, and coryza. The diagnosis is best achieved by immunofluorescent antigen assays, as rapid culture and serologic assays are not available. Like that of RSV, treatment of parainfluenza virus is usually supportive, but patients with severe disease should quickly be referred to a center experienced in treatment of this infection.

HERPES SIMPLEX VIRUS

Viral pneumonia caused by herpes simplex virus (HSV) or varicella zoster virus (VZV) can be a devastating disease in both immunocompetent and immunocompromised hosts.[5] Symptoms include fever, cough, dyspnea, wheezing, chest pain, and hemoptysis. Cutaneous or oral lesions may be present, although the pneumonia is the result of disseminated disease and not of the spread of cutaneous infection. In VZV pneumonia, the pulmonary findings correlate with the severity of the rash. Unlike viral pneumonia from other causes, HSV/VZV pneumonia may start as a focal process, then spread into diffuse infiltrates. Mortality is high, and infection must be treated aggressively with intravenous acyclovir.

CYTOMEGALOVIRUS

Cytomegalovirus (CMV) is a common pathogen in organ transplant recipients, particularly those who have had a bone marrow, lung, or heart transplant. Lung involvement has the highest mortality and is associated with increased immunosuppression or with transplantation of CMV-colonized tissue into a seronegative recipient. Symptoms are often subacute, with a nonproductive cough, fever, and malaise.

The diagnosis can be made using CMV antigen assays but may require bronchoscopy with biopsy. When inclusion bodies suggestive of CMV infection are found only on bronchoalveolar lavage, it is difficult to be sure of the significance because CMV may be found on bronchoalveolar lavage without disease or in the presence of other pathogens. When CMV pneumonia is suspected, quick referral to an experienced center is indicated because of the high morbidity and mortality associated with this infection.

Chlamydia and Mycoplasma

Chlamydia and *Mycoplasma* are common causes of community-acquired pneumonia. Typically they present with cough, fever, headache, and minimal physical examination abnormalities, but significant radiographic findings of pneumonia. The onset of infection may be insidious and recovery prolonged. Illness can be severe in the immunocompromised host. The diagnosis is made based on clinical criteria, but can be helped by the judicious use of laboratory tests, including serologic testing for *Mycoplasma.* Serologic studies are not available on-site at most institutions and are not useful in the acute care of the patient.

Treatment of these infections in the immunocompromised patient should include a fluoroquinolone active against atypical pathogens or a newer macrolide such as azithromycin or clarith-romycin. Caution is necessary when using macrolides in the transplant population, since these drugs alter the metabolism of cyclosporine. Cyclosporine levels must be monitored when macrolides are used.

Bacteria

GRAM-NEGATIVE BACILLI (GNB)

In the normal host, the bacterial flora of the oropharynx is predominantly gram-positive, whereas the oropharynx of the immunocompromised host is frequently colonized with Enterobacteriaceae (*Klebsiella pneumoniae, Enterobacter* spp., and *Escherichia coli*), *P. aeruginosa*, and gram-negative organisms. Alteration in the surface characteristics of the mucosal epithelium in the immunosuppressed host facilitates the attachment of these pathogens. As aspiration of oral-pharyngeal secretions is the first step in developing pneumonia, the alteration in mucosal colonization is important in the pathogenesis of gram-negative bacillary pneumonia. A decrease in stomach acidity also facilitates colonization with gram-negative bacilli.

Typically patients with GNB pneumonia present with significant fever, cough productive of purulent sputum, and a chest radiograph showing a broncho- or lobar pneumonia pattern. While the chest radiograph is useful in diagnosis, it is less helpful in following recovery, as the radiographic findings lag behind clinical improvement. Sputum Gram stain often makes the diagnosis.

Treatment success is dependent on the patient's receiving effective antimicrobials as initial therapy. Because many of the gram-negative pathogens are highly resistant to multiple classes of antibiotics, therapy should be initiated with two antibiotics effective according to local resistance patterns against GNB. Often, a quinolone and a beta-lactam antibiotic given intravenously will be effective against most organisms.

Every immunocompromised patient with a suspected GNB pneumonia should be hospitalized. As the patient improves and bacterial antibiotic sensitivities are known, therapy may be tapered to a single agent. The optimal duration of antibiotic therapy is unknown for many infections, but generally the treatment duration in GNB pneumonia is a minimum of 14 days, with a 21-day course often being appropriate for patients with severe infections. HIV-infected patients with *P. aeruginosa* pneumonia may require more prolonged therapy and often never clear the pathogen. A similar problem exists in patients with cystic fibrosis, who may require frequent courses of intravenous antibiotics to decrease the bacterial load in their respiratory tract.

GRAM-POSITIVE COCCI

Gram-positive cocci, especially *Streptococcus pneumoniae* and *Staphylococcus aureus*, are common causes of pneumonia. The Gram stain may be useful in determining if these organisms are present in the sputum of the patient with pneumonia. A good microbiology technician will often be able to discriminate between the sheets of diplococci from pneumococcus and the clusters of a staphylococcus. Since pneumococcus may not be seen in culture, the Gram stain should be evidence enough of a pneumococcal infection even if the sputum culture returns no growth or "oral flora." Although classically pneumococcus has a lobar pattern and *S. aureus* has a nodular pattern on chest radiograph, any presentation is possible. Thus, chest radiograph is helpful in making a diagnosis of pneumonia but not helpful in determining the pathogen in gram-positive cocci pneumonia.

Appropriate treatment of pneumococcal pneumonia is unclear at this time because breakpoints for antibiotic sensitivity and resistance will soon be revised. If an institution has a high percentage of penicillin-resistant pneumococcus, initial treatment with a third-generation cephalosporin plus vancomycin is appropriate until bacterial sensitivities are known. Other treatment options include fluoroquinolones, third-generation cephalosporins, or macrolides.

For *S. aureus*, treatment with a beta-lactamase-resistant penicillin (e.g., nafcillin) is appropriate unless there is a high percentage of methicillin-resistant *S. aureus* (MRSA) in the community, or in the hospital if the patient was recently hospitalized. In this case, vancomycin should be used until sensitivities are known. A note of caution when using vancomycin for treatment of *S. aureus* infections: vancomycin does not appear to be as effective as a beta-lactam in treating non-methicillin-resistant *S. aureus*, so it should not be substituted solely for convenience of administration in the treatment of *S. aureus* pneumonia. The overuse of vancomycin also leads to increased incidence of vancomycin-resistant enterococci. The role of newer agents such as linezolid and quinupristin-dalfopristin for treatment of *S. aureus* pneumonia is still not clear.

LEGIONELLA

The incidence of *Legionella* pneumonia seems highly dependent on geographic location. Some institutions seldom diagnose *Legionella* pneumonia, whereas it is endemic in others. One explanation for this difference is how frequently clinicians consider this organism in their differential diagnosis and the ability of the laboratory to detect *Legionella*. Patients present with fever and a productive cough. The original suggestion that *Legionella* pneumonia is associated with gastrointestinal symptoms has not been substantiated in further studies.

Chest radiographs of patients with *Legionella* pneumonia may have interstitial, lobar, or nodular infiltrates. The Gram stain is negative in *Legionella* disease. The diagnosis can be made by *Legionella* urinary antigen, special *Legionella* cultures, and, if bronchoscopy is performed, direct fluorescent antibody (DFA) staining of bronchial secretions. Either a macrolide or a quinolone is effective against *Legionella*. Tetracyclines are alternative agents, but beta-lactams are not effective. The duration of treatment should be 14 to 21 days.

MYCOBACTERIA

Mycobacterium tuberculosis pneumonia still presents as a surprise to many clinicians. Patients often present with a chronic cough productive of purulent sputum, fever, night sweats, and weight loss, but commonly tuberculosis (TB) is not considered in the initial differential diagnosis of pneumonia. This leads to placing the patient in a hospital room without negative-pressure ventilation and exposing other patients and staff to the TB organism.

Typically *M. tuberculosis* pneumonia in immunocompromised patients is a reactivation disease; the tubercular bacilli have been inactive for years, then break through after immunosuppression. Thus, *M. tuberculosis* pneumonia is often a preventable disease if a history of tuberculous exposure is obtained and tuberculin skin testing and prophylactic therapy are used prior to beginning immunosuppression. Prophylaxis with 6 months of isoniazid is 75 percent effective in preventing reactivation during the lifetime of the patient.

If all patients presented with typical symptoms, the clinical diagnosis would not be difficult. Instead, patients may present with fever, cough, or weight loss and are not diagnosed with tuberculosis until the organism has spread to hospital staff and others. The chest radiograph classically shows a cavitary lesion, but immunosuppression may inhibit granuloma and cavity formation. If the immunocompromised patient is at high risk and has any findings consistent with tuberculosis, the patient should be presumed to have tuberculosis and should be placed in respiratory isolation until acid-fast bacillus (AFB) smears document the absence of mycobacteria.

Since isoniazid resistance is common in many areas of the country and therapy with less than two effective antitubercular drugs will quickly lead to the development of resistance, patients usually are started on four-drug therapy. Isoniazid, rifampin, ethambutol, and pyrazinamide are used for 2 months; then, after sensitivities are known, therapy is changed to two effective drugs for an additional period of time depending on which drugs are used. Rifabutin should be substituted for rifampin in patients receiving protease inhibitor therapy for HIV infection. Directly observed therapy by the local health department is very effective.

Mycoses

NOCARDIA

Nocardia are fungal organisms that are ubiquitous in the environment and that occasionally cause pneumonia in immunosuppressed hosts. The organism is inhaled, and when cell-mediated immunity and/or neutrophil function is depressed, the organism proliferates. Patients present with fever, malaise, cough, and dyspnea. *Nocardia* often disseminate to the central nervous system, skin, or bone.

Sputum staining is often positive for grampositive branching filamentous rods. The organism is differentiated from actinomyces by its growth in aerobic conditions and staining acid-fast using a modified Kinyoun stain. Chest radiographs may demonstrate lobar infiltrates or the presence of single or multiple nodules with or without cavity formation. Diagnostic serology is not available, so the diagnosis is made by isolation of the organism in culture.

Treatment is usually initiated with intravenous trimethoprim-sulfamethoxazole (TMP-SMX), changing to an oral formulation after the patient is stabilized. Patients should complete a 6- to 12-month course of therapy. Speciation and susceptibility testing often are useful in making treatment decisions, as patients may be intolerant of long-term sulfa drug therapy.

ASPERGILLUS

Clinical findings of *Aspergillus* pneumonia are often nonspecific. *Aspergillus* pulmonary infections may present with pleuritic chest pain and hemoptysis, with nodular, cavitary, or interstitial infiltrates on chest radiographs. One clue to a fungal infection, however, is that the patient's fever does not respond to antibiotic therapy.

The organism may be isolated from sputum or bronchial secretions. Although a single isolate of an aspergillus species is commonly ignored in an immunocompetent host, isolation of *Aspergillus* in the granulocytopenic or immunosuppressed host is significant and should prompt a thorough examination of the chest. CT scanning of the chest often shows more extensive disease, nodules, cavities, and halo signs not seen by chest radiographs. The presence of radiographic findings mandates the institution of appropriate therapy.

Other Fungi

The endemic and opportunistic fungi are not infrequent causes of pneumonia in immunosuppressed patients. Diagnosis of deep-seated fungal infection mandates decreasing immunosuppression to the lowest possible level. Reactivation of endemic fungi, such as histoplasmosis, coccidioidomycosis, and cryptococcus, may occur in less immunocompromised hosts, while *Aspergillus* and *Mucor* more often occur in highly immunosuppressed patients. *Candida* species, although commonly isolated from skin, mucous membranes, respiratory secretions, and blood, should not be considered a cause of pneumonia in the immunocompromised host.

CRYPTOCOCCAL PNEUMONIA

Cryptococcal pneumonia often goes unnoticed. Chest radiographs may demonstrate localized or nodular infiltrate. Diagnosis can be made by isolating the organism from sputum or detect-ing cryptococcal antigen in blood. Immunosuppressed patients diagnosed with cryptococcal pneumonia should undergo lumbar puncture to test for the presence of cryptococcal meningitis by antigen assays.

HISTOPLASMOSIS

Histoplasmosis is disseminated at diagnosis in most immunosuppressed patients. Clinically, patients complain of fever, cough, weight loss, and malaise. On chest radiographs, histoplasmosis appears as diffuse or miliary infiltrates. On physical examination, hepatosplenomegaly may be found. A careful history looking for residence or travel in areas of endemic histoplasmosis (Mississippi River valley) is important in making the diagnosis of pulmonary histoplasmosis. Once suggested by history and clinical presentation, the diagnosis can be confirmed by isolating the organism or by detection of histoplasma antigen in blood or urine. Current guidelines suggest that amphotericin B should be used as initial therapy. Itraconazole is an alternative agent but must be used with caution because it interacts with multiple other medications, including cyclosporine.

COCCIDIOIDOMYCOSIS

Coccidioidomycosis is endemic in the southwest United States. Infection in immunocompromised hosts is often caused by reactivation of old foci of infection. Thus, as with histoplasmosis, an exposure history is important in making the diagnosis. Diagnosis is made by the histology showing the presence of the organism or culture. Serologic tests may also be useful.

TREATMENT OF FUNGAL PNEUMONIA

Treatment of aspergillus or any fungal pneumonia should be undertaken in consultation with an experienced specialist. Pulmonary mucormycosis is clinically similar to aspergillosis but is more commonly involved in rhinocerebral infections. Patients present with nasal discharge, proptosis, and ophthalmoplegia. Any suggestion of rhinocerebral mucor in an immunocompromised patient or in a diabetic patient in diabetic ketoacidosis should prompt diagnostic scanning by CT or magnetic resonance imaging (MRI) and consultation with an otolaryngologist for diagnostic specimens and, if mucor is present, wide debridement of infected tissues. Aggressive treatment with amphotericin B is indicated.

Other Organisms

PNEUMOCYSTIS CARINII

Pneumocystis carinii is a pathogen made infamous by the acquired immunodeficiency syndrome (AIDS) epidemic. The increased number of cases of *P. carinii* pneumonia (PCP) taught clinicians about its presentation and encouraged the development of treatment and prevention strategies. Most high-risk transplant or HIV-infected patients are now placed on PCP prophylaxis, usually TMP-SMX, which is very effective at preventing disease.

Patients with PCP present with fever, nonproductive cough, and dyspnea on exertion. Sputum, when induced, is usually clear; the presence of purulent sputum argues against the diagnosis of PCP. Classically, the chest radiograph shows bilateral interstitial infiltrates, but nodular infiltrates or a clear chest radiograph are sometimes seen.

An alveolar blood gas (ABG) is especially helpful in determining the prognosis in these patients. While an ABG in almost every patient with PCP pneumonia will show hypoxia and an arterial-alveolar (A-a) gradient, those with a high A-a gradient or a Pa_{O_2} less than 70 mmHg are at highest risk of respiratory compromise. Respiratory function in most patients will continue to decline for the first 3 to 5 days of therapy. While the diagnosis can be made clinically, patients often require a bronchoalveolar lavage for definitive diagnosis.

Treatment of PCP pneumonia is usually initiated with TMP-SMX, with the most common significant side effects being rash and neutropenia. Multiple other regimens are available, including intravenous pentamidine and dapsone-TMP. Treatment should be continued for 21 days.

STRONGYLOIDES

Strongyloides stercoralis is a nematode that lives in the soil in warm areas. In most cases, the organism is acquired through skin contact with the infective larvae in the soil. In addition, transmission of larvae from the feces of infected individuals to others can occur. In temperate areas, fecal-oral transmission is the more common mode of infection.

Strongyloides is of concern to immunosuppressed patients because its life cycle allows for chronic asymptomatic colonization after exposure. With immunosuppression, a hyperinfection syndrome with systemic invasion may occur. Individuals at highest risk for *Strongyloides* infection include those on chronic corticosteroids, renal transplantation recipients, patients with Hodgkin's disease and other lymphomas, and patients with leukemia.

The history in these patients is usually not helpful in identifying *Strongyloides* as the causative agent. Clinically, patients have pneumonitis with bronchospasm, possibly central nervous system (CNS) involvement, polymicrobial bloodstream infections with gut organisms carried by the nematode, and transient rashes or skin lesions. Symptoms of pulmonary involvement include fever, dyspnea, productive cough, and hemoptysis. The expected findings of eosinophilia may not be found in the immunocompromised host. Chest radiographs show diffuse bilateral infiltrates that may progress to consolidation and cavity formation. The diagnosis can be made by demonstrating the filariform larvae in stools or sputum. However, negative stool examinations do not rule out the disease.

Treatment is with ivermectin or thiabendazole for 2 to 7 days, although longer treatment may be necessary to clear involved tissues of larvae. Often, pneumonia may be refractory or recurrent. Mortality with disseminated infection is high.

Caring for Patients with Specific Types of Immune Deficiencies

Approach to the Elderly Patient with Pneumonia

Pneumonia is still the leading infectious cause of death in the elderly. Decreases in immune function occur with age as a result of the loss of thymus-mediated T-cell differentiation and function, and a diminution of the humoral response to vaccines. Although there is a loss of both cell-mediated and humoral competence with age, it does not progress to such a level that one sees the onset of infections, such as *P. carinii* pneumonia, that are normally noted with significant immune disease.

In the immunocompetent patient, pneumonia typically presents with fever and productive cough, and often with pleuritic chest pain. It is accompanied by physical findings such as rales and signs of consolidation that are found in areas of radiographic abnormality.[6] In the elderly, many if not all of these findings may be absent.[7] Elderly patients with pneumonia may present with a change in mental status as a symptom. Dyspnea or tachypnea may replace cough as the most prominent sign, and delirium is often present. The physical findings associated with pneumonia are often lacking in the elderly patient, and signs of lobar consolidation are typically absent. As fever is often absent, tachypnea

and tachycardia are often the most sensitive, if nonspecific, signs.[8]

Although commonly believed, there is little evidence to support the notion that leukocytosis is blunted or absent in most cases of geriatric pneumonia. At least two-thirds of older patients will mount an increased white blood cell count in response to a pulmonary infection. A depressed neutrophil count in the face of serious infection in the elderly is a poor prognostic sign, just as it is in other populations.[9]

Chest radiograph results will usually reveal an infiltrate, but the initial study may be negative, with an infiltrate evident only after hospitalization and hydration.[10] A high degree of awareness of the prevalence of pneumonia in older patients coupled with a willingness to obtain a chest radiograph in the absence of physical findings is often necessary to make the diagnosis.

The etiology of pneumonia in the elderly can be divided into that acquired in the community and that acquired in the nursing home or another institution (Tables 12-7 and 12-8). Institutionally acquired pneumonia has a case fatality rate of 50 percent. Chronic disease, altered mental status, and problems with aspiration all contribute to the high mortality rate.[11] Management of these patients begins with accurate diagnosis and, if possible, isolation of the organism. Sputum studies are useful when they yield a clear causative organism; when that is absent, empiric treatment must be considered. Table 12-2

Table 12-7

Community-Acquired Pneumonia in Elderly

PATHOGEN	FREQUENCY
Streptococcus pneumoniae	35–70%
Gram-negative bacilli	5–30%
Haemophilus influenzae	5–20%
Legionella pneumophila	0–30%
Staphylococcus aureus	2–10%

Table 12-8

Institutionally Acquired Pneumonia in Elderly

PATHOGEN	FREQUENCY
Gram-negative bacilli	40–50%
Klebsiella pneumoniae	14%
Pseudomonas aeruginosa	10–15%
Enterobacter spp.	6–10%
Escherichia coli	6–9%
Serratia marcescens	4–6%
Proteus spp.	4–6%
Gram-positive cocci	13–33%
Streptococcus pneumoniae	10–20%
Staphylococcus aureus	3–13%
Legionella pneumophila	0–15%

suggests diagnostic studies useful in the management of pneumonia in the geriatric patient.

In the geriatric population, patients who are in otherwise good health, without risk factors such as diabetes, coronary artery disease, chronic pulmonary disease, neurologic disease, or dementia, and who have no hypoxia associated with their pneumonia may be considered for treatment as outpatients. However, close follow-up and home supervision are usually required.

Empiric antibiotic treatment must be initiated when the causative organism is not known. When treating community-acquired pneumonia, coverage for *S. pneumoniae, Haemophilus influenzae,* and gram-negative bacilli should be included. Adding coverage for *Legionella pneumophila* and *S. aureus* should be considered for patients residing in institutional settings. In all elderly individuals, but especially in patients with cognitive disturbances, aspiration is a common cause of nosocomial-like pneumonia, and coverage for gram-negative bacilli, aerobic gram-positive organisms, and some anaerobic organisms is appropriate. Adequate respiratory support and fluid and electrolyte management are of course important. Nutritional assessment and early nutritional support may be essential.

Approach to the Cancer Patient with Pneumonia

In patients undergoing chemotherapy, neutropenia is common and places the patient at greater risk of opportunistic infections. Neutropenia is defined as an absolute neutrophil count of less than $1000/mm^3$. In the neutropenic patient with a fever, the lung and oropharynx account for 50 percent of infections. Nose and sinus infections account for another 5 percent.[12] Consequently, respiratory infections should always be considered when a cancer patient with neutropenia has a febrile illness.

Fever is a common presenting sign of infection in neutropenic patients. In patients with leukemia, fever may be mistakenly assumed to be caused by the underlying disease process. Typical signs of respiratory infections, such as a cough and/or purulent sputum, may not be present. A chest radiograph may not show an infiltrate even with pneumonia. Additional radiographs of the sinuses should be performed if facial tenderness or swelling is present. There should be a low threshold for obtaining CT scans of the chest or sinuses to document the extent of infection or the presence of cavities, findings that are often missed with plain radiographs. In patients with very low neutrophil counts, i.e., under $500/mm^3$, empiric use of broad-spectrum antibiotics is warranted even if no signs of infection are present on the initial evaluation.

The most important bacterial organisms causing infections in these patients include gram-positive cocci (*Staphylococcus epidermidis,* alpha-hemolytic streptococci, and *S. aureus*) and gram-negative bacilli. Fungal infections are also important in neutropenic patients, with *Aspergillus* spp. and *Candida* spp. heading this list. *Aspergillus* species often cause necrotizing infections in the lung or sinuses.[13] *Legionella* infections are frequent in patients with solid tumors and lymphoma. Clinical and radiologic manifestations of *Legionella* infection in the immunocompromised patient may be atypical.

P. carinii is more common in AIDS patients, but it also occurs in patients with leukemia and lymphoma and in patients with solid tumors who are taking high doses of corticosteroids.

Approach to the Transplant Patient with Pneumonia

Cell-mediated immunity is impaired as a result of chemotherapy or steroid treatment in cancer and transplant patients. Whether the patient is taking chronic high doses of corticosteroids for the prevention of rejection of a transplant or the management of a chronic disease like asthma or connective tissue disorder, the results to the cell-mediated immune system are the same. Inhibition of migration of lymphocytes to the site of antigen challenge, inhibition of lymphokine production, and consequent inhibition of lymphocyte proliferation all increase the risk for opportunistic infection.[14] Although this is a significant reduction in the function of the cell-mediated immune system, patients on chronic corticosteroid therapy generally have few infections associated with this. Often, previously dormant infections (e.g., tuberculosis, severe or disseminated varicella zoster, and herpes simplex viral infections) become active. The infectious complications secondary to corticosteroid use increase with doses of prednisone over 20 mg/day and treatments longer than 30 days.[15]

Table 12-4 provides a list of organisms involved in respiratory infections in patients with cell-mediated immune impairment. Patients who have impaired cell-mediated immunity from other conditions, especially cancers, may have other respiratory diseases (see Table 12-3). Renal, liver, and lung transplant recipients are at particular risk for *Legionella*, although heart transplant recipients are not.[16] The incidence of *Nocardia* has decreased with the use of TMP-SMX prophylaxis; previously it was commonly seen in renal transplant and steroid-treated patients.[17] Fever, cough, and weight loss should suggest mycobacterial infection.

Reactivation and dissemination of *Histoplasma capsulatum* or *Coccidioides immitis* may occur with impairment of cellular immunity, so determining previous places of residence and obtaining a detailed travel history is important. *Candida, Aspergillus,* and *Strongyloides* infections may occur in patients with primarily compromised cell-mediated immunity but are much less common than in patients with neutropenia.[18]

Viral infections also are important in cell-mediated immunocompromised patients. Disseminated varicella, herpes simplex, and cytomegalovirus may result in pneumonia.[18]

Approach to the HIV-Infected Patient with Pneumonia

In patients with HIV with a suspected respiratory infection, the approach is adjusted based upon the patient's CD4 count. With a CD4 count above 400 cells/mm^3, the patient can be considered a normal host, and the usual community-acquired pathogens are the most likely cause of infection. As the CD4 count continues to drop below 400 cells/mm^3, however, different pathogens need to be addressed. Below 400 cells/mm^3, the clinician may see reactivation of tuberculosis and an increased incidence of pneumococcal pneumonia. Also, as the CD4 count drops, pneumonia is less likely to present with common signs and symptoms. When the CD4 count falls below 200 cells/mm^3, PCP becomes more common. At still lower CD4 counts, cryptococcal pneumonia and gram-negative pneumonia, especially *Pseudomonas* pneumonia, are more likely.

Although the list of pathogens that may cause pneumonia in HIV-infected patients is long, the most important pathogens to consider in the initial evaluation are *S. pneumoniae, H. influenzae, S. aureus, P. aeruginosa, M. tuberculosis,* and *P. carinii.* When an HIV-infected patient presents with a suspected pneumonia, a chest radiograph, sputum cultures for bacteria and mycobacteria, and an ABG should be obtained. A chest radiograph with a localized infiltrate and an ABG without an A-a gradient can be useful in ruling out PCP as a diagnosis.

Initial therapy should be directed against the most likely organisms, given the patient's CD4 counts. Additionally, whenever tuberculosis is in the differential, respiratory isolation is indicated until the diagnosis is confirmed.

Prevention of infection in patients with low CD4 counts also is important. TMP-SMX is highly effective in preventing PCP even taken three times a week.

Approach to the Diabetic Patient with Pneumonia

Although there is a widely held belief that diabetes is associated with increased susceptibility to infection, there is little evidence to support this.[19] However, once a patient with diabetes becomes ill, the ability to combat infection may be hampered by impairments in neutrophil function. In patients with diabetes, there is decreased adherence to bacteria along with impairment of chemotaxis and phagocytosis that reduces the neutrophils' ability to kill bacteria. Further impairment in immune function occurs through glucose binding to complement C3, which reduces opsonization. Complement C4 also is reduced in some diabetics. These defects are exacerbated by poor glycemic control and, it is believed, predispose the diabetic to purulent bacterial infections with both gram-positive and gram-negative organisms (Table 12-9).[20]

Diabetes is a risk factor for increased mortality and bacteremia in patients with pneumococcal pneumonia.[6] Pneumococcal vaccine offers some but not complete protection. There is a higher incidence of staphylococcal pneumonia in diabetic patients, thought to be secondary to a

Table 12-9

Respiratory Infections in Diabetic Patients

INFECTION	CAUSATIVE AGENT
Pneumonia	*Streptococcus pneumoniae*
	Staphylococcus aureus
	Haemophilus influenzae
	Influenza virus
	Gram-negative bacilli
Malignant otitis externa	*Pseudomonas aeruginosa*
Rhinocerebral mucormycosis	*Rhizopus* and *Mucor* species

high incidence of nasal infection with *S. aureus.* Increased frequency of pneumonia caused by gram-negative organisms and tuberculosis also occurs in diabetics. Influenza is known to cause increased mortality in diabetic patients.[20]

Two upper respiratory infections occur most commonly in diabetics. Malignant otitis externa, an invasive form of otitis externa that extends beyond the external auditory canal, is almost always caused by *P. aeruginosa.* It may be life-threatening and presents with purulent otorrhea, hearing loss, and intense pain. Fever is not usually present, but there is typically edema and cellulitis of the ear canal, and potentially osteomyelitis and CNS involvement.[21] Hospital admission for debridement of the ear canal and topical and parental antibiotics for *P. aeruginosa* is necessary.

Rhinocerebral mucormycosis is another severe upper respiratory infection that often occurs in diabetic patients with diabetic ketoacidosis (DKA). Patients present with facial or ocular pain and with fever and headache along with their DKA. On examination of the nasal cavity, a black eschar on the turbinates may suggest the diagnosis.[22]

Rhizopus and *Mucor* species are the causative organisms. Sinus cavernosus, carotid, or jugular thrombosis may occur as well as cerebral abscesses. Amphotericin B is the standard treatment, but mortality rates are high and increase with any complications. Late recurrences can occur even in successfully treated individuals, so long-term observation is required for early detection of recurrent infection.

Approach to the Alcoholic Patient with Pneumonia

Alcoholics are more susceptible to pulmonary infections and are likely to have a poorer prognosis than nonalcoholic patients.[23] Acute intoxication inhibits chemotaxis in neutrophils.[24] There is depressed complement activity and an inhibition of the antibody response, and alveolar macrophages have impaired phagocytosis. Transient neutropenia may develop from the direct toxic effect of alcohol on the bone marrow. Malnutrition, also common in chronic alcoholism, further damages the immune response.

In addition to the effect on the immune system, there is an increased incidence of oropharyngeal colonization by gram-negative bacteria, and aspiration is more common in alcoholics because of loss of reflexive glottic closure during intoxication or seizures.[23] Intoxication also interferes with respiratory tract defense mechanisms, with suppressed cough reflex and decreased ciliary motility and aspiration. Nicotine addiction, a co-morbid condition in 85 percent of alcoholics, can impair respiratory defenses even further.

Gram-negative bacteria frequently complicate aspiration pneumonia in alcoholism and must be considered in the antibiotic coverage for community-acquired pneumonia. Tuberculosis is also more common in this population. There is increasing evidence that vaccination with pneumococcal vaccine is not as effective in alcoholics.[25,26] Consequently, pneumococcus must be considered as a causative agent in these patients even if they have been vaccinated.

Conclusion

Respiratory infections in the immunocompromised patient are different and require a more comprehensive approach to diagnosis and management than infections that occur in immunocompetent individuals. Knowing the type of immune impairment may prepare the clinician to consider specific etiologies that one would not normally think of in dealing with a patient with an intact immune system. Recognition of the atypical presentation of serious respiratory infections in the immunosuppressed patient requires that diagnostic testing be done early and with more thoroughness than is required in the patient with a normal immune system.

The immunocompromised patient may have a causative organism that is not effectively treated with empiric antimicrobial regimens, which heightens the need to find the actual cause of the infection. Hospitalization is often necessary to effectively treat these patients. Early use of cultures, imaging studies, and invasive diagnostic studies may improve the yield in the search for a treatable cause. Finally, these patients often have co-morbid conditions that may require extra attention during their care.

References

1. Sickles EA, Greene WH, Wiernik PH: Clinical presentation of infection in granulocytopenic patients. *Arch Intern Med* 135:715, 1975.
2. Collin BA, Ramphal R: Pneumonia in the immunocompromised patient including cancer and transplant patients. *Infect Dis Clin North Am* 12(3): 781–805, 1998.
3. Chendrasekhar A: Are routine blood cultures effective in the evaluation of patients clinically diagnosed to have nosocomial pneumonia? *Am Surg* 62(5):373–376, 1996.
4. Bartlett JG, Dowell SF, Mandell LA, et al: Practice guidelines for the management of community-

acquired pneumonia in adults. *Clin Infect Dis* 31:347–382, 2000.

5. Feldman S, Stokes DC: Varicella zoster and herpes simplex pneumonias. *Semin Respir Infect* 2:84–94, 1987.

6. Levison ME: Pneumonia, including necrotizing pulmonary infections (lung abscess), in Braunwald E, Fauci AS, Isselbacher KJ, et al (eds): *Harrison's Principles of Internal Medicine*, 14th ed. New York, McGraw-Hill, 2001.

7. Marrie TJ: Community-acquired pneumonia in the elderly. *Clin Infect Dis* 31(4):1066–1078, 2000.

8. McFadden JP, Price RC, Eastwood HD, et al: Raised respiratory rate in elderly patients: a valuable physical sign. *Br Med J* 284:626–627, 1982.

9. Berman P, Hogan DB, Fox RA: The atypical presentation of infection in old age. *Age Ageing* 16:201–207, 1987.

10. Millard RL, Simons RJ: Pneumonia in the geriatric patient, in Bone RC (ed): *Pulmonary and Critical Care Medicine*. St. Louis, Mosby-Year Book, 1998.

11. Simons RJ, Reynolds HY: Altered immune status in the elderly. *Semin Respir Infect* 5:251–259, 1990.

12. Giamarellou H: Empiric therapy for infections in the febrile, neutropenic, compromised host. *Med Clin North Am* 79:559, 1995.

13. Saral R: *Candida* and *Aspergillus* infections in immunocompromised patients: an overview. *Rev Infect Dis* 13:487, 1991.

14. Boumpas DT, Paliogianni F, Anastassiou ED, et al: Glucocorticosteroid action on the immune system: molecular and cellular aspects. *Clin Exp Rheumatol* 9:413, 1991.

15. Axelrod L: Glucocorticoids, in Kelley WN, Harris ED, Ruddy S, et al (eds): *Textbook of Rheumatology*, 4th ed. Philadelphia, WB Saunders, 1993.

16. Singh N, Gayowski T, Wagener M, et al: Pulmonary infections in liver transplant recipients receiving tacrolimus. *Transplantation* 61:396–401, 1996.

17. Wilson JP, Turner HR, Kirschner KA, et al: Nocardial infections in renal transplant recipients. *Medicine* 68:38–57, 1989.

18. Rosenberg AS, Brown AE: Infection in the cancer patient. *Dis Mon* 39:507, 1993.

19. Joshi N, Caputo GM, Weitekamp MR, Karchmer AW: Infections in patients with diabetes mellitus. *N Engl J Med* 341:1906–1912, 1999.

20. Moutschen MP, Scheen AJ, Lefebvre PJ: Impaired immune response in diabetes mellitus: analysis of the factors and mechanisms involved. Relevance to the increased susceptibility of diabetic patients to specific infections. *Diabetes Metab* 18:187, 1992.

21. Slattery WH III, Brackmann DE: Skull base osteomyelitis: malignant external otitis. *Otolaryngol Clin North Am* 29:795–806, 1996.

22. Tierney MR, Baker AS: Infections of the head and neck in diabetes mellitus. *Infect Dis Clin North Am* 9:195–216, 1995.

23. Skerrett SJ: Host defenses against respiratory infection. *Med Clin North Am* 78:941, 1994.

24. Jaysinghe R, Gianutsos G, Hubbard AK: Ethanol-induced suppression of cell-mediated immunity in the mouse. *Alcohol Clin Exp Res* 16:331, 1992.

25. Hanna JN, Wenck DJ, Murphy DN: Three fatal pneumococcal polysaccharide vaccine failures. *Med J Aust* 173(6):305–307, 2000.

26. McMahon BJ, Parkinson AJ, Rudolph K, et al: Sepsis due to *Streptococcus pneumoniae* in a patient with alcoholism who received pneumococcal vaccine. *Clin Infect Dis* 28(5):1162–1163, 1999.

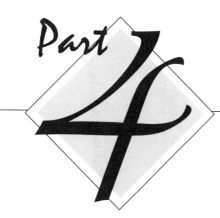

Noninfectious Acute Pulmonary Problems

Kesh Hebbar

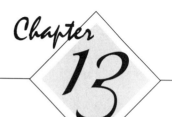

Pulmonary Embolism

Pulmonary embolism (PE) usually results from a deep vein thrombosis (DVT) in the lower extremities and should be considered a part of the same pathologic process. Both conditions are frequently unsuspected, which can lead to significant delays in the diagnosis and contribute to the morbidity and mortality associated with these conditions. The prevalence of PE at autopsy has not changed over the last three decades, with approximately 15 percent of hospitalized patients suffering a PE.[1] Despite advances in imaging techniques, the clinical diagnosis of PE remains difficult, and the postmortem data contrast sharply with the ante-mortem diagnosis. A meta-analysis of 12 postmortem studies carried out from 1971 through 1995 showed that more than 70 percent of fatal PEs are missed by clinicians.[2,3]

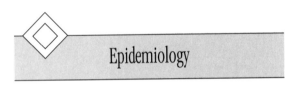

Epidemiology

An estimated 250,000 patients in the United States are diagnosed each year with venous thromboembolism. The number of undiagnosed and clinically silent cases cannot be accurately determined but is estimated to be an additional 250,000.[4] The annual incidence of DVT and PE in the general population of the Western world has been estimated at 1.0 and 0.5 per 1000, respectively.[5]

Mortality rates for PE are high. In the PIOPED (Prospective Investigation of Pulmonary Embolism Diagnosis) study, the overall 3-month mortality rate was about 15 percent.[6] In untreated PE the mortality rate is approximately 30 percent, but with treatment this can be reduced to 2 to 8 percent. Recurrent pulmonary embolism is especially dangerous, with a death rate of 40 to 45 percent.[6] Men have higher fatality rates than women (13.7 percent vs. 12.8 percent), and blacks have higher rates than whites (16.1 percent vs. 12.9 percent).[7] Pregnant women have

the highest mortality rates. In fact, PE is the most common medical cause of maternal deaths associated with live births in the United States.[8]

Risk Factors

The majority of pulmonary emboli originate from thrombi in the leg veins. Risk factors associated with venous thromboembolism are summarized in Table 13-1.[9,10] The primary factors that promote DVT are referred to as Virchow's triad and include venous stasis, abnormalities of the venous wall, and alterations in the coagulation system. Other factors that promote thrombosis include smoking, certain cancers, and invasive venous procedures.

VENOUS STASIS

Stasis of venous blood is promoted by immobilization from any cause. Congestive heart failure, stroke, and acute myocardial infarction are common conditions that promote venous stasis and thrombosis. Abdominal, pelvic, hip, and spine surgery are the procedures that carry the highest risk for venous thrombosis. Surgery predisposes patients to pulmonary embolism even as late as 1 month following the procedure, based on evidence that 25 percent of PEs occur between the 15th and 30th postoperative day.[11]

HYPERCOAGULATION DISORDERS

Hypercoagulability is seen in a variety of disease states. Activated protein C is a potent natural anticoagulant, and resistance to this protein is the most common cause of hypercoagulability. The defect, called factor V Leiden mutation, appears to be inherited as an autosomal dominant trait and is a result of a point mutation of coagulant factor V.[12] Deficiencies of antithrombin III, protein C, and protein S also have been associated with thromboembolism.

Homocysteinemia also contributes to hypercoagulability. The presence of hyperhomocys-

Table 13-1

Risk Factors for Venous Thromboembolism

A. PRIMARY RISK FACTORS	
Antithrombin deficiency	Factor V Leiden
Hyperhomocysteinemia	Protein S deficiency
Anticardiolipin antibodies	Factor XII deficiency
Protein C deficiency	

B. SECONDARY RISK FACTORS	
Trauma/fatigue	Surgery
Stroke	Immobilization
Advanced age	Malignancy + chemotherapy
Central venous catheters	Obesity
Chronic venous insufficiency	Heart failure
Smoking	Long-distance travel
Pregnancy/puerperium	Oral contraceptives
Nephrotic syndrome	Lupus anticoagulant
Hyperviscosity (polycythemia, Waldenström's macroglobulinemia)	Prosthetic surfaces

SOURCE: Guidelines on diagnosis and management of acute pulmonary embolism: Task Force on Pulmonary Embolism, European Society of Cardiology. *Eur Heart J* 21:1301–1336, 2000, with permission.

teinemia triples the risk of idiopathic venous thrombosis. The presence of hyperhomocysteinemia and factor V Leiden together in the same patient increases the risk of venous thrombosis by a factor of 10.[13]

Hypercoagulation also occurs with medication use. Patients taking oral contraceptives are at three times the risk of developing DVT, but the incidence is generally low in young women.[14] The risk of thrombosis with oral contraceptives appears to be higher during the start of therapy than after long-term use.[15] Smoking is an independent risk factor for thrombosis and is compounded in patients taking oral contraceptives. Like oral contraceptives, postmenopausal hormone replacement therapy (HRT) also is associated with a threefold increase in the risk of a DVT. The effects of HRT on DVT risk are accentuated in the presence of factor V Leiden mutation.[16]

CANCER

There is a clear association between thromboembolism and cancer. PE or DVT may be the first presentation of an occult cancer. However, searching for an occult malignancy in a patient who presents with a DVT is usually not productive.[17] A particular migratory thrombophlebitis, referred to as Trousseau's syndrome, however, is frequently associated with deep-seated cancers such as pancreatic and lung cancer.

VENOUS TRAUMA FROM INVASIVE PROCEDURES

Finally, upper extremity venous thrombosis due to multiple invasive procedures such as internal jugular and subclavian vein cannulation recently has been associated with an increased risk for PE.[18]

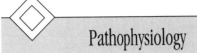

Pathophysiology

PEs are usually caused by thrombi from the deep veins of the legs, arms, and pelvis that dislodge and embolize to the pulmonary arteries. The incidence of PE seems to be lowest if the thrombus is confined to the calf veins. Unfortunately, in many patients thrombi that originally start in the calf veins progress into the proximal veins, increasing the risk for embolization.[19]

The embolization of thrombi into the pulmonary arterial system causes mechanical obstruction of arterial outflow and increases the right ventricular afterload. Vasoactive substances are released that cause pulmonary vasoconstriction and further increase pulmonary vascular resistance. Right-sided heart pressures increase, leading to right ventricular dilatation, dyskinesia, and decreased left ventricular filling. This leads to a low cardiac index and hypotension.

If there is a persistent patent foramen ovale, the increased right ventricular pressures cause right-to-left shunting of blood and severe hypoxemia. A patent foramen ovale or other atrial septal defect also can result in the embolus passing from the venous circulation into the arterial circulation. This can result in emboli showering the cerebral arterial system or other organs.

Areas of poor pulmonary arterial perfusion cause ventilation/perfusion mismatch and hypoxia. Reflex bronchoconstriction and hypoxia result in hyperventilation.

thrombus to the popliteal and femoral veins is not clearly understood. Furthermore, an inadequately treated proximal DVT has a high rate of recurrence.

If untreated, PE has a mortality rate of 25 to 30 percent.[21] The short-term outcome is considerably improved with anticoagulation, which reduces the otherwise high risk of recurrent embolization in the first 4 to 6 weeks after the initial PE.[22] The long-term prognosis is influenced by a number of factors. A history of cancer, advanced age, immobility, congestive heart failure, and congenital clotting factor deficiencies are associated with a higher mortality.

Recently, the right ventricular (RV) dysfunction seen with PE has been linked to adverse clinical outcomes. RV dyskinesia detected by echocardiogram has been reported to be present in about 40 percent of patients, including those patients who have normal systemic arterial pressure. The finding of RV dysfunction was associated with a doubling of the mortality from PE at 14 days.[23] Additionally, the mortality rate at 1 year was three times higher in patients with right ventricular dysfunction than in those with normal right ventricular function.[24]

Some long-term survivors of PE have developed severe pulmonary hypertension with chronic thromboembolic disease. The mechanism of chronic thromboembolic pulmonary hypertension is either silent recurrent PE or inadequate resolution of a large thrombus.[25] Some patients develop chronic PE, which, if untreated, is usually fatal in 2 to 3 years.[26]

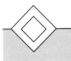

Natural History

If DVT is confined to the calf veins, the risk for local recurrence and PE is low.[20] Unfortunately, the risk for proximal extension of the calf vein

Diagnosis of Venous Thromboembolism

Algorithms for the diagnosis of a DVT and PE are shown in Figs. 13-1 and 13-2. Since the symp-

Figure 13-1

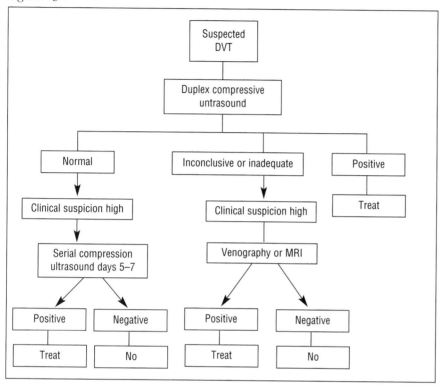

ABBREVIATIONS: DVT, deep vein thrombosis; MRI, magnetic resonance imaging.

toms and signs of DVT and PE can be nonspecific, clinicians need to maintain a high index of
suspicion and be willing to obtain initial diagnostic tests even when classic indicators of a
DVT or PE are absent. For both these disorders,
the initial test should be noninvasive and very
sensitive, so that only patients without disease
are ruled out by a negative test. When equivocal
results are obtained, follow-up with more invasive testing such as a venogram or pulmonary
arteriogram may be needed to confirm the diagnosis.

Symptoms and Signs

As noted, the clinical diagnosis of PE is difficult,
as symptoms and signs often mimic those of

other cardiopulmonary diseases. When evaluating the patient with a suspected PE, it is important for the clinician to categorize the clinical
suspicion as low or high risk. This clinical assessment helps to select and interpret the diagnostic
tests. The lack of specificity of the symptoms and
signs mandates further testing even when the
clinical suspicion is high.

Dyspnea and pleuritic chest pain are present
in a majority of patients with PE. Sometimes the
sudden onset of unexplained dyspnea is the only
symptom of PE. Pleuritic chest pain from emboli
in the distal branches of the pulmonary arterial
circulation causing pleural irritation is a frequent
symptom. Chest pain is sometimes substernal in
location and can mimic angina pectoris. Substernal chest pain and dyspnea due to PE are

Figure 13-2

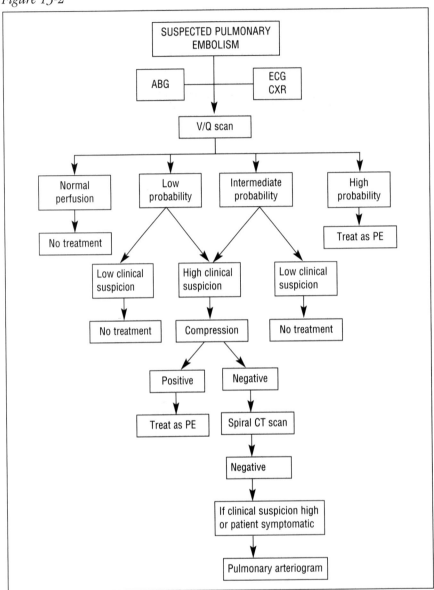

ABBREVIATIONS: ABG, arterial blood gas; ECG, electrocardiogram; CXR, chest x-ray; V/Q, ventilation/perfusion; PE, pulmonary embolism; CT, computed tomography.

indicative of the involvement of "central" blood vessels. The hemodynamic consequences of this type of PE are more prominent than those of a "peripheral" PE, which involves smaller blood vessels. Lightheadedness, hypotension, and syncope from PE are indications of a major episode.

Physical Examination

The physical examination of the patient is often normal. PE should always be suspected in the setting of unexplained acute hypotension, syncope, or hypoxemia.

In patients with an acute PE, tachypnea and tachycardia are consistent findings. Only patients with a massive PE will have signs such as a prominent jugular venous pulse, a right ventricular "heave" (over the left sternal border), a loud pulmonary closure sound (P_2), and an ejection systolic murmur. These are due to an acute increase in right-sided heart pressures and pulmonary hypertension.

The frequency of the most common symptoms and signs encountered in patients in whom PE is eventually proved by pulmonary angiography is summarized in Table 13-2.

The detection of a DVT is an excellent clue to the presence of PE in the appropriate clinical setting. However, the clinical diagnosis of DVT is very inaccurate and needs objective evaluation for confirmation. In six studies that included evaluation for calf tenderness, the range for sensitivity for detection of DVT was 56 to 82 percent, and specificity varied from 26 to 74 per-cent.[27] Swelling of the leg or calf was also a poor indicator of a DVT, with sensitivities ranging from 35 to 97 percent and specificity from 8 to 88 percent.[27]

Thus the clinical evaluation alone cannot be relied on to confirm or exclude DVT even in high-risk patients. Further work-up with laboratory testing and imaging studies is invariably needed if DVT or PE is suspected

Laboratory and Imaging

Routine laboratory studies contribute little to the diagnosis of PE or DVT. Leukocytosis and increased erythrocyte sedimentation rate are seen only in a major pulmonary infarction. Laboratory testing can be useful in establishing hypoxemia and evaluating patients for coagulopathies. However, the mainstay of testing for patients with a DVT or PE is imaging studies.

ARTERIAL BLOOD GAS

Pulmonary embolism is commonly associated with arterial hypoxemia, hypocapnia, and respiratory alkalosis. However, hypoxia is not present

Table 13-2

Common Symptoms and Signs in Patients with Pulmonary Embolism Confirmed by Pulmonary Angiography

SYMPTOM OR SIGN	% OF CONFIRMED PE CASES WITH SYMPTOM
Dyspnea	73%
Pleuritic chest pain	66%
Cough	37%
Leg pain	26%
Hemoptysis	13%
Tachypnea (RR ≥ 100 breaths/min)	70%
Rales	51%
Tachycardia (HR > 100 beats/min)	30%
Increased S_2P	23%
Pleural friction rub	3%

ABBREVIATIONS: RR, respiratory rate; HR, heart rate.
SOURCE: Reprinted with permission from Ryu JH, Olson EJ, Pellikka PA: Clinical recognition of pulmonary embolism: problem of unrecognized cases. *Mayo Clin Proc* 73:873–879, 1998, with permission.

universally, and young patients with no underlying lung disease may have a normal Pa_{O_2}. Therefore, the diagnosis of PE cannot be excluded solely on the basis of a normal Pa_{O_2}.

COAGULATION TESTS

Laboratory testing to evaluate patients for a hypercoagulable state is indicated in a patient with a history of recurrent DVT or PE. These tests include evaluations for factor V Leiden deficiency, antiphospholipid antibody, assays of protein C and S, and homocysteine levels.

Factor V Leiden mutation is the most common procoagulant abnormality associated with recurrent venous thrombosis. In the Physicians Health Study the relative risk for thrombosis in men with the mutation was 2.7.[28] The defect appears to be most common in Europe and least common in Africa and Southeast Asia.[29] Discontinuation of anticoagulant therapy for PE in patients with factor V Leiden mutation increases the risk of recurrent pulmonary embolism by a factor of 2 to 4.[30]

Antiphospholipid anticoagulant is an acquired abnormality associated with recurrent miscarriage, stroke, pulmonary hypertension, and venous thrombosis.[31] It is important to note that although antiphospholipid antibodies are associated with systemic lupus erythematosus, many patients who are antibody positive do not have the disease.

Other tests that can be helpful are assays of protein C, protein S, antithrombin III, and homocysteine. Levels of protein C, protein S, and antithrombin III are difficult to interpret, as these levels drop during an acute thrombotic event and heparin also depresses the levels of antithrombin III.[32] Routine testing for these procoagulants may be misleading.

D-DIMER

D-dimer is a degradation product that is released when fibrin undergoes fibrinolysis. An enzyme-linked immunosorbent assay (ELISA) and the more rapid latex agglutination test are currently used to measure D-dimer levels. Elevated D-dimer value is a very sensitive test for the diagnosis of DVT and PE.[33] However, D-dimer levels are nonspecific and are also elevated in myocardial infarction, pneumonia, and heart failure and in patients who have had recent surgery. So the positive predictive value is limited in the presence of other conditions.

On the other hand, the negative predictive value for D-dimer alone was 97.2 percent to 99 percent in two separate studies.[34] If this can be validated in larger studies, D-dimer measurement could be a powerful tool for ruling out PE or DVT.

One obstacle to the use of D-dimer is the variation in the assays.[35] Inconsistency in individual lab performance makes this test difficult to use in the clinical setting.

CHEST X-RAY

The majority of patients with PE have an abnormal chest x-ray, but the common abnormalities are usually nonspecific. Common findings are atelectasis, pleural effusion, pulmonary infiltrates, and elevation of the hemidiaphragm. Classic findings of abnormal wedge-shaped peripheral opacities or decreased vascularity are suggestive but infrequent. Thus, an abnormal chest x-ray cannot confirm the diagnosis of PE, and a normal chest x-ray does not exclude the diagnosis. The chest x-ray is more useful for excluding other disorders that can mimic PE, such as pneumonia, pneumothorax, rib fracture, pneumomediastinum, and aortic dissection.

ELECTROCARDIOGRAM

While many electrocardiographic (ECG) changes have been observed in patients with a proven PE, none of these changes are specific. In the Urokinase Pulmonary Embolism Trial (UPET), ECG changes were observed in 87 percent of patients with proven PE.[36] Sinus tachycardia and nonspecific T-wave changes are commonly seen. New-onset right axis deviation, right bundle branch block, and T-wave inversion in the V_1, V_2, and V_3 chest leads may indicate a massive pulmonary embolus, right ventricular strain, and the development of pulmonary hypertension.

SPIRAL (HELICAL) COMPUTED TOMOGRAPHY

Spiral computed tomography (sCT) technology is a new noninvasive tool that can make a rapid diagnosis of PE. This technique involves continuous movement of the patient through a CT scanner while the x-ray tube rotates in the spiral direction. This technique produces an image in a much shorter time with less breath holding than a conventional CT scanner.

Of the noninvasive tests available, sCT has the best sensitivity for main lobar and segmental pulmonary artery thrombi (95 to 100 percent).[37,38] However, subsegmental thrombi are not well visualized by sCT. The clinical significance of subsegmental thrombi is not clear and is currently being debated. If the clinical suspicion for PE is high and sCT is negative, pulmonary angiogram remains the gold standard for detection of peripheral thrombi, but the validity of a pulmonary angiogram diagnosis of subsegmental thrombi also has been questioned.[39]

Algorithms for the diagnosis of PE have incorporated sCT for patients with an abnormal chest x-ray or preexisting pulmonary disease.[40,41] These patients are most likely to have nondiagnostic and intermediate-probability ventilation/perfusion (V/Q) scans when investigated for possible PE. Patients who are negative for both sCT and lower extremity ultrasound should have a conventional pulmonary angiogram if the clinical suspicion remains high.

The other limitations of sCT are poor visualization of horizontal pulmonary vessels in the right middle lobe and lingula. Intersegmental lymph nodes may result in false positive scans. Advantages of spiral CT include the ability to visualize other nonvascular structures and condi-tions, such as lymph nodes, tumors, emphysema, and pleural and pericardial diseases.

VENTILATION/PERFUSION SCAN

V/Q scan is commonly performed for evaluating patients with suspected PE, but it is being performed less often with the development of sCT.

Evidence for the usefulness of the V/Q scan is based on the PIOPED study, which was designed to determine the sensitivity and specificity of the V/Q scan in patients with suspected PE.[39] The trial found that it is important to combine clinical suspicion with the V/Q scan in order to make an accurate diagnosis.

The study found that PE was present in 40 percent of "low-probability" scans if the clinical suspicion was high. With a "high-probability" lung scan and clinical probability that is "uncertain" or "unlikely," the likelihood of PE is only 88 percent and 56 percent, respectively. The PIOPED data are summarized in Table 13-3.

Perfusion lung scan remains a useful screening test to rule out clinically acute PE. A totally normal perfusion scan is almost never found with acute PE.[42,43]

Intermediate-probability V/Q scans are the most commonly reported abnormalities, especially in patients with cardiopulmonary diseases (e.g., chronic obstructive pulmonary disease). If clinical suspicion is moderate to high, further diagnostic steps are needed to rule out acute PE.

PULMONARY ANGIOGRAPHY

Pulmonary angiogram is considered the gold standard for the diagnosis of PE and until recently was considered the next step in the case of a nondiagnostic V/Q scan. In the PIOPED study, 1111 patients underwent pulmonary angiograms and 35 percent had positive studies. Interobserver agreement for identifying a PE by angiography was 98 percent for a lobar PE and 90 percent for a segmental PE, but only 66 percent for a subsegmental PE.[44]

Table 13-3

Clinical Assessment and Ventilation/Perfusion Scan Probability in PIOPED

V/Q Scan (Probability)	CLINICAL PROBABILITY		
	HIGHLY LIKELY (80–100%)	UNCERTAIN (20–79%)	UNLIKELY (0–19%)
High	96%	88%	56%
Intermediate	66%	28%	16%
Low	40%	16%	4%
Near normal/normal	0%	6%	2%

ABBREVIATION: PIOPED, Prospective Investigation of Pulmonary Embolism Diagnosis.
SOURCE: Tapson VF, Carroll BA, Davidson BL, et al: The diagnostic approach to acute venous thromboembolism: clinical practice guideline. American Thoracic Society. *Am J Respir Crit Care Med* 160:1043–1066, 1999, with permission.

When an arteriogram is performed, the most frequent site of access for the catheter is the femoral vein. Relative contraindications for the procedure include low platelet count, renal insufficiency, and diabetic renal disease. Patients should be well hydrated before the procedure to reduce the risk of acute tubular necrosis.

Complications related to pulmonary arteriography were well documented in the PIOPED trial. Deaths occurred in 5 of 1111 patients (0.5 percent), contrast-induced renal failure in 3 patients (0.3 percent), and severe cardiopulmonary compromise in 4 patients. Other complications include arrhythmias, bleeding from the venipuncture site, a rise in serum creatinine, and allergic reactions.

MAGNETIC RESONANCE ANGIOGRAPHY

Magnetic resonance angiography (MRA) can be used to evaluate PE. In a prospective, blinded study using gadolinium-enhanced MRA in 30 patients with suspected PE, the sensitivities for MRA were 100 percent, 87 percent, and 75 percent with specificities of 95 percent, 100 percent, and 95 percent, with conventional pulmonary angiography used as the gold standard. The advantages of MRA over angiography are that MRA is rapid and accurate and does not involve the use of nephrotoxic agents. A drawback is that, as with spiral CT, the sensitivity of MRA is low for subsegmental thrombi. With the increasing use of magnetic resonance imaging (MRI) for detecting proximal lower limb and pelvic DVT, as described later, there is the possibility that MRI imaging can be used to detect clots in both lungs and legs simultaneously.[45]

ECHOCARDIOGRAM

Right ventricular dysfunction is common in acute PE, but its role in the diagnosis of PE remains undefined. However, right ventricular hypokinesia has been shown to predict adverse outcomes, so evaluation of right ventricular function may play a role in evaluating overall prognosis in a patient with recent PE. In a Swedish study in which 126 patients with PE underwent echocardiography, the mortality rate at 1 year was found to be three times higher in patients with right ventricular dysfunction than in those with normal right ventricular function.[25] In the MAPPET (Management Strategy and Prognosis of Pulmonary Embolism) Registry, of 1001 patients with PE and right ventricular dysfunction, the mortality rate increased as right ventricular failure worsened.[46] Given these findings, it is possible that echocardiography can develop into a tool that can be used to estimate future risk and/or prognosis from PE.

In critically ill patients, echocardiogram can also help identify other conditions (myocardial infarction, dissection of aorta, and pericardial tamponade) that may mimic PE or be associated with it.

DIAGNOSIS OF PE BASED ON FINDING A DVT

When the V/Q scan is nondiagnostic, other studies are equivocal, and a pulmonary angiogram is not advisable, sometimes the diagnosis of a PE can be presumed in a patient with a DVT. In these cases, the diagnosis of a DVT should be actively pursued in the clinical setting of PE.

Since 90 percent of PE arise from thrombi in the deep veins, if a DVT is detected, invasive diagnostic tests for PE are not warranted and the patient can be commenced on anticoagulation. Unfortunately, DVT is diagnosed only in 70 percent of cases even by contrast venogram in angiographically proven PE.[47]

VENOGRAM   Venogram remains the gold standard for diagnosing a DVT, but it is rarely performed today because it is an invasive test and the contrast agent can cause phlebitis. Instead, a variety of noninvasive means are used to detect a DVT. These include compression ultrasonography and MRI.

COMPRESSION ULTRASONOGRAPHY   Duplex lower limb B mode compression ultrasonography (US) allows direct visualization of the femoral and popliteal veins and their compression by the ultrasound probe. A noncompressible vein is highly specific for proximal DVT with a sensitivity > 95 percent.[48]

One problem with US is that it cannot exclude calf vein and iliac vein thrombosis.[49] In symptomatic patients with isolated calf DVT, the sensitivity of US is only 73 percent for compression US and 81 percent for duplex US.[50] In asymptomatic patients the sensitivity for detecting calf

vein thrombosis is even lower, ranging from 33 to 58 percent.[51]

Overall, several studies have shown that US shows a DVT in approximately 30 to 50 percent of patients with confirmed PE.[52,53] Thus, while US-documented DVT is highly suggestive of PE in a patient suspected of having a PE, a normal US of the lower extremities should not be relied upon to rule out a PE.

The sensitivity of US can be improved by performing serial ultrasound. After an initially negative US, a repeat US 5 to 7 days later can improve the detection of proximal extension of a calf DVT. A second negative study a week after the first test is reassuring enough to withhold anticoagulation for suspected DVT.[54] However, this may not be useful in deciding whether to treat the patient with a suspected PE, since outcomes are improved only with early recognition and treatment.

MAGNETIC RESONANCE IMAGING   MRI directly images the thrombus and is a logical choice for detection of DVT. Some studies have shown sensitivity of 90 to 100 percent in symptomatic proximal DVT.[55] Diagnosis of calf DVT with MRI is less sensitive than with a contrast venogram, but sensitivity and specificity comparable to venography have been observed for pelvic vein DVT.[56]

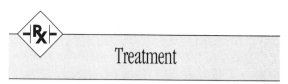

Treatment

Treatment of PE includes reducing the risk of recurrent embolism through rapid anticoagulation followed by long-term anticoagulation, reduction of ongoing risk factors, and, in selected cases, clot lysis or surgical removal. The vast majority of patients who are stable are treated with anticoagulation only. Rapid anticoagulation can be achieved using a heparin product, with long-term anticoagulation continued with warfarin.

Heparin

Heparin promotes the action of antithrombin III and prevents additional thrombi from forming. Heparin should be withheld only when contraindicated, such as with active bleeding, hemostatic disorders, severe uncontrolled hypertension, or recent stroke.

LOW-MOLECULAR-WEIGHT HEPARIN

Low-molecular-weight heparin (LMWH) preparations have been approved for prevention and treatment of venous thrombosis, for treatment of PE, and for the early treatment of unstable angina. LMWHs are derived from heparin by enzymatic depolymerization, yielding fragments that are one-third the size of unfractionated heparin. Like unfractionated heparin, LMWH produces its anticoagulant effect by activating antithrombin. LMWH preparations have a longer plasma half-life, better bioavailability, and a more predictable dose response than the traditional unfractionated heparin.[57] The various LMWHs approved for use in Europe and the United States are shown in Table 13-4.

Currently, enoxaparin sodium is the only LMWH product approved for use in the United States. In a study using doses of 1 mg/kg and 1.5 mg/kg once a day, both doses were equivalent to unfractionated heparin in patients with

Table 13-4

Commercially Available Low-Molecular-Weight Heparin Products in Europe and the United States

AGENTS
Nadroparin calcium (Fraxiparin)
Enoxaparin sodium (Lovenox/Clexane)
Dalteparin (Fragmin)
Ardeparin (Normiflo)
Tinzaparin (Innohep)
Reviparin (Clivarine)

DVT or PE. The biggest advantage of LMWH is the ability for patients to be discharged from the hospital much earlier than with unfractionated heparin.[58] In another study, 72 percent of patients treated with LMWH were able to be discharged within 48 h of admission on 1 mg/kg a day of enoxaparin; patients who were discharged had similar outcomes to those who were maintained in the hospital on standard unfractionated heparin therapy.[59]

Laboratory monitoring of LMWH is usually not necessary. Monitoring may be needed in very obese patients and in patients with renal failure. If monitoring is needed, anti-Xa assay is indicated, usually 4 h after a subcutaneous injection of LMWH. A conservative therapeutic range is 0.6 to 1.2 international units (IU)/mL.[60]

Because of its ease of administration and its safety profile, LMWH has become the anticoagulant of choice for prevention of venous thrombosis. Approaches to prevention of venous thrombosis following major orthopedic surgery are summarized in Table 13-5. In general surgical patients and in high-risk medical patients, LMWH is at least as effective and definitely more convenient than conventional heparin. A meta-analysis of 11 randomized studies comparing intravenous heparin and subcutaneous LMWH in about 3500 patients with acute DVT found less major bleeding with LMWH; the frequency of recurrent thromboembolism did not differ between the treatment groups.[61]

Complications from LMWH use include bleeding and immune-mediated thrombocytopenia. LMWH should not be used, or should be used cautiously, in patients at risk for bleeding events. Patients who have had heparin-associated thrombocytopenia in the past with unfractionated heparin remain at high risk for thrombocytopenia when using LMWH.

UNFRACTIONATED HEPARIN

Since LMWH has not been approved for use in patients with recurrent PE, unfractionated

Table 13-5

Approaches to Prevention of Venous Thrombosis

CONDITION OR PROCEDURE	PROPHYLAXIS*
General surgery	Unfractionated heparin, 5000 U two or three times a day
	Enoxaparin, 40 mg/day SC
	Dalteparin, 2500 or 5000 U/day SC
	Nadroparin, 3100 U/day SC
	Tinzaparin, 3500 U/day SC, with or without graduated-compression stockings
Total hip replacement	Warfarin (target INR 2.5)
	Intermittent pneumatic compression
	Enoxaparin, 30 mg SC twice daily
	Danaparoid, 750 U SC twice daily
Total knee replacement	Enoxaparin, 30 mg SC twice daily
	Ardeparin, 50 U/kg SC twice daily
General medical condition requiring hospitalization	Graduated-compression stockings, intermittent pneumatic compression, or unfractionated heparin, 5000 U two or three times daily
Condition requiring hospitalization in the intensive care unit	Graduated-compression stockings and intermittent pneumatic compression, with or without unfractionated heparin, 5000 U two or three times daily
Pregnancy in high-risk patient*	Dalteparin, 5000 U/day SC
	Enoxaparin, 40 mg/day SC

* High risk includes patients with previous pulmonary embolism or DVT.
ABBREVIATIONS: SC, subcutaneously; INR, international normalized ratio; DVT, deep vein thrombosis.
SOURCE: Goldhaber SZ: Pulmonary embolism. *N Engl J Med* 339:93–104, 1998, with permission.

heparin remains the treatment for these patients. Unfractionated heparin is given with an initial intravenous bolus at a dose of 5000 to 10,000 IU, followed by a continuous infusion. The infusion rate is guided by body weight according to nomograms.[62] The infusion rate is usually 18 IU/kg/h up to 1600 IU/h. This usually rapidly results in a therapeutic activated partial thromboplastin time (aPTT).

Monitoring of anticoagulation is performed using the aPTT. The aPTT should be maintained at 1.5 to 2 times control with heparin infusion. The first aPTT should be done 4 to 6 h after initiation of heparin infusion. Because of the variability of aPTT results with various reagents,

it is recommended that each laboratory determine the range of aPTT ratio. At least 5 days of heparin therapy is required because true anticoagulation requires the depletion of factor II (thrombin), which takes about 5 days.[63,64]

In addition to bleeding problems resulting from overaggressive anticoagulation, use of unfractionated heparin is associated with an immune-mediated thrombocytopenia.

Warfarin

Warfarin can be started on the first or second day of heparin treatment. Warfarin should be started at an initial dose of 5 mg, with the pro-thrombin time (PT) and international normalized ratio (INR) monitored daily until a therapeutic INR of 2.0 to 3.0 is achieved. Administering a loading dose of warfarin does not achieve a faster therapeutic INR and does not shorten the duration of intravenous heparin therapy.[65]

The duration of anticoagulation for pulmonary embolism should depend on whether the event was related to an acute event, such as an injury or surgery; is associated with an ongoing risk for recurrent thrombosis, such as a coagulopathy; or was idiopathic. If the event was precipitated by a reversible risk factor or acute event, such as surgery or trauma, there is evidence that treatment for 6 months results in significantly fewer recurrences than if patients are treated for only 6 weeks.[66] Likewise, patients with idiopathic PE also should be treated with anticoagulants for 6 months. Indefinite anticoagulation is recommended for patients with continuing risk factors, such as cancer, a hypercoagulable condition, or recurrent PE.

The most common complication associated with warfarin usage is hemorrhage. Evidence shows that the risk of bleeding is minimal below an INR of 3.0.[67] However, some patients, such as those with antiphospholipid syndrome, need to be maintained on a higher INR for prevention of recurrent thrombosis,[68] and their risk of bleeding is higher. Serious bleeding should be treated with fresh frozen plasma; less serious bleeding is managed by holding warfarin therapy, reducing maintenance doses of warfarin, and giving oral or subcutaneous vitamin K.[69]

Thrombolytic Agents

The use of thrombolytic agents for PE is not well defined. Thrombolytic agents are usually reserved for a presumed massive PE when the patient exhibits hemodynamic instability and looks as if he or she is going to die.

Currently available agents include urokinase, streptokinase, tPA, and reteplase. All four drugs convert plasma protein plasminogen to plasmin. Plasmin breaks down fibrin, which dissolves clots. Thrombolytic agents result in superior resolution of lung scan abnormalities, and there is evidence of rapid hemodynamic improvement in patients presenting with shock.[70] However, thrombolytic therapy for a PE does not have convincing mortality reduction data, as have been observed for patients with acute myocardial infarction. It is suspected that with PE, in contrast to coronary artery thrombi, thrombolytic therapy does not result in the complete dissolution of the clot because these emboli are older, larger, and more organized than coronary thrombi.[71,72]

All thrombolytic agents are administered intravenously. For PE, tPA is recommended in a 100-mg infusion over 2 h. Streptokinase is given as a 250,000-IU loading dose followed by 100,000 IU/h for 24 h. Once the infusion is completed, intravenous heparin therapy can be continued as long as the aPTT is less than twice the normal.

Inferior Vena Caval Filters

Inferior vena caval (IVC) filters have become commonplace in the management of PE despite scant evidence supporting any long-term efficacy. For example, one study in which 400 patients were followed over 2 years showed that filters did not reduce the mortality rates compared to oral anticoagulation alone.[73]

Filters are useful for short-term use in patients who have a PE and are actively bleeding. There is some rationale for using IVC filters in patients who have recurrent emboli despite intensive anticoagulation.

The long-term impact of IVC filters has not been studied extensively. In one study of IVC recipients for DVT, recurrent DVTs occurred in 12 percent of patients who were not anticoagulated and 15 percent of those who were on anticoagulants.[74] About 2 percent of patients had recurrent PEs; anticoagulation did not alter the rate of recurrent PE. Another study of 100 patients with IVCs who were followed for a mean of 38 months showed a DVT rate of 23 percent and asymptomatic complications related to the IVC, such as thrombi trapped in the filter or the filter tilting, malpositioning, or migrating, in nearly 50 percent of those who survived 3 years.[75] Given the high mortality rates from recurrent PE, the complications rates from long-term IVC insertion appear to be a worthwhile trade-off in high-risk patients.

Prevention

Prevention of venous thrombosis and pulmonary embolism is important in high-risk medical settings. The specific settings in which there is a high risk for DVT include patients with fractures of the pelvis and lower extremities; patients undergoing abdominal, pelvic, or gynecological surgery; patients with acute myocardial infarction/severe congestive heart failure; patients with certain malignancies, especially breast cancer patients undergoing chemotherapy and those taking tamoxifen therapy;[76] and upper extremity thrombosis in patients with indwelling central venous catheters. Additionally, patients in whom prolonged bed rest is anticipated derive some benefit from preventive therapy for DVT until they are able to ambulate again.

For the prevention of DVT, graduated compression stockings and intermittent pneumatic compression have been used alone or in combination. These are mechanical approaches that promote venous blood flow in the lower extremities. Foot pumps have also been used for prophylaxis, but they are not as widely available.

Subcutaneous LMWH has increasingly replaced the traditional subcutaneous unfractionated heparin because of its superior bioavailabilty, lower complication rate, and decreased frequency of administration. There has been some controversy as to the duration of prophylaxis after surgical procedures. It has been suggested that 4 to 6 weeks of LMWH following total hip replacement is safer and more effective than restricting LMWH to the initial period of hospitalization.[77] A Canadian collaborative group proposed limiting the postoperative anticoagulation to 10 days following surgery.[78] This decision may have to be taken on an individual basis depending on co-morbid risk factors.

References

1. Stein PD, Henry JW: Prevalence of acute pulmonary embolism among patients in a general hospital and at autopsy. *Chest* 108:78–81, 1995.
2. Mandelli V, Schmid C, Zogno C, et al: False negatives and false positives in acute pulmonary embolism: a clinical post-mortem comparison. *Cardiologia* 42:205–210, 1997.
3. Morpugo M, Schmid C, Mandelli V: Factors influencing the clinical diagnosis of pulmonary embolism: analysis of 229 postmortem cases. *Int J Cardiol* 65(suppl I):S79–S82, 1998.
4. Anderson FA Jr, Wheeler HB, Goldberg RJ, et al: A population-based perspective of the hospital incidence and fatality of deep vein thrombosis and pulmonary embolism. *Arch Intern Med* 151: 933–938, 1991.
5. Van Beek EJR, ten Cate JW: The diagnosis of venous thromboembolism: an overview, in Hull RD, Raskob GE, Pineo GF (eds): *Venous Thromboembolism: An Evidence Based Atlas.* Armonk, NY, Futura, 1996; pp 93–99.
6. Carson JL, Kelley MA, Duff A, et al: The clinical course of pulmonary embolism. *N Engl J Med* 326:1240–1245, 1992.
7. Siddique RM, Siddique MI, Connors AF Jr, Rimm AA: Thirty day case-fatality rates for pulmonary embolism in the elderly. *Arch Intern Med* 156:2343–2347, 1996.
8. Turkstra F, Kuijer PMM, van Beek EJR, et al: Diagnostic utility of ultrasonography of leg veins in patients suspected of having pulmonary embolism. *Ann Intern Med* 12:775–781, 1997.

9. Lane DA, Mannucci PM, Bauer KA, et al: Inherited thrombophilia: part I. *Thromb Haemost* 76:651–662, 1996.

10. Lane DA, Mannucci PM, Bauer KA, et al: Inherited thrombophilia: part 2. *Thromb Haemost* 76:824–834, 1996.

11. Bergqvist D, Lindbald B: A 30-year survey of pulmonary embolism verified at autopsy: an analysis of 1274 surgical patients. *Br J Surg* 72:105–108, 1985.

12. Svensson PJ, Dahlback B: Resistance to activated protein C as a basis for venous thrombosis. *N Engl J Med* 330:517–522, 1994.

13. Ridker PM, Hennekens CH, Selhub J, et al: Interrelation of hyperhomocystinemia, factor V Leiden and risk of future venous thromboembolism. *Circulation* 95:1777–1782, 1997.

14. World Health Organization: Venous thromboembolic disease and combined oral contraceptives: results of international multicenter case-control study. *Lancet* 346:983–987, 1995.

15. Vandenbroucke JP, Helmerhorst FM: Risk of venous thrombosis with hormone-replacement therapy. *Lancet* 348:972, 1996.

16. Grodstein F, Stampfer MJ, Goldhaber SZ, et al: Prospective study of exogenous hormones and risk of pulmonary embolism in women. *Lancet* 348:983–987, 1996.

17. Soren HT, Mallemkjaer L, Steffensen FH, et al: The risk of diagnosis of cancer after primary deep vein thrombosis or pulmonary embolism. *N Engl J Med* 338:1169–1173, 1998.

18. Monreal M, Lafoz E, Ruiz J, et al: Upper-extremity deep vein thrombosis and pulmonary embolism. *Chest* 99:280–283, 1991.

19. Kakkar VV, Flanc C, Howe CT, Clarke MB: Natural history of postoperative deep-vein thrombosis. *Lancet* 2:230–232, 1969.

20. Leclerc JR: Natural history of venous thromboembolism, in Leclerc JR (ed): *Venous Thromboembolic Disorders.* Philadelphia, Lea & Febiger, 1991; pp 166–175.

21. Barritt DW, Jordan SC: Clinical features of pulmonary embolism. *Lancet* 1:729–732, 1961.

22. Pacouret G, Alison D, Pottier JM, et al: Free-floating thrombus and embolic risk in patients with angiographically confirmed proximal deep vein thrombosis: a prospective study. *Arch Intern Med* 157:305–308, 1997.

23. Goldhaber SZ, De Rosa M, Visani L: International Cooperative Pulmonary Embolism Registry detects high mortality rate (abstract). *Circulation* 96(suppl I):1–159, 1997.

24. Ribero A, Lindmarker P, Juhlin-Dannfelt A, et al: Echocardiography Doppler in pulmonary embolism: right ventricular dysfunction as a predictor of mortality rate. *Am Heart J* 134:479–487, 1997.

25. Palla A, Donnamaria V, Petrizzelli S, et al: Enlargement of the right descending pulmonary artery in pulmonary embolism. *Am J Roentgenol* 141:513–517, 1983.

26. Riedal M, Stanek V, Widimsky J, Prerovsky I: Long-term follow-up of patients with pulmonary thromboembolism. Late prognosis and evaluation of hemodynamic and respiratory data. *Chest* 81:151–158, 1982.

27. Leclerc JR, Illescas F, Jarzem P: Diagnosis of deep vein thrombosis, in Leclerc JR (ed): *Venous Thromboembolic Disorders.* Philadelphia, Lea & Febiger; 1991: pp 176–228.

28. Ridker PM, Hennekens CH, Lindpainter K, et al: Mutation in the gene coding for coagulation factor V and the risks of myocardial infarction, stroke, and venous thrombosis in apparently healthy men. *N Engl J Med* 332:912–917, 1995.

29. Rees DC, Cox M, Clegg JB: World distribution of factor V Leiden. *Lancet* 346:1133–1134, 1995.

30. Simioni P, Prandoni P, Lensing AWA, et al: The risk of recurrent venous thromboembolism in patients with an Arg506 Gln mutation in the gene for factor V (factor V Leiden). *N Engl J Med* 92:2800–2802, 1995.

31. Hughes GRV: The antiphospholipid syndrome: ten years on. *Lancet* 342:341–344, 1998.

32. Comp PC, Thurnau GR, Welsh J, Esmon CT: Functional and immunologic protein S levels are decreased during pregnancy. *Blood* 68:881–885, 1986.

33. Bounameaux H, de Moerloose P, Perrier A, Miron MJ: D-dimer testing in suspected venous thromboembolism: an update. *Q J Med* 90:437–442, 1997.

34. Ginsberg JS, Kearon C, Douketis J, et al: The use of D-dimer testing and impedance plethysmographic examination in patients with clinical indications of deep vein thrombosis. *Arch Intern Med* 157:1077–1081, 1997.

35. Becker DM, Philbrick JT, Bachhuber TL, Humphries JE: D-dimer testing and acute venous thromboembolism: a short-cut to accurate diagnosis? *Arch Intern Med* 156:939–946, 1996.

36. The Urokinase Pulmonary Embolism Trial: a national cooperative study. *Circulation* 47(suppl II):1–108, 1973.

37. Remy-Jardin MJ, Remy J, Deschildre F, et al: Diagnosis of acute pulmonary embolism with spiral CT: comparison with pulmonary angiography and scintigraphy. *Radiology* 200:699–706, 1996.

38. van Rossum AB, Treuniat FE, Kieft GJ, et al: Role of spiral volumetric computed tomographic scanning in the assessment of patients with clinical suspicion of pulmonary embolism and abnormal ventilation perfusion scan. *Thorax* 51:23–28, 1996.

39. PIOPED Investigators: Value of the ventilation-perfusion scan in acute pulmonary embolism: results of the Prospective Investigation of Pulmonary Embolism Diagnosis (PIOPED). *JAMA* 263:2753–2759, 1990.

40. Remy-Jardin M, Remy J, Artaud D, et al: Spiral CT of pulmonary embolism: technical considerations and interpretive pitfalls. *J Thorac Imaging* 12:103–117, 1997.

41. Goodman LR, Lipchik RJ: Diagnosis of acute pulmonary embolism: time for a new approach. *Radiology* 199:25–27, 1996.

42. Hull RD, Raskob GE, Coates G, Panju AA: Clinical validity of a normal perfusion lung scan in patients with suspected pulmonary embolism. *Chest* 97:23–26, 1990.

43. Van Beck EJR, Kuyer PMM, Schenk BE, et al: A normal perfusion lung scan in patients with clinically suspected pulmonary embolism: frequency and clinical validity. *Chest* 108:170–173, 1995.

44. Stein PD, Athanasoulis C, Alavi A, et al: Complications and validity of pulmonary angiography in acute pulmonary embolism. *Circulation* 85:462–469, 1992.

45. Tapson VF: Pulmonary embolism: new diagnostic approaches. *N Engl J Med* 336:1449–1451, 1997.

46. Kasper W, Konstantinidis S, Giebel A, et al: Management strategies and outcome in acute major pulmonary embolism: results of a multi-center registry. *J Am Coll Cardiol* 30:1165–1171, 1997.

47. Hull RD, Hirsh J, Carter CJ, et al: Pulmonary angiography, ventilation lung scanning, and venography for clinically suspected pulmonary embolism and abnormal perfusion lung scan. *Ann Intern Med* 98:891–899, 1983.

48. Becker DM, Philbrick JT, Abbitt PL: Real-time ultrasonography for the diagnosis of lower extremity deep vein thrombosis. The wave of the future? *Arch Intern Med* 149:1731–1734, 1989.

49. Wells PS, Lensing AWA, Davidson BL, et al: Accuracy of ultrasound for the diagnosis of deep vein thrombosis in asymptomatic patients after orthopedic surgery: a meta-analysis. *Ann Intern Med* 122:47–53, 1995.

50. Rose SC, Zwiebel WJ, Nelson BD, et al: Symptomatic lower extremity deep vein thrombosis: accuracy limitations, and role of color duplex flow imaging in diagnosis. *Radiology* 175:639–644, 1990.

51. Agnelli G, Volpato R, Radicchia S, et al: Detection of asymptomatic deep vein thrombosis by real-time B-mode compressive ultrasound in hip surgery patients. *Thromb Haemost* 68:257–260, 1992.

52. Killewick LA, Bedford GR, Beach KW, Strandness DE: Diagnosis of deep vein thrombosis. A prospective study comparing duplex scanning to contrast venography. *Circulation* 78:810–814, 1989.

53. Beecham RP, Dorfman GS, Cronan JJ, et al: Is bilateral lower extremity compression sonography useful and cost-effective in the evaluation of suspected pulmonary embolism? *Am J Roentgenol* 161:1289–1292, 1993.

54. Cogo A, Lensing LW, Koopman MM, et al: Compression ultrasonography for the diagnostic management of patients with clinically suspected deep vein thrombosis: prospective cohort study. *Br Med J* 316(7124):2–3, 1998.

55. Erdman WA, Jayson HT, Redman HC, et al: Deep vein thrombosis of extremities: role of MRI in the diagnosis. *Radiology* 174:425–431, 1990.

56. Laissy JP, Cinqualbre A, Loshkajian A, et al: Assessment of deep vein thrombosis in the lower limbs and pelvis: MR venography versus duplex Doppler sonography. *Am J Roentgenol* 167:971–975, 1996.

57. Handeland GF, Abidgaard GF, Holm U, et al: Dose adjusted heparin treatment of deep vein thrombosis: a comparison of unfractionated and low molecular weight heparin. *Eur J Clin Pharmacol* 39:107–112, 1990.

58. The COLUMBUS Investigators: Low-molecular-weight heparin in the treatment of patients with thrombo-embolism. *N Engl J Med* 337:657–662, 1997.

59. Simonneau G, Sors H, Charbonnier B, et al, for the Thesee Study Group: A comparison of low-molecular-weight heparin and unfractionated heparin for acute pulmonary embolism. *N Engl J Med* 337:663–669, 1997.

60. Boneu B: Low molecular weight heparin therapy: is monitoring needed? *Thromb Haemost* 72:330–334, 1994.

61. Gould MK, Dembitzer AD, Doyle RL, et al: Low molecular weight heparins compared with unfractionated heparin for the treatment of acute deep vein thrombosis: a meta analysis of randomized controlled trials. *Ann Intern Med* 130:800–809, 1999.

62. Raschke RA, Reilly BM, Guidry JR, et al: The weight-based heparin dosing nomogram compared with a "standard care" nomogram: a randomized controlled trial. *Ann Intern Med* 119:874–881, 1993.

63. Hyers TM, Agnelli G, Hull RD, et al: Anti-thrombin therapy for venous thrombolic disease. *Chest* 114/115(suppl):561S–578S, 1998.

64. Gallus A, Jackman J, Tillet J, et al: Safety and efficacy of warfarin started early after submassive venous thrombosis or pulmonary embolism. *Lancet* 2:1293–1296, 1986.

65. Harrison L, Johnston M, Massicotte MP, et al: Comparison of 5 mg and 10 mg loading doses in the initiation of warfarin therapy. *Ann Intern Med* 126:133–136, 1997.

66. Schulman S, Rhedin AS, Lindmarker P, et al: A comparison of six weeks of anticoagulation therapy after a first episode of venous thromboembolism. *N Engl J Med* 332:1661–1665, 1995.

67. Coon WW, Willis PW III: Hemorrhagic complications of anticoagulant therapy. *Arch Intern Med* 133:386–392, 1974.

68. Khamashta MA, Cuadrado MJ, Mujic R, et al: The management of thrombosis in the antiphospholipid-antibody syndrome. *N Engl J Med* 332:993–997, 1995.

69. Crowther MA, Donovan D, Harrison L, et al: Low-dose oral vitamin K reliably reverses over anticoagulation due to warfarin. *Thromb Haemost* 79:1116–1118, 1998.

70. Dalen JE, Alpert JS: Thromboembolytic therapy for pulmonary embolism; is it effective? Is it safe? When is it indicated? *Arch Intern Med* 157:2550–2556, 1997.

71. Marder VJ: The use of thrombolytic agents; choice of patient, drug administration, laboratory monitoring. *Ann Intern Med* 90:802–808, 1979.

72. Goldhaber SZ, Kessler CM, Heitt J, et al: Randomized controlled trial of recombinant tissue plasminogen activator versus urokinase in the treatment of acute pulmonary embolism. *Lancet* 2:293–298, 1988.

73. Decousus H, Leizorowicz A, Parent F, et al: A clinical trial of vena-caval filters in the prevention of pulmonary embolism in patients with proximal deep vein thrombosis. *N Engl J Med* 338:409–415, 1998.

74. Greenfield LJ, Proctor MC: Recurrent thromboembolism in patients with vena cava filters. *J Vasc Surgery* 33:510–514, 2001.

75. Schleich JM, Morla O, Laurent M, et al: Long-term follow-up of percutaneous vena cava filters: a prospective study in 100 consecutive patients. *Eur J Vasc Endovasc Surg* 21:450–457, 2001.

76. Pritchard KI, Paterson AH, Paul NA, et al: Increased thrombo-embolic complications with concurrent tamoxifen and chemotherapy in a randomized trial of adjuvant therapy for women with breast cancer. *J Clin Oncol* 14:2731–2737, 1996.

77. Planes A, Vochelle N, Darmon JY, et al: Risk of deep vein thrombosis after hospital discharge in patients having undergone total hip replacement: double blind randomized comparison of enoxaparin versus placebo. *Lancet* 348:234–238, 1996.

78. Leclerc JR, Gent M, Hirsh J, et al: Canadian collaborative group. The incidence of symptomatic venous thromboembolism during and after prophylaxis with enoxaparin: a multi-national cohort study in patients who underwent hip or knee arthroplasty. *Arch Intern Med* 158:873–878, 1998.

Kevin C. Oeffinger

Lung Cancer

In the past, screening and treatment for lung cancer have generally been associated with dismal outcomes. Consequently, primary care clinicians have focused on methods of primary and secondary prevention of tobacco use to combat lung cancer. Despite these efforts, the burden of smoking-related cancers in current smokers is considerable and is likely to increase in the coming decades. Encouragingly, recently developed screening techniques now provide the potential for early diagnosis and more favorable outcomes. Coupled with this, several novel chemotherapeutic agents may improve the prognosis of patients with more advanced lung cancer.

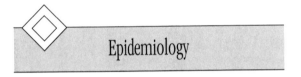

Epidemiology

Incidence and Mortality

Lung cancer is the second most common cancer and the leading cause of cancer mortality in the United States. In 2001, an estimated 169,500 new cases of lung cancer will be diagnosed, representing 13.4 percent of all cancers. Approximately 157,400 persons will die from lung cancer in 2001, which is more than triple the number who will die from the second most common fatal cancer, colorectal carcinoma. Lung cancer will account for 32 percent of male cancer deaths and 25 percent of female cancer deaths in the United States in 2001.[1]

The overall age- and race-adjusted incidence of lung cancer in the United States is 54.2 per 100,000 population. The incidence of lung cancer is higher in males than in females and in African Americans than in Caucasians. In black males, the age-adjusted incidence is 101.4 per 100,000, versus 68.4 per 100,000 in white males. The age-adjusted incidence in black and white females is 47.2 and 43.7 per 100,000, respectively. While the incidence of lung cancer in men

has steadily decreased since the 1970s by about 2.5 percent, it has increased by 123 percent in women over the same time period.

The peak incidence of lung cancer diagnosis is between the ages of 65 and 79, with a median age at diagnosis of 68. It is rare for someone to be diagnosed with lung cancer prior to the age of 40.

Histology

Lung cancer is generally divided into two groups. Small cell lung cancer (SCLC), previously referred to as oat cell carcinoma, comprises about 20 percent of lung cancer cases. The remaining 80 percent consist of three other cell types: squamous cell, large cell undifferentiated, and adenocarcinoma. These three cancers are generally grouped together and called non-small cell lung cancer (NSCLC) because they commonly coexist within a tumor, can be difficult to distinguish, and have similar treatment regimens and prognoses.

Etiologic Factors

Tobacco smoke is the primary etiologic agent that promotes the development of lung cancer. It is estimated that smoking contributes to the development of almost 90 percent of all lung cancers,[2] and one in five cigarette smokers ultimately develop lung cancer. Several studies suggest that females may be more susceptible to the carcinogenic effects of tobacco smoke than males.

While the prevalence of smoking in adults in the United States has decreased from 42.3 percent to 23.2 percent, adolescent smoking rates have increased. From 1991 to 1997, tobacco consumption increased 32 percent among high school students, resulting in about 3 million adolescents who smoke regularly. Because of the increase in smoking among younger individuals, it is estimated that cigarette smoking will contribute to about 10 million premature deaths worldwide from lung cancer and other smoking-related illnesses by the year 2030.

Tobacco-induced lung carcinogenesis is complex and involves induction of multiple gene mutations that affect the various and overlapping components of detoxification metabolism and that are probably amplified by genetic polymorphisms.[3] The model of tobacco-induced lung carcinogenesis provides the opportunity for investigators to study the role of dose exposure, early response of normal cells, alteration in structure and function, and the ultimate development of cancer cells. In the next one or two decades, ongoing work in this area will provide a much more detailed model of lung carcinogenesis and provide concepts that will enhance our understanding of how cancer develops.

Radon, an inert gas that is formed during the natural decay of uranium-238, is the second most common etiologic agent implicated in the development of lung cancer.[4] The most common source of exposure is from soil beneath homes and buildings. There is a significant synergism in the development of lung cancer in individuals who both smoke and are exposed to radon. About 14,000 lung cancer deaths per year are caused by radon, but most of these occur in cigarette smokers.

Other occupational exposures known to increase the risk of lung cancer include asbestos, arsenic, chloromethyl ethers, chromium, coke oven emissions, iron and steel founding, nickel, and vinyl chloride (Table 14-1). As with radon, cigarette smoking is generally synergistic with these exposures in the development of lung cancer.

Table 14-1

Exposures Associated with Lung Cancer

- Tobacco
- Radon
- Asbestos
- Arsenic
- Chloromethyl esters
- Chromium
- Coke oven emissions
- Iron and steel foundries
- Nickel
- Vinyl chloride

risk of lung cancer in comparison with current smokers. Reducing current levels of smoking by 50 percent, therefore, would prevent 20 to 30 million premature deaths over the next 25 years. Thus, continued efforts to prevent the onset of smoking and promote smoking cessation are critical. A recent Cochrane publication presented an excellent review of the effectiveness of different methods to promote smoking cessation.[5] Effective interventions included advice from doctors, structured interventions from nurses, individual and group counseling, and nicotine replacement.

Chemoprevention

In the past few years, much interest in chemoprevention for lung cancer in current and past smokers has been generated. Two large randomized clinical trials did not show a benefit with beta-carotene chemoprevention. Recent studies suggest that 13-*cis* retinoic acid, selenium, and vitamin E may alter some of the tobacco-induced cytopathologic changes and thus may be useful in chemoprevention.[6] Three large randomized clinical trials to assess the use of different methods of chemoprevention on early and late endpoints are in process.

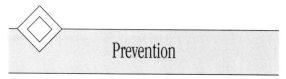

Prevention

Primary and Secondary Prevention

Former smokers who are abstinent for more than 15 years have an 80 to 90 percent reduction in

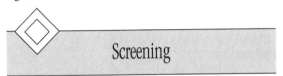

Screening

Because the 5-year survival rate of lung cancer still hovers around 10 percent, there has been much interest in identifying early cancer that may be amenable to treatment. With the advent of new radiographic tests and molecular markers, a number of studies are investigating different methods of screening for early cancer in high-risk populations.

In the 1970s and 1980s, four randomized trials determined that chest radiographs (CXR) alone or in combination with sputum cytology were not effective screening tools for early lung cancer.[7–10] These studies showed that most cases of lung cancer detected by chest radiograph already have regional or distant metastatic disease.

These findings led to further study of strategies involving newer technologies. The three primary tools of interest have been low-dose helical (spiral) chest computed tomography (CT), autofluorescence bronchoscopy, and advanced sputum analysis with molecular markers. A brief description of each tool is provided here (Table 14-2).

Low-Dose Helical CT

Three recent clinical trials reported that helical CT was superior to CXR in finding lung cancer.[11–13] In a study of 1000 asymptomatic adults older than 60 years who had a greater than 10-pack-a-year history of smoking, the Early Lung Cancer Action Project reported that 27 subjects (2.7 percent) were found to have lung cancer by helical CT, in comparison with 7 (0.7 percent) by CXR.[13] Patients with lung cancer who were detected by CT were significantly more likely to have resectable or stage I disease than those discovered with CXR. However, this study lacked a control population to compare whether early detection translates into reduction in mortality rates versus an increased lead-time survival.

An important limitation of helical CT is the high false positive rate, leading to increased costs for serial CT scans and other diagnostic studies. In the Early Lung Cancer Action Project, 233 (23.3 percent) subjects were found to have noncalcified nodules on helical CT, but in only 27 did these prove to be malignant.[13] The protocol used to categorize nodules needing to be biopsied was quite accurate, with only one subject having a biopsy for a nonmalignant nodule. The percentage of unnecessary biopsies may be

Table 14-2

Potential Screening Techniques for Identification of Early Lung Cancer

SCREENING TOOL	LOCATION OF CANCER IDENTIFIED
Imaging Techniques	
Low-dose helical CT scan (with CAD)	Peripheral
PET-FDG scan	Central and peripheral
Autofluorescence bronchoscopy	Central
Sputum Biomarkers	
hnRNP A2/B1	Central
K-*ras*	Central
p53	Central
CpG islands of p16	Central

ABBREVIATIONS: CT, computed tomography; CAD, computer-aided three-dimensional imaging; PET-FDG, positron emission tomography with fluoro-deoxyglucose; hnRNP, heterogeneous nuclear ribonucleoprotein.

a greater problem in areas where granulomatous disease is more prevalent. Methods such as nodule enhancement and positron emission tomography using fluoro-deoxyglucose (PET-FDG) are being studied to determine ways to better distinguish between granulomatous and malignant nodules prior to biopsy.

A second potential limitation of helical CT is the accurate assessment of growth rates of small malignant nodules.[14] A doubling in the volume of a 5-mm nodule results in a 1.25-mm increase in nodule diameter, a change that can be difficult to detect with serial CT. Sophisticated software to enhance computer-aided three-dimensional measurements of nodule volume rather than diameter is likely to reduce this limitation.

Finally, helical CT detects peripheral cancers much better than central ones, thus biasing toward early detection of adenocarcinoma, which tends to occur peripherally. To be effective, a screening strategy will need to combine methods of detecting both peripheral and central cancers.

Autofluorescence Bronchoscopy

Conventional bronchoscopy is a valuable tool in detecting preinvasive lung cancer but has not been shown to be an effective screening test. By illuminating the bronchial surface with violet or blue light, autofluorescence bronchoscopy enhances the detection of the dysplastic lesions or carcinoma in situ. This method requires extensive training, but once someone is proficient at the technique, it adds only a few minutes to a standard bronchoscopy. Studies are ongoing to compare the detection rate of premalignant and preinvasive lesions with autofluorescence bronchoscopy to that with conventional bronchoscopy and other techniques.

The cost and invasiveness of the autofluorescence bronchoscopy will limit its usefulness in widespread screening, but it may well serve as an invaluable step following noninvasive techniques in a screening algorithm for high-risk populations.

Sputum Cytology and Molecular Biomarkers

The sensitivity of standard sputum cytology for detecting lung cancer is low, ranging from 20 to 30 percent in screening studies. Sensitivity is highest for central cancers, particularly squamous cell carcinoma. Recent techniques for enhancing sputum cytology are promising.[15]

Sputum immunostaining for heterogeneous nuclear ribonucleoprotein A2/B1 (hnRNP A2/B1), a ribonucleoprotein that is overexpressed in most lung cancer cell types, increases the sensitivity of cytologic screening to a range of 77 to 91 percent, with a specificity of 65 to 88 percent.[16,17] This overexpression of hnRNP A2/B1 appears to occur in preneoplastic cells and thus may serve as a method to stratify risk in subjects in the precancer phases. Two trials are in process in large populations to determine the role of hnRNP A2/B1 in the diagnosis of preclinical and early lung cancer.

Polymerase chain reaction (PCR) assays have been developed to test for tumor-specific gene mutations, including oncogene K-ras and p53 mutations. K-ras mutations appear to be associated with adenocarcinomas, with the codon-12 mutation of K-ras being associated with smoking-related adenocarcinomas.[18] An increased genomic instability, including allelic imbalance on the short arms of chromosomes 3, 9, and 17, appears to be associated with the early stages of lung cancer development and can be measured by PCR amplification. Also, hypermethylation of the CpG islands of the p16 gene can be measured in the sputum and appears to be highly associated with early stages of NSCLC.

Future Directions in Screening

Helical CT has a higher sensitivity for small peripheral neoplasms, whereas sputum immunodiagnosis is more sensitive for small central lung cancers. Systematic approaches combining helical CT with a panel of sputum immunoassays in high-risk patients are being studied.

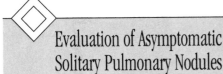

Evaluation of Asymptomatic Solitary Pulmonary Nodules

Asymptomatic solitary pulmonary nodules (SPNs) are seen in 0.09 to 0.2 percent of chest radiographs. An SPN is defined as a single spherical lesion completely surrounded by lung without associated atelectasis or adenopathy.[19] The prevalence of lung cancer in SPNs varies significantly with risk factors, including age, smoking history, and characteristics of the nodule. Because the 5-year survival of a stage IA NSCLC approaches 80 percent, it is important to systematically evaluate an SPN in order to detect and treat a cancer, if one is present. Integral in the decision-making process is the need to balance early diagnosis of a potentially treatable cancer with avoidance of unnecessary cost and invasive procedures.

Initial Evaluation

Evaluating the appearance of an SPN on CXR is the first step in assessing the likelihood of a malignant versus a benign etiology. Consulting a previous CXR, if available, allows one to ascertain whether the lesion was present in the past and whether it has increased in size over time. SPNs that were present in the past and have not changed size for more than 2 years are generally benign. Next, one should assess the absolute size of the nodule. Nodules greater than 3 cm in diameter are almost always malignant. Third, evaluation of associated features of the nodule should be noted. The presence of fine linear strands extending outward from the nodule, referred to as the *corona radiata* sign, has a high positive predictive value for malignancy. Laminated, central, popcorn, and diffuse calcifications within nodules are generally associated with benign etiologies. In contrast, stippled or eccentric calcifications are associated with malignancies.

Chest CT generally provides useful supplementary information in the evaluation of a patient with an SPN. The nodule is better visualized, and CT scans are more sensitive for identifying nodular calcifications and other nodules. Computer-aided diagnosis by an artificial neural network may further improve the diagnostic accuracy in distinguishing benign from malignant nodules.[20]

Low- and High-Risk Groups

Following CXR and chest CT, a patient can be categorized into a low-, indeterminate-, or high-risk group. To date, though, there has not been a prospective, randomized clinical trial comparing different methods of risk stratification or evaluation. The following recommendations represent the traditional approach, which is based on small retrospective studies and clinical experience.[19] Low-risk nodules include those that are stable in size (≥ 2 years), have benign-type calcifications (laminated, central, popcorn, or diffuse), and occur in younger individuals (< 35 years old) who have no history of pro-neoplastic exposures (tobacco, radon, asbestos). Traditional methods of follow-up for patients in the low-risk group, which have not been subjected to the rigors of an evidence-based approach, recommend serial CXR every 3 months for a year followed by one every 4 to 6 months for another year.

High-risk patients, including those with a larger nodule (> 3 cm), those with abnormal radiographic or calcification patterns (*corona radiata*, eccentric/stippled calcifications), and older patients who smoke and have a new nodule, should be aggressively managed. If not contraindicated by other co-morbid conditions, high-risk patients should have prompt video-assisted thoracoscopy. Video-assisted thoracoscopic surgery (VATS) is a minimally invasive technique in which a video-optical tube is introduced through a small intercostal incision to provide a panoramic view of the thoracic cavity. It is less invasive than an open thoracotomy and can be converted to an open procedure if the nodule is found to be malignant on frozen section.

Indeterminate-Risk Group

Most patients cannot be categorized into either of these two groups and are considered at indeterminate risk. Optimum approaches to this group have not been prospectively and systematically evaluated. Encouragingly, recent advances in technology provide some alternatives that are under investigation. PET scanning may provide a useful, noninvasive step in the evaluation of patients with an SPN and indeterminate risk. Because lesions with low uptake on PET-FDG scanning are almost always benign, it is anticipated that research will confirm a high negative predictive value of PET scanning for evaluating an intermediate-risk SPN.

Bronchoscopic biopsy is useful for nodules that are > 2 cm and are near the bronchial tree. However, most SPNs that are evaluated either are smaller or are located peripherally. Complications of bronchoscopy are infrequent, with an incidence of pneumothorax < 5 percent. CT-guided transthoracic fine needle biopsy is useful in detecting cancer in peripheral nodules, including smaller lesions. The sensitivity and specificity of fine needle biopsy for peripheral nodules ranges from 80 to 95 percent and from 50 to 88 percent, respectively.[19] In a study of 222 patients, the positive predictive value of transthoracic fine needle biopsy was 98.6 percent with a negative predictive value of 96.6 percent.[21] Depending on the institution and the radiologist, false negative rates can range from 3 to 28 percent. Transthoracic needle biopsy is invasive, with pneumothorax occurring in almost a third of patients, although most do not require chest tube placement.

When biopsy by bronchoscopy or transthoracic fine needle is indeterminate, there are two management options: careful radiographic follow-up or thoracotomy. The decision should be individualized and should be a shared decision by the patient and the physician. Thoracotomy is the most definitive method of determining etiology. In this case, VATS may be ideal, since it is most successful with peripheral or central nodules.

Clinical Manifestations of Lung Cancer

Clinical manifestations of lung cancer generally connote advanced disease. Presenting signs and symptoms can be grouped into pulmonary/local manifestations and extrapulmonary manifestations (Table 14-3).

Pulmonary/Local Invasion

Local growth of the lung cancer can cause a cough, hemoptysis, or airway obstruction. Cough is the most common presenting symptom, occurring in almost 75 percent of patients and characterized by production of copious thin secretions. The patient may present with a new cough or a change in the character of a chronic cough. Hemoptysis, occurring in less than a third of patients at presentation, can manifest as either sputum streaked with blood or gross, larger amounts of blood. Though bronchitis is the most common etiology of hemoptysis, patients with a history of smoking or other lung cancer exposures should be promptly investigated. Unilateral wheezing, more common in squamous cell carcinoma, occurs from obstruction of a major airway. Obstruction can also be present as a postobstructive pneumonia or abscess.

Invasion of adjacent structures can cause a variety of signs and symptoms. Vague chest pain is common and is often due to invasion of the chest wall or mediastinum. Recurrent laryngeal paralysis, resulting in hoarseness, can occur with tumor extension into the mediastinum. Invasion of the pleura can lead to an effusion, resulting in progressive dyspnea. Pericardial invasion can

Table 14-3

Clinical Manifestations of Lung Cancer

Pulmonary	**Paraneoplastic syndromes**
Cough	*Endocrine system*
Hemoptysis	SIADH
Unilateral wheezing	Cushing's syndrome
Postobstructive pneumonia/abscess	Hypercalcemia
	Gonadotropin-induced gynecomastia
Local invasion	*Nervous system*
Chest pain	Cerebellar degeneration
Hoarseness	Encephalomyelitis
Pleural effusion	Lambert-Eaton myasthenic syndrome
Cardiac tamponade/arrhythmia	Sensorimotor peripheral neuropathy
Dysphagia	Dermatomyositis
Superior vena cava syndrome	Osteoarthropathy
Pancoast tumor with invasion of	Thromboembolic disease
cervical (Horner's syndrome)	Acantosis nigricans
or brachial nerve	

ABBREVIATION: SIADH, syndrome of inappropriate secretion of antidiuretic hormone.

result in cardiac tamponade or an arrhythmia, while esophageal invasion can present as dysphagia.

Superior vena cava syndrome is caused by obstruction by the tumor of venous return from jugular veins into the superior vena cava. The syndrome is characterized by periorbital and facial edema and eventually blue discoloration and new-vessel formation on the anterior chest wall. The edema is usually worse in the morning or after lying in a horizontal position for several hours, and it improves upon standing.

Tumors involving the superior sulcus or apex of the lung, referred to as Pancoast tumors, can cause cervical and brachial plexopathies. Horner syndrome results from disruption of the cervical sympathetic nerves by tumor invasion and is characterized by unilateral facial anhidrosis, ptosis, and miosis. Tumor invasion of the brachial plexus is generally manifested by shoulder and arm pain.

Extrapulmonary Manifestations

Extrapulmonary manifestations can be further subdivided into those due to metastatic disease and those caused by paraneoplastic syndromes. Signs and symptoms of metastatic disease include cervical and supraclavicular adenopathy, bone pain, headaches, and seizures resulting from the spread of cancer to the lymph nodes, brain, bone, and bone marrow. Liver and adrenal metastases are generally asymptomatic. Systemic symptoms, such as anorexia and weight loss, are common in patients with metastatic disease.

About 10 percent of patients with lung cancer have a paraneoplastic syndrome, an extrapulmonary complication of lung cancer not caused by metastases. SCLC is the classic example. Small cell cancer often is associated with ectopic hormone production that results in distant manifestations. The two systems most commonly affected by SCLC are the endocrine and nervous systems. Cushing's syndrome, resulting from ectopic production of adrenocorticotropic hormone, occurs in about 5 percent of patients with SCLC. Rather than the overt Cushing's that is commonly seen with exogenous steroid use, patients with SCLC generally have milder and more subtle symptoms, manifested by increased pigmentation, hypokalemia, and frequent infections. Another common endocrinopathy associated with SCLC is the syndrome of inappropriate secretion of antidiuretic hormone (SIADH), manifested by chronic hyponatremia and inappropriately elevated urine osmolality. Hypercalcemia, which occurs from ectopic secretion of parathyroid-like hormone, is associated with squamous cell carcinoma. Neurologic paraneoplastic syndromes associated with SCLC include myasthenic Lambert-Eaton syndrome (proximal muscle weakness), subacute cerebellar degeneration (ataxia, dysarthria, dementia), and peripheral neuropathy. Other paraneoplastic syndromes that are associated with NSCLC include hypertrophic osteoarthropathy (digital clubbing and tenderness over the distal aspect of long bones) and a hypercoagulable state (thromboembolic disease).

Diagnosis and Staging

Diagnosis

If lung cancer is suspected, either because of an evaluation of an asymptomatic solitary nodule or because of overt signs or symptoms, sampling of lung tissue is necessary for definitive diagnosis. Tissue for biopsy can be obtained via bronchoscopy, CT-guided transthoracic fine needle aspiration, thoracentesis, mediastinoscopy, or thoracoscopy/thoracotomy. The first two were noted earlier. Pleural fluid obtained through tho-

racentesis is positive for malignant cells in about 30 percent of patients with a malignant pleural effusion.[22]

Cervical mediastinoscopy is generally not necessary for diagnosis, but is useful in staging for paratracheal and hilar nodal involvement. Mediastinoscopy by left parasternal approach (Chamberlain) allows sampling of nodes in the aorticopulmonary window and paratracheal area. Alternatively, endoscopic ultrasonography-guided fine needle aspiration via the esophagus can be used to sample subcarinal, paraaortic, and aorticopulmonary window nodes.

VATS has also become a popular method of staging invasive disease, allowing easy access to the inferior mediastinal nodes in addition to the paraaortic and aorticopulmonary window nodes. Use of VATS also allows for exploration of the chest cavity to determine if any pleural seeding is evident and can reveal the presence of inoperable cancer without the need for a thoracotomy.

Staging Small Cell Lung Cancer

SCLC is generally disseminated at the time of diagnosis, and thus surgical cure is not an option. The most commonly used classification system for SCLC was proposed by the Veterans Administration Lung Cancer Study Group. This system categorizes patients into two stages: limited and extensive disease. Limited-stage SCLC is found in about 30 to 40 percent of patients and includes those with disease confined to (1) a hemithorax, (2) a primary site with ipsilateral hilar or supraclavicular nodes, or (3) a primary site with ipsilateral or contralateral supraclavicular nodes. All other patients are classified as having extensive-stage SCLC.

To assist in the staging of a patient with SCLC, a primary care clinician should perform a thorough history and physical and obtain a complete blood count, liver enzymes (alanine aminotransferase and aspartate aminotransferase), and a serum alkaline phosphatase. Because 15 percent of patients without central nervous system (CNS) symptoms have brain metastases, a head CT is usually included in the staging evaluation. Similarly, almost a third of patients who have a normal alkaline phosphatase and are asymptomatic are found to have a positive bone scan. However, the value of these tests to stratify treatment alternatives has not been shown to improve survival in patients treated for SCLC.

Staging Non-Small Cell Lung Cancer

The 1997 revised International Staging System is used to determine prognosis and treatment options for patients with NSCLC. The burden of disease is classified with the TNM system, where T refers to the primary tumor size and the presence/absence of local invasion, N refers to the presence/absence of regional lymph node involvement, and M refers to the presence/absence of metastases. Stages IA (< 3 cm) and IB (> 3 cm) correlate with locally confined disease, IIA and IIB with local disease with regional nodal involvement, IIIA and IIIB with regional invasion, and IV with distant metastasis.

The primary goal of staging patients with NSCLC is to determine which patients may be cured by surgical resection of the tumor. To accomplish this goal, assessment for intrathoracic involvement and distant metastasis is needed.[23] If CT scanning of the chest was not obtained in the initial evaluation, it is useful at this juncture to assess hilar and mediastinal nodes. However, 13 percent of lymph nodes smaller than 1 cm by CT scan have pathologic involvement, necessitating more invasive methods of nodal assessment, including mediastinoscopy or VATS. PET scanning appears to be superior to CT scanning for detecting mediastinal lymph nodes, with a sensitivity ranging from 89 to 93 percent and a specificity of 94 to 100 percent, and thus may provide a noninvasive method of evaluation of lymph node involvement. Further studies are necessary to compare PET-FDG with invasive procedures to assess its role in staging algorithms. Presence of a malignant pleural effusion precludes an operative cure, so if the patient has a pleural effusion, a thoracentesis for cytology is warranted.

A search for metastatic disease should start with a thorough history and physical examination, focusing on signs or symptoms of CNS, bone, and liver involvement. A complete blood count, liver enzymes, calcium, alkaline phosphatase, albumin, creatinine, and electrolytes are generally obtained. CT scanning should also include the liver and adrenal glands because 3 to 6 percent and 5 to 10 percent of patients with NSCLC have metastases to these two organs, respectively. Suspicious lesions should be biopsied. The role of further radiographic testing is controversial, and to date there is no evidence to suggest that use of CT scans of the head or bone scans in asymptomatic individuals without nodal involvement affects the prognosis.

Treatment

Small Cell Lung Cancer

SCLC is very aggressive, and median survival without treatment is about 1 to 3 months after diagnosis. Initially, SCLC is very responsive to chemotherapy, with initial responses in 70 to 90 percent of patients. Unfortunately, most patients relapse; the 5-year survival in 1997 was 6.2 percent.[1]

Patients with limited-stage disease are treated with combined chemotherapy and radiotherapy. Standard treatment consists of four to six courses of cisplatin and etoposide, resulting in a median survival of about 14 to 16 months and a five-year survival rate of less than 15 percent.[24] Studies are in progress to assess the response/toxicity of high-dose chemotherapy with and without autologous bone marrow transplantation. Concurrent thoracic radiotherapy, starting with the onset of chemotherapy, is recommended, either as a total dose of 45 Gy given twice a day over 3 weeks or as 50.4 Gy given once a day over 5 weeks. The twice-a-day regimen appears to be associated with a longer median survival.

Following completion of chemotherapy and thoracic radiotherapy, prophylactic cranial irradiation is sometimes administered, although its role is still controversial. A recent meta-analysis reported a 5.4 percent increase in absolute survival at 3 years with the use of cranial irradiation.[25] The primary complication of cranial irradiation is late-onset neurotoxicity, including dementia and ataxia.

If a patient has extensive-stage disease, carboplatin is used instead of cisplatin, and since the disease is diffuse, thoracic radiotherapy is omitted. Median survival of patients with extensive disease is about 8 to 11 months, with a long-term survival rate of below 3 percent.

New groups of chemotherapeutic agents, including taxanes (paclitaxel), topo-isomerase I inhibitors (topotecan), and vinorelbine, may be effective in patients with SCLC, with initial response rates of 23 percent in extensive disease and 88 percent in limited disease.[26] Relapse rates are still very high, though, and different methods to intensify or time treatment are being studied. Other novel therapies being investigated include anti-angiogenesis agents, signal transduction inhibitors, and cell cycle targeting agents.

Non-Small Cell Lung Cancer

Patients with stage IA or IB disease are potentially curable with surgical resection of the tumor. Radical resection with lobectomy or pneumonectomy is superior to limited resection, with 5-year survival rates ranging between 60 and 80 percent.[27] Addition of adjuvant chemotherapy to increase the survival rate is being studied.

Stage II and III patients are generally treated with a combination of radical surgical resection

plus adjuvant chemotherapy with etoposide and cisplatin.[28] Studies assessing the addition of adjuvant thoracic radiotherapy with newer chemotherapeutic agents such as taxanes and vinorelbine are in progress. Treatment of stage IV disease has been uniformly dismal.

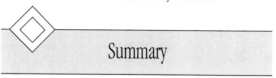

Summary

The financial and quality of life burdens of lung cancer to both the individual and society are considerable. Recognizing the prevalence of this problem and the poor outcomes of this disease, the National Institutes of Health and other granting agencies have provided a great deal of support to investigations aimed at improving methods for screening, chemoprevention, and treatment of lung cancer. Early results are promising, suggesting that our view of lung cancer may change in the near future. The role of the primary care physician in chemoprevention and screening will be critical.

Currently, though, it is important for the primary care clinician to recognize that early-stage non-small cell lung cancer is quite treatable and thus warrants aggressive management in potentially curable patients. Further, increased efforts in primary and secondary prevention through education regarding tobacco use are necessary.

References

1. Ries LAG, Eisner MP, Kosary CL, et al: SEER cancer statistics review, 1973–1998. Bethesda, MD, National Cancer Institute; 2001.
2. Smith RA, Glynn TJ: Epidemiology of lung cancer. *Radiol Clin North Am* 38:453–470, 2000.
3. Christiani DC: Smoking and the molecular epidemiology of lung cancer. *Clin Chest Med* 21:87–93, 2000.
4. Samet JM, Eradze GR: Radon and lung cancer risk: taking stock at the millennium. *Environ Health Perspect* 108(suppl 4):635–641, 2000.

5. Lancaster T, Stead L, Silagy C, et al: Effectiveness of interventions to help people stop smoking: findings from the Cochrane Library. *Br Med J* 321: 355–358, 2000.

6. Khuri FR, Lippman SM: Lung cancer chemoprevention. *Semin Surg Oncol* 18:100–105, 2000.

7. Frost JK, Ball WC Jr, Levin ML, et al: Early lung cancer detection: results of the initial (prevalence) radiologic and cytologic screening in the Johns Hopkins study. *Am Rev Respir Dis* 130:549–554, 1984.

8. Flehinger BJ, Melamed MR, Zaman MB, et al: Early lung cancer detection: results of the initial (prevalence) radiologic and cytologic screening in the Memorial Sloan-Kettering study. *Am Rev Respir Dis* 130:555–560, 1984.

9. Fontana RS, Sanderson DR, Taylor WF, et al: Early lung cancer detection: results of the initial (prevalence) radiologic and cytologic screening in the Mayo Clinic study. *Am Rev Respir Dis* 130:561–565, 1984.

10. Kubik A, Polak J: Lung cancer detection. Results of a randomized prospective study in Czechoslovakia. *Cancer* 57:2427–2437, 1986.

11. Kaneko M, Eguchi K, Ohmatsu H, et al: Peripheral lung cancer: screening and detection with low-dose spiral CT versus radiography. *Radiology* 201:798–802, 1996.

12. Sone S, Takashima S, Li F, et al: Mass screening for lung cancer with mobile spiral computed tomography scanner. *Lancet* 351:1242–1245, 1998.

13. Henschke CI, McCauley DI, Yankelevitz DF, et al: Early Lung Cancer Action Project: overall design and findings from baseline screening. *Lancet* 354:99–105, 1999.

14. Boiselle PM, Ernst A, Karp DD: Lung cancer detection in the 21st century: potential contributions and challenges of emerging technologies. *Am J Roentgenol* 175:1215–1221, 2000.

15. Mulshine JL: Reducing lung cancer risk: early detection. *Chest* 116:493S–496S, 1999.

16. Zhou J, Mulshine JL, Unsworth EJ, et al: Purification and characterization of a protein that permits early detection of lung cancer. Identification of heterogeneous nuclear ribonucleoprotein-A2/B1 as the antigen for monoclonal antibody 703D4. *J Biol Chem* 271:10760–10766, 1996.

17. Tockman MS, Mulshine JL, Piantadosi S, et al: Prospective detection of preclinical lung cancer: results from two studies of heterogeneous nuclear ribonucleoprotein A2/B1 overexpression. *Clin Cancer Res* 3:2237–2246, 1997.

18. Montuenga LM, Mulshine JL: New molecular strategies for early lung cancer detection. *Cancer Invest* 18:555–563, 2000.

19. Ost D, Fein A: Evaluation and management of the solitary pulmonary nodule. *Am J Respir Crit Care Med* 162:782–787, 2000.

20. Nakamura K, Yoshida H, Engelmann R, et al: Computerized analysis of the likelihood of malignancy in solitary pulmonary nodules with use of artificial neural networks. *Radiology* 214:823–830, 2000.

21. Conces DJ, Schwenk GR, Doering PR, et al: Thoracic needle biopsy. Improved results utilizing a team approach. *Chest* 91:813–816, 1987.

22. Light RW, Erozan YS, Ball WC Jr: Cells in pleural fluid. Their value in differential diagnosis. *Arch Intern Med* 132:854–860, 1973.

23. Hyer JD, Silvestri G: Diagnosis and staging of lung cancer. *Clin Chest Med* 21:95–106, 2000.

24. Johnson DH: Management of small cell lung cancer. *Chest* 116:525S–530S, 1999.

25. Auperin A, Arriagada R, Pignon JP, et al: Prophylactic cranial irradiation for patients with small-cell lung cancer in complete remission. Prophylactic Cranial Irradiation Overview Collaborative Group. *N Engl J Med* 341:524–526, 1999.

26. Adjei A: Management of small cell cancer of the lung. *Curr Opin Pulmonary Med* 6:384–390, 2000.

27. Dominioni L, Imperatori A, Rovera F, et al: Stage I non-small cell lung carcinoma: analysis of survival and implications for screening. *Cancer* 89: 2334–2344, 2000.

28. Bunn PA Jr, Mault J, Kelly K: Adjuvant and neoadjuvant chemotherapy for non-small cell lung cancer. *Chest* 117:119S–122S, 2000.

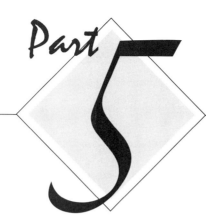

Chronic
Respiratory
Problems

Peter J. Carek
Lori M. Dickerson

Chapter

15

Allergic Rhinitis: Mechanisms, Evaluation, and Treatment

Rhinitis is defined as inflammation of the mucous membranes that line the nose. This condition is characterized by nasal congestion, rhinorrhea, sneezing, itching of the nose, and/or postnasal drainage.[1] Rhinitis is often associated with asthma, eustachian tube dysfunction, otitis media, rhinosinusitis, nasal polyps, allergic conjunctivitis, and atopic dermatitis.

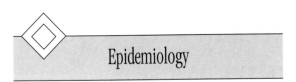

Epidemiology

Allergic rhinitis is the most common nasal problem and the sixth most common chronic disease in the United States, affecting as many as one in five adults and children.[2] The prevalence of allergic rhinitis in the United States varies from region to region, depending upon the amount and type of airborne allergens present. Evidence exists that the prevalence of allergic rhinitis is increasing worldwide.[3,4]

The onset of allergic rhinitis is typically in childhood, adolescence, or early adulthood. In a study based in Tucson, Arizona, 42 percent of children evaluated had allergic rhinitis by 6 years of age,[5] but the onset of symptoms most commonly occurs between the ages of 10 and 20 years. Allergic rhinitis develops before the age of 20 years in 80 percent of cases.[1] During the first 10 years after onset, about one-third of adults improve and approximately half experience worsening symptoms.

Because of the large number of individuals affected, allergic rhinitis creates a burden in terms of expenditures for medical care and lost productivity from work. The annual direct economic impact of allergic rhinitis is nearly $1.2 billion.[6] Most of these costs (> 90 percent) are attributed to direct medical expenses, with medications emerging as the single largest component of these costs.[7] Furthermore, allergic rhinitis accounts for approximately 811,000 missed workdays, 824,000 missed school days, and 4,230,000 days of reduced activity.[7] The combined impact of health care services and lost productivity is estimated to be $5.6 billion annually.[8]

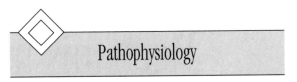

Pathophysiology

Allergic rhinitis may be seasonal or perennial, and both types may coexist in the same individual. Both the seasonal and perennial forms of allergic rhinitis are the result of an IgE-mediated reaction of the nasal mucosa to an allergen, and each type has identifiable characteristics (Table 15-1).[2]

The most common seasonal allergens are pollens. Tree pollens are released mostly during the early to mid-spring. The height of the grass pollen season is late spring to early summer. Weed pollen is present during the late summer to early fall. Pollination may occur year round in the southern United States.[9] The heavy, sticky pollens of brightly colored flowers seldom cause allergy symptoms, as these pollens are spread by insects and not by wind currents.

Perennial allergic rhinitis is caused by an IgE-mediated reaction to perennial environmental allergens. These allergens include dust mites, animal dander, and molds. Additionally, cockroaches and other insects, certain occupational substances, and other plants may produce allergens responsible for perennial allergic rhinitis.

Common Allergens

In most areas of the world, house dust mites are a major source of allergens in the indoor environment.[10] House dust is a mixture of lint, mites, mite-derived feces, dander, insect parts, fibers, and other particulate materials.[11] Mites live in

Table 15-1

Differentiating Characteristics of Seasonal and Perennial Allergic Rhinitis

CHARACTERISTIC	SEASONAL	PERENNIAL
Timing of allergen	One or more seasonal allergens	Allergens show little or no seasonal variation
Timing of symptoms	Period correlating with seasonal variation in aeroallergens	Intermittent or continuous throughout the year
Characteristic symptoms	Watery rhinorrhea Nasal congestion Repetitive sneezing Pruritus of eyes, nose, ears, and throat Watery eyes	Prominent and severe nasal blockage and congestion Postnasal drainage
Common allergens	Grass pollens Tree pollens Weed pollens Fungal (mold) pollens	House-dust mite Animal dander Cockroach Mold

SOURCE: Adapted from American Academy of Allergy, Asthma, and Immunology,[2] with permission.

bedding, mattresses, and carpets and feed on human skin dander. Ordinary vacuuming and dusting have little effect on reducing dust mites; in fact, vacuuming may lead to a brief episode of airborne mite feces, leading to inhalation and initiation of the allergic reaction.

Animal dander is another common allergen. The major source of allergens in animal dander is proteins secreted by animal skin glands.[9] These allergens accumulate in carpets, bedding, upholstered furniture, and clothing. Since skin glands secrete these proteins, short-haired and long-haired breeds may be equally allergenic. Cats are a greater source of indoor allergens than dogs and other pets.

Molds and fungi are also important indoor and outdoor allergens.[11] While pollen allergens typically become windborne during dry weather and are removed from the air during rain, high mold-spore counts are found in clouds and mist. Many upper respiratory tract allergy symptoms that occur during periods of high humidity are probably attributable to favorable conditions for mold growth.

The Allergic Reaction

The allergic reaction begins when airborne particles are deposited on the respiratory mucous membranes during normal inhalation. Particles the size of most pollen grains and the larger mold spores are deposited on the nasal mucosa.[11]

The mast cell, found in the superficial mucosal tissues of the nose and coated with IgE antibodies, is the pivotal cell of the acute allergic reaction.[12] Mast cell degranulation is the most important initiating event in the acute allergic reaction.[7] Eosinophils and lymphocytes also contribute to the allergic reaction.

The IgE-mediated allergic response occurs in three steps: sensitization, early-phase reaction, and late-phase reaction.[2] In sensitization, the initial exposure to an allergen leads to synthesis of allergen-specific IgE antibodies. These specific antibodies are released into circulation and accumulate on the surface of mast cells. On subsequent exposure, reaction with the specific IgE on the surface of mast cells results in the early-phase reaction, with degranulation of mast cells induced by allergens leading to the release of a complex cascade of mediators (Table 15-2).[13] This reaction occurs within minutes of exposure as preformed mediators (i.e., histamine, tryptase, and heparin) and newly synthesized mediators (i.e., leukotrienes) are released as a result of the antigen's cross-linking adjacent IgE.[14] Histamine is an important mediator of mast cell degranulation and is thought to account for approximately half of the symptoms associated with allergic rhinitis.[13]

Histamine causes vascular permeability, sneezing, and pruritus, and stimulates reflex-mediated glandular secretions.[15] Histamine is capable of stimulating almost every end organ in the nasal tissue and producing every symptom of the constellation that constitutes allergic rhinitis.[12]

The late-phase reaction occurs 4 to 6 h after the early-phase reaction. In the late-phase reaction, allergen stimulation of immune cells (i.e., mast cells, lymphocytes, and epithelial cells) results in the release of cytokines.[14] These substances prolong and enhance the allergic reaction, with resulting edema and infiltration of tissues by eosinophils, basophils, and neutrophils. Clinically, an increase in nasal mucosal thickness can be detected as increased nasal airflow resistance occurs with minimal if any change in other nasal symptoms.[13] Further synthesis and release of inflammatory mediators may occur over the subsequent hours.

In addition to the chemical mediators of the allergic reaction, the activation of sensory nerves during the allergic reaction is also an important element in the generation of the acute symptoms of rhinitis.[12] Via the parasympathetic nervous system, this activation causes the stimulation of submucosal glands, resulting in sneezing and itching—typical symptoms of allergic rhinitis.

In addition to the IgE-mediated allergic response, mucosal hyperresponsiveness may occur. Hyperresponsiveness is a characteristic of mucosal surfaces during inflammation.[13] Hyperresponsiveness indicates an increased mucosal response to nonspecific irritants such as histamine, methacholine, bradykinin, hypertonic saline solution, and other provocational agents.[7] In addition, repeated allergen exposure results in hyperresponsiveness, as symptoms occur at lower allergen levels and in response to nonspecific irritants.

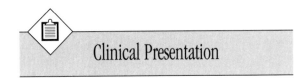

Clinical Presentation

History

A detailed and accurate history is important in the initial evaluation of individuals with allergic rhinitis. The patient's clinical presentation should

Table 15-2

Common Symptoms of Allergic Rhinitis and the Associated Mediators

Symptom	Mediator
Tickling, itching, nose rubbing, allergic salute	Histamine, prostaglandins
Sneezing	Histamine
Nasal congestion, stuffy nose, mouth breathing, snoring	Histamine, leukotrienes, bradykinin
Runny nose, postnasal drip, throat clearing	Histamine, leukotrienes

Source: Adapted from Pearlman,[15] with permission.

be noted, and any family and personal history of atopy (e.g., allergic rhinitis, asthma, atopic eczema) during infancy or childhood should be determined.[16]

Questions about symptoms and symptom pattern, including onset, progression, severity, duration, relationship to seasons, and casual and exacerbating factors, should be asked.[13] In addition to these questions, other important questions to ask during the initial evaluation of the patient presenting with allergic-type symptoms include the following:[16]

1. Does the house environment include pets? What are the bedding materials, the source of heat? Are air conditioners used in the summer?

2. Are there increasing symptoms during a particular season, during activity such as vacuuming, or in the presence of irritants and pollutants such as tobacco smoke, air fresheners, or household chemicals?

3. What are the person's occupational and leisure activities, particularly those that may aggravate symptoms?

4. Are the nasal symptoms isolated, or are there concomitant signs from other parts of the upper airways, such as sinuses or ears? Is there a history of lower airway, ocular, or dermatologic disease such as asthma symptoms, conjunctivitis, eczema, or contact urticaria?

Symptoms of allergic rhinitis may include sneezing; itching of the nose, eyes, palate, or pharynx; nasal stuffiness with partial or total obstruction of airflow; and rhinorrhea, often accompanied by postnasal drainage. Tearing and soreness of the eyes coupled with a gelatinous conjunctival discharge in the mornings and loss of well-being with irritability, fatigue, and depression may also occur during peak symptom periods.[11]

A personal history of other atopic diseases, a strong family history of allergy, or a regular seasonal pattern of compatible symptoms strongly suggests an allergic cause. Other risk factors for allergic rhinitis include higher socioeconomic class and exposure to indoor allergens such as animals and dust mites.[1]

Physical Examination

The physical examination should focus on the nose, eyes, throat, and ears (Table 15-3).[1] The lungs and skin also should be closely examined. Several findings on physical examination are characteristic of allergic rhinitis (Table 15-4).[2,11,17]

Patients with active allergic rhinitis typically demonstrate pale, swollen, inflamed nasal mucosa; clear rhinorrhea; and, occasionally, injected sclera with edematous eyelids.[17] The nasopharynx may show clear to creamy discharge and lymphoid hypertrophy. Upper airway edema and compression of local venous and lymphatic flow frequently create allergic shiners. A transverse crease across the nasal bridge caused by repeated upward nasal rubbing is often present. This "allergic salute" is a by-product of intense, intolerable pruritus. Some of these typical signs are shown in Fig. 15-1.

Purulent rhinorrhea is characteristic of infectious rhinitis, which may reflect a viral upper respiratory tract infection or a bacterial rhinosinusitis.[17] The presence of purulent secretions does not exclude the possibility of allergic rhinitis, however; allergic rhinitis is a frequent predisposing factor for sinusitis.

Foreign bodies, tumors, polyps, and other abnormalities should be sought on direct visual examination of the nose. Nasal polyps in children should raise the possibility of cystic fibrosis.[17] Adults with nasal polyps invariably have eosinophilic rhinitis with coexisting recurrent bacterial sinusitis and moderate to severe persistent asthma.

Laboratory Testing

Several laboratory tests are available to assist with the diagnosis of allergic rhinitis.

Table 15-3

Areas of Focus in the Physical Examination for Patients Presenting with Symptoms Suggestive of Allergic Rhinitis

AREA	FINDING(S)
General observations	Facial pallor, mouth breathing, nasal crease
Eyes	Evidence of conjunctivitis, Dennie-Morgan lines (accentuated lines or folds below the margin of the inferior eyelid)
Nose	Presence or absence of external deformity, nasal mucosal swelling, nasal polyps, deviated septum, septal perforation, discharge, blood
Ears	Abnormalities of tympanic membranes (pneumatic otoscopy), including abnormal mobility patterns, retraction, air-fluid levels, bubbles behind tympanic membrane; consider tympanometry to confirm the presence or absence of effusion and middle ear under- or overpressure
Mouth	Malocclusion or high arched palate associated with chronic mouth breathing, tonsillar hypertrophy, lymphoid "streaking" in the oropharynx, pharyngeal postnasal discharge, halitosis, and pain upon mouth occlusion suggestive of temporomandibular joint syndrome
Neck	Lymphadenopathy, thyroid enlargement
Chest	Signs of asthma
Skin	Eczema, skin dryness, dermatographism

SOURCE: Adapted from Joint Task Force on Practice Parameters in Allergy, Asthma and Immunology,[1] with permission.

Table 15-4

Specific Findings on Physical Examination Characteristic of Allergic Rhinitis

FINDING	DESCRIPTION	COMMENT
Allergic crease	Hyperpigmented or hypopigmented groove at the junction of the tip of the nose and the more rigid nasal bone	See allergic salute
Allergic gape	Continuous open-mouth breathing	Nasal blockage
Allergic salute	Using the palm of a hand for an upward thrust of the nares, thereby relieving itching and opening the nasal airway	Nasal blockage
Allergic shiners	Dark discoloration in the orbital-palpebral grooves beneath the lower eyelids	Venous stasis caused by mucosal edema of the nose and sinuses
Cobblestoning	Bands of lymphoid hyperplasia of the posterior pharynx	Chronic postnasal drainage
Dennie-Morgan lines	Wrinkle just beneath the lower eyelids that may be present from early infancy	Associated with atopic dermatitis and allergic rhinitis

SOURCE: Adapted from American Academy of Allergy, Asthma, and Immunology,[2] Kaliner and Lemanske,[11] and Variant,[17] with permission.

Figure 15-1   Presentation of Allergic Rhinitis: Clues

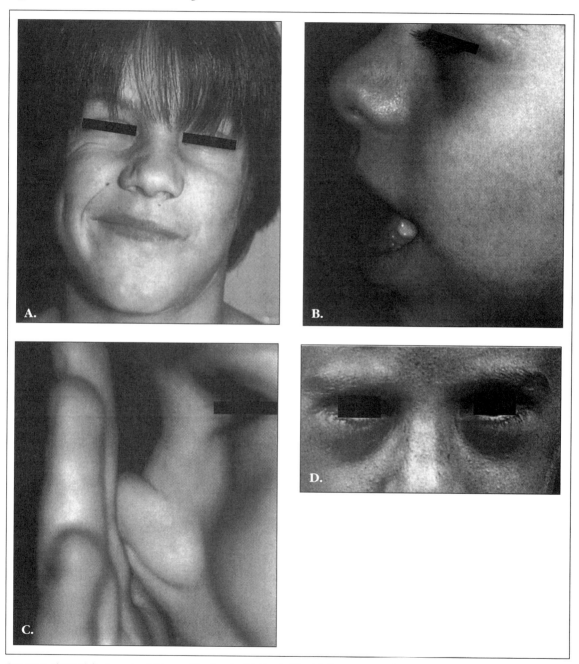

Common physical findings in children with allergic rhinitis. **A.** Nasal itching. **B.** Mouth breathing. **C.** "Allergic salute." **D.** "Allergic shiners." Source: Reprinted from Skoner et al: Allergy and immunology, in Zitelli et al: *Atlas of Pediatric Physical Diagnosis.* St. Louis, Mosby-Wolfe; 1997, by permission.

EOSINOPHIL COUNT AND TOTAL IgE

A moderate peripheral blood eosinophilia may be present, particularly in the presence of an accompanying allergic disease such as asthma. Although suggestive of an allergic etiology, blood eosinophilia is also associated with numerous other problems (i.e., dermatitis, parasitic infestations, malignant diseases, irradiation, hypereosinophilic syndrome, and other miscellaneous conditions).

Total IgE levels are elevated in only 30 to 40 percent of patients with allergic rhinitis, and they are also elevated in several nonallergic conditions. Therefore, a normal IgE level does not exclude the diagnosis and an elevated IgE level does not make a diagnosis of allergy. Certain immunodeficiency diseases, IgE myeloma, drug-induced interstitial nephritis, graft versus host disease, parasitic diseases, and hyper-IgE syndrome are nonatopic syndromes with elevated serum IgE.[9] Total IgE levels contribute less to the evaluation and care of the potentially allergic patient than a well-performed history and physical examination, complemented by specific allergy testing.[18]

NASAL CYTOLOGY

The examination of nasal secretions for inflammatory cells is a useful adjunct. In allergic rhinitis, the nasal secretions demonstrate a significant percentage of eosinophils.[17] The presence of eosinophils in clumps or eosinophils constituting more than 10 percent of the total white cells counted indicates a probable allergic cause. On the other hand, an elevation in the total neutrophil count with a low percentage of eosinophils suggests an infectious etiology.

SKIN TESTS

Skin tests are the preferred method for diagnosing IgE-mediated sensitivity, as test positivity is closely associated with the symptoms of nasal allergy.[9,19] In patients with perennial symptoms, testing should include antigens for dust mites, animal danders, and molds. Seasonal symptoms should prompt investigation of appropriate regional tree, grass, and weed pollens. In small children, particularly those with asthma or eczema, certain food allergens (e.g., egg, peanut, milk, wheat, soy, tree nuts, fin fish, and shellfish) also may be significant.[20]

Skin testing involves exposing a small group of mast cells to a suspected allergen via percutaneous or intradermal injection of the allergen.[18] If IgE molecules specific for the particular allergen are present on mast cells, the mast cells will degranulate, leading to a wheal (localized swelling) and flare (localized redness).

Prick or scratch (epicutaneous) tests are the preferred initial method of skin testing. In this test, a small amount of antigen is placed on the skin surface and a sharp point from a needle or another similar device is used to minimally puncture or scratch the skin.[18] After 15 min, the test sites are examined and the results interpreted. These specific tests are sensitive and safe and involve minimal discomfort.

Intradermal tests are the secondary method applied for allergens that were negative on prick punctures when 100 percent sensitivity is important. These tests are used more often to identify allergies to environmental allergens such as dust mites, animals, or indoor molds, or to provide a comprehensive evaluation of a patient who is likely to initiate allergen-specific immunotherapy.[18] In this test, a volume of antigen extract is injected just under the skin surface to create a distinct 2- to 3-mm-diameter bleb. After 15 min, the puncture sites are examined for urticaria or erythema.

The prick test has several advantages compared to the intradermal test and is usually the initial test performed.[9,18] The prick test exposes the patient to a smaller amount of antigen and therefore is less likely to lead to severe allergic reactions. In addition, the prick test is less painful and is easier and faster to perform. Prick testing results also correlate better with clinical allergy history than do the results of intradermal testing.

Because it is designed to expose the patient to a minimal amount of allergen, however, the prick test is somewhat limited in its ability to identify all patients who are allergic to a given substance.[18] In contrast, the intradermal test, because it exposes the patient to a larger dose of antigen, is believed to be more sensitive, though it is less specific.

RADIOALLERGOSORBENT TESTS

There are various in vitro methods of measuring specific IgE antibodies. Of the several methods available, the radioallergosorbent test (RAST) is most useful clinically. RAST is an alternative to skin tests. This test is a useful screen that involves combining the patient's serum with a mixture of common inhalant allergens bound to a matrix or disk.[21,22] The correlation of the findings with prick testing for pollens is approximately 80 percent. Further, specific IgE measurement and skin testing may be considered complementary to one another in diagnosing allergic rhinitis.[19] In vitro IgE immunoassays should be considered in patients with the following characteristics: severe dermatographism, ichthyosis, and generalized eczema; use of long-acting antihistamines and tricyclic antidepressants; risk for anaphylaxis with skin testing to a particular allergen; or high risks associated with discontinuation of current medications.[9]

OTHER TESTS

Plain radiographs and computed tomography (CT) are rarely useful in the diagnosis of allergic rhinitis. CT or magnetic resonance imaging (MRI) is useful when chronic or recurrent rhinosinusitis is suspected as a complicating factor.

In selected cases, special techniques such as fiber-optic nasal endoscopy and/or rhinomanometry may be useful in evaluating patients presenting with rhinitis symptoms.[1] Fiber-optic nasal endoscopy (rhinolaryngoscopy) is the most useful diagnostic procedure in an evaluation for anatomic factors causing upper airway symptoms. Endoscopy provides a clear view of the nasal cavity and allows for detailed examination of the middle meatus, superior meatus, sphenoethmoidal recess, and posterior nasopharynx, as well as the structures of the oropharynx and larynx.[23]

Rhinomanometry measures the resistance (or conductance, the inverse of resistance) to airflow through the nose.[1] Rhinomanometry is a test of functional obstruction to airflow in the upper airway. The objective information obtained from rhinomanometry may be particularly important when it is suspected that an occupational exposure is causing nasal congestion.

Differential Diagnosis

Several conditions should be considered in the evaluation of a patient presenting with allergic symptoms (Table 15-5).[16,24] Vasomotor rhinitis, infectious rhinitis, and rhinitis medicamentosa often present a diagnostic dilemma.

Vasomotor Rhinitis

Vasomotor rhinitis, a result of "nasal hyperresponsiveness," produces persistent nasal congestion and rhinorrhea. Symptoms increase with nonspecific stimuli, such as rapid temperature or humidity changes, strong smells, ingestion of alcoholic beverages, emotional changes, or air pollution. While a specific etiology for vasomotor rhinitis has not been determined, an imbalance in the autonomic innervation of the nose that favors parasympathetic vasodilatation and nasal congestion is felt to be the cause.

Infectious Rhinitis

Infectious rhinitis caused by viral agents is very common, especially in childhood. Occasionally,

Table 15-5

Differential Diagnosis of Rhinitis

Infectious rhinitis
Allergic rhinitis
Seasonal
Perennial
Drug-induced rhinitis
Hormonal rhinitis
Nonallergic rhinitis with eosinophilia syndrome (NARES)
Nonallergic rhinitis without eosinophilia
Occupational rhinitis
Rhinitis medicamentosa
Rhinitis of pregnancy
Vasomotor rhinitis
Disturbed nasal function associated with the following:
Adenoidal hypertrophy
Ciliary dyskinesia
Hypothyroidism
Horner's syndrome
Hypertrophy of the nasal turbinates
Foreign body
Nasal polyps
Nasal septal deviation
Enlarged tonsils and adenoids
Sinusitis
Tumors
Wegener's granulomatosis
Cerebral spinal fluid rhinorrhea
Aspirin intolerance

SOURCE: Adapted from Urval[16] and Matthews,[24] with permission.

a bacterial infection (e.g., *Streptococcus pneumoniae* or *Haemophilus influenzae*) with sinus involvement may be present. An average child has three to six viral upper respiratory tract infections per year. As these illnesses often occur in rapid succession over relatively short periods of time, differentiating infectious from allergic rhinitis is often difficult.

Rhinitis Medicamentosa

Rhinitis medicamentosa is a condition of nasal hypersensitivity, mucosal swelling, and tolerance that is induced or aggravated by the overuse of topical vasoconstrictors.[25] This condition most commonly results from excessive use of topical nasal decongestants, such as oxymetazoline, naphazoline, phenylephrine, and xylometazoline. Rhinitis medicamentosa may also occur in patients taking ovarian hormonal agents (i.e., oral contraceptives), aspirin, and some antihypertensive medications (i.e., clonidine, reserpine, hydralazine, or alpha and beta blockers). Cocaine, a recreational drug, is also known to cause nasal congestion and rhinorrhea.

Treatment

Several general principles should be followed in the management of allergic rhinitis. Initially, allergens that cause symptoms should be avoided if at all possible. If symptoms persist despite allergen avoidance, pharmacotherapy may be instituted and directed at relief of symptoms. Finally, the patient may be evaluated for allergen immunotherapy if allergen avoidance and pharmacotherapy do not provide sufficient relief of symptoms.

Allergen Avoidance

When possible, environmental control measures for allergens should be applied (Table 15-6).[9,10] Even if the effect of these measures is not complete, they generally improve the patient's symptoms and reduce the need for pharmacologic treatment. While most of these measures can be accomplished, reducing exposure to pollens and outdoor allergens is extremely difficult, and the

Table 15-6

Environmental Control of Allergen Exposure

ALLERGEN	RECOMMENDATIONS FOR REDUCING EXPOSURE
Animal dander	Remove animal from house or, at minimum, keep animal out of patient's bedroom.
	Seal (or cover with a filter) air ducts that lead to bedroom.
	Wash pet weekly.
	Remove carpet or other reservoirs for allergens from bedroom.
	Install room air filters (HEPA type).
Dust mites	Encase mattress, pillow, and box springs in an allergen-impermeable cover.
	Remove stuffed animals, toys, or both from bedroom.
	Wash bedding weekly in hot water (>130°F).
	Reduce indoor humidity to < 50 percent.
	Remove carpets from the bedroom and from other rooms where they are laid on concrete.
	Minimize upholstered furniture.
	Vacuum weekly (vacuum cleaner should have good-quality bags).
Pollens and outdoor molds	Limit exposure during season by staying indoors with windows closed, especially when pollen levels are elevated.
	Use air conditioning.
Indoor mold	Prevent spore infiltration by closing doors and windows.
	Use air conditioning.
	Control moisture by means of dehumidification; seal water leaks and use dehumidifiers.
	Clean and remove contaminated materials by applying fungicides.
	Maintain heating and air conditioning systems.
	Install room air filters (HEPA type).
Tobacco smoke	Stop all smoking and do not allow smoking in house or car.
	Avoid all exposure to secondhand tobacco smoke.
Indoor/outdoor pollutants and irritants	Reduce exposure to wood-burning stoves or fireplaces, unvented stoves or heaters, and other irritants, such as perfumes and cleaners.

ABBREVIATION: HEPA = high-efficiency particulate air.

SOURCE: Adapted from American Academy of Allergy, Asthma, and Immunology[2] and Eggleston and Bush,[10] with permission.

benefit of allergen source removal may take several weeks or months to be perceived.

Pharmacotherapy

Pharmacotherapy for allergic rhinitis includes antihistamines, intranasal corticosteroids, decongestants, mast cell stabilizers, and anticholinergic agents. When choosing appropriate therapy, the pathophysiology of the condition should be considered. For example, if it is possible to anticipate the onset of symptoms (i.e., seasonal allergic rhinitis), prophylactic therapy can be initiated prior to exposure.

ANTIHISTAMINES

Histamine$_1$-receptor antagonists, or antihistamines, are first-line therapy in the treatment of allergic rhinitis.[1,2] Overall, antihistamines are most effective in reducing itching, sneezing, and rhinorrhea (Table 15-7).[1,2] They are generally ineffective in relieving nasal congestion in patients with allergic rhinitis and are often combined with an oral decongestant (e.g., phenylpropanolamine or pseudoephedrine) or intranasal corticosteroid.[1]

The first-generation antihistamines (i.e., diphenhydramine, brompheniramine, chlorpheniramine, etc.) are highly sedating and are available without a prescription. The second-generation agents are typically referred to as the nonsedating antihistamines (e.g., cetirizine, fexofenadine, loratadine) and are currently available only by prescription (Table 15-8).[1,26,27]

Azelastine is a nonsedating second-generation antihistamine available for intranasal inhalation. The newer agents are approved for use in adults and children; individual dosing and age recommendations vary with each product (Table 15-8).

Antihistamines reduce or prevent the signs and symptoms of allergic rhinitis by competitive antagonism of histamine, the primary mediator of allergic rhinitis symptoms, at H$_1$ receptors in the vasculature and airway smooth muscle.[1,26] Binding of the antihistamine to the receptor is reversible and may be overcome by excessive exposure to allergen. As other inflammatory mediators play a role in the symptoms of allergic rhinitis, antihistamines do not completely prevent all symptoms. First-generation antihistamines also have affinity for peripheral H$_1$, cholinergic, dopaminergic, serotoninergic, and alpha-adrenergic receptors and cross the blood-brain barrier.[28] Nonsedating antihistamines do

Table 15-7

Overview of Effectiveness of Pharmacotherapy for Allergic Rhinitis

AGENT	SNEEZING	ITCHING	CONGESTION	RHINORRHEA	EYE SYMPTOMS	APPROVED FOR USE IN CHILDREN < 12 YEARS OF AGE
Oral antihistamines	++	++	+/−	++	++	Yes
Nasal antihistamines	+	+	+/−	+	−	No
Intranasal corticosteroids	++	++	++	++	+	Yes
Oral decongestants	−	−	+	−	−	Yes
Intranasal decongestants	−	−	++	−	−	Yes
Intranasal mast cell stabilizers	+	+	+	+	−	Yes
Topical anticholinergics	−	−	−	++	−	Yes

ABBREVIATIONS: −, provides no benefit; +/−, provides little or minimal benefit; +, provides modest benefit; ++, provides substantial benefit.
SOURCE: Adapted from American Academy of Allergy, Asthma, and Immunology,[2] with permission.

Table 15-8.

Comparison of Antihistamines for Allergic Rhinitis

DRUG	FORMULATION	AVAILABLE WITH DECONGESTANT	DOSAGE	COMMENTS
FIRST-GENERATION ANTIHISTAMINES				
Brompheniramine (Dimetapp Allergy, generic)	Capsules (4 mg)	Yes	2–6 years: 0.5 mg/kg/day divided QID 6–12 years: 4 mg TID > 12 years: 4–8 mg QID up to 24 mg/day	As a class, the first-generation antihistamines have the following characteristics: Side effects are due to anticholinergic and antihistaminic activity, and include somnolence, dry mouth, dry eyes, urinary retention, impaired psychomotor performance, decreased concentration.
Chlorpheniramine (Chlor-Trimeton, generic)	Tablets (4 mg) Chewable tablets (2 mg) Time-release tablets (8 mg, 12 mg) Syrup (2 mg/5 mL)	Yes	2–6 years: 1 mg QID 6–12 years: 2 mg QID up to 12 mg/day > 12 years: 4 mg QID up to 24 mg/day	Central nervous system effects may persist until morning after use and decrease learning/work productivity.
Clemastine (Tavist)	Tablets (1.34 mg, 2.68 mg) Syrup (0.67 mg/5 mL)	Yes	6–12 years: 0.67 mg BID up to 2.25 mg/day > 12 years: 1.34 mg BID up to 8.04 mg/day	May cause paradoxical excitation in children and the elderly. Contraindicated in patients with narrow-angle glaucoma, symptomatic prostatic hypertrophy, bladder obstruction.
Diphenhydramine (Benadryl, generic)	Tablets (25 mg, 50 mg) Chewable tablets (12.5 mg) Capsules (25 mg, 50 mg) Syrup (6.25 mg/5 mL, 12.5 mg/5 mL)	Yes	Infants > 10 kg: 12.5–25 mg T-QID or 5 mg/kg/day divided QID Adults: 25–50 mg T-QID	Pregnancy category B/C; avoid in breastfeeding mothers.
Hydroxyzine (Atarax, Vistaril, generic)	Tablets (10 mg, 25 mg, 50 mg, 100 mg) Capsules (50 mg, 100 mg) Syrup (10 mg/5 mL)	No	< 6 years: 5–10 mg QID 6–12 years: 10–25 mg QID > 12 years: 25 mg QID	
SECOND-GENERATION ANTIHISTAMINES				
Azelastine (Astelin)	Nasal spray (137 µg/spray)	No	> 12 years: 2 sprays per nostril BID	With first use, prime the pump with 4 sprays until a fine mist appears. Repeat with 2 sprays if > 3 days have passed since last use.
Cetirizine (Zyrtec)	Tablets (5 mg, 10 mg) Syrup (5 mg/5 mL)	No	2–5 years: 2.5–5 mg QD or 2.5 mg BID 6–11 years: 5–10 mg QD > 11 years: 5–10 mg QD	Active metabolite of hydroxyzine. May be sedating even at recommended doses. Pregnancy category B.
Fexofenadine (Allegra)	Tablets (30 mg, 60 mg, 180 mg) Capsules (60 mg)	Yes	6–11 years: 30 mg BID > 11 years: 60 mg BID or 180 mg QD	Relatively free of sedative side effects even in high doses. Pregnancy category C.
Loratadine (Claritin)	Tablets (10 mg) Syrup (5 mg/5 mL) Reditabs (10 mg)	Yes	2–5 years: 5 mg QD 6–11 years: 10 mg QD > 11 years: 10 mg QD	In low doses is nonsedating; sedation increases with dosage increase. May be less effective than cetirizine and fexofenadine. Pregnancy category B.

ABBREVIATIONS: QID, four times daily; TID, three times daily; BID, twice daily; QD, once daily.

not share these properties, a characteristic that may explain the lack of significant adverse reactions when compared to the older agents.[28]

Onset of action of oral antihistamines is an important factor when considering the management of an acute allergic response. Overall, the currently available nonsedating antihistamines have a rapid onset of action (i.e., 15 to 30 min), comparable to that of the first-generation agents. The first-generation agents have a shorter duration of action (i.e., 4 to 6 h) and require multiple daily doses. The nonsedating antihistamines have a duration of action ranging from 8 to 24 h, allowing dosing only once or twice a day.[26] All oral agents are hepatically metabolized and excreted in the urine.

Symptom improvement with antihistamine therapy is typically noted within 1 to 2 h after the initial dose, but maximum effects may not be noted for several weeks. Treatment should be continued for 2 to 3 weeks before a decision is made to change medication because of lack of effectiveness. Once-daily preparations should be taken at bedtime, to minimize any sedative effects. For optimal results, antihistamines should be taken on a regular basis.

Drug interactions are common with the older sedating antihistamines, particularly when used in combination with central nervous system depressants, alcohol, or monoamine oxidase inhibitors. Azole antifungals (i.e., fluconazole, itraconazole, ketoconazole, etc.) and macrolide antibiotics (i.e., azithromycin, clarithromycin, erythromycin) can increase serum concentrations of loratadine, but the clinical importance of this interaction is minimal.

Sedation and performance impairment are the primary adverse effects associated with antihistamines, particularly the first-generation agents. Some patients experience tolerance to the sedative effects of the older antihistamines, but recent evidence suggests that performance impairment persists even without associated sedation.[1,2,28] Using a sedating antihistamine at night and a nonsedating antihistamine during the day may still affect daytime functioning and is currently

not recommended.[2,28] The risk of work impairment with sedative antihistamines has been compared to that with other centrally acting substances like alcohol, benzodiazepines, and narcotic analgesics.[29,30] The risk of this impairment includes automobile accidents, occupational accidents, decreased work performance and productivity, and impaired learning and academic performance. Workers in the transportation industry should avoid first-generation antihistamines to reduce the risk of work-associated injuries and accidents.[1] Currently, more than 30 states in the United States have laws that impose a fine, license suspension or revocation, or a jail sentence on persons convicted of driving under the influence of sedating antihistamines.[1] These agents also negatively affect school performance in children, reinforcing the preference for using second-generation antihistamines in this group.[31] Other side effects associated with first-generation antihistamines include dry mouth, dry eyes, and urinary retention (Table 15-8).[1,26,27]

Second-generation antihistamines poorly penetrate the central nervous system and are associated with much less sedation than the older agents. Of the second-generation antihistamines, cetirizine is the most sedating, often referred to as a "low-sedating" rather than a nonsedating antihistamine. Azelastine nasal spray may be systemically absorbed, and therefore has an incidence of somnolence similar to that of the oral second-generation antihistamines.

Although significant differences in tolerability exist, the clinical efficacy of both groups of antihistamines is similar (Table 15-7).[2] In clinical practice, patients usually express a definite preference for one drug over another.

DECONGESTANTS

Decongestants are alpha-adrenergic agonists that cause nasal vasoconstriction, reducing the blood supply to the mucosa and inhibiting nasal obstruction.[2,28] These sympathomimetic agents are available over the counter in oral and intranasal formulations. While decongestants are not effective in relieving sneezing, itching, or ocular symptoms, they may provide relief from nasal congestion (Table 15-7).[2] The primary oral decongestant used is pseudoephedrine. Phenylpropanolamine was previously available in many products but was removed from the market because of an association with hemorrhagic stroke.[32]

Oral decongestants are associated with multiple side effects, including restlessness, agitation, tremor, insomnia, loss of appetite, headache, dry mucous membranes, urinary retention, increased intraocular pressure, and cardiovascular effects, such as increased blood pressure, palpitations, and tachycardia.[1,2,28] Oral decongestants should not be used in patients with arrhythmias, angina, poorly controlled hypertension, or hyperthyroidism. They should be used cautiously in elderly patients at increased risk for side effects. Pseudoephedrine is approved for use in adults and children over 3 months of age.[26]

Oral decongestants are often used in combination with oral antihistamines (Table 15-8).[1,26,27] These combination products have been found to be more effective than either agent alone.[1,2] The stimulatory effects of decongestants may counteract the sedative properties of the first-generation antihistamines, improving tolerability.

Intranasal decongestants (i.e., oxymetazoline, naphazoline, phenylephrine, xylometazoline) are available for short-term relief of nasal congestion in patients with allergic rhinitis.[1,2,26] In addition to a faster onset of action and greater effectiveness than oral decongestants, these agents have fewer systemic side effects. Topical sympathomimetics are recommended for short-term use only (i.e., less than 3 to 5 days) to minimize the risk of rhinitis medicamentosa. Topical decongestants are approved for use in children 2 years of age and older.[26]

CORTICOSTEROIDS

Intranasal corticosteroids are the most effective pharmacologic agents for treating allergic rhinitis.[1,2] Several intranasal corticosteroids are currently available, including beclomethasone, budesonide, flunisolide, fluticasone, mometasone, and triamcinolone (Table 15-9).[2,26]

These agents are most useful when nasal obstruction is the patient's most significant symptom. Their efficacy is related to several factors. These agents reduce endothelial and epithelial permeability, minimizing nasal mucosal edema. Furthermore, they reduce inflammatory cell infiltration in the nasal mucosa, minimize nonspecific nasal hyperreactivity, and decrease the response of mucous glands to cholinergic stimulation. Local administration has the greatest effect on these properties, supporting the administration of corticosteroids intranasally. Prophylactic use reduces congestion, sneezing, rhinorrhea, and itching (Table 15-7).[1,2] Because a clear nasal passage is necessary for delivery of corticosteroids, topical decongestants may need to be used for a few days prior to initiation of intranasal corticosteroids.

Intranasal corticosteroids produce significantly greater relief than oral antihistamines for nasal blockage, discharge, sneezing, nasal itch, and postnasal drip.[33] However, the time needed to achieve symptom relief and to reach maximum benefit appears to be longer than with the antihistamines. Initial relief may occur within 12 h of initiation of therapy, and the maximum therapeutic benefit occurs by the second week of use. To maintain efficacy, intranasal corticosteroids must be used regularly, even in the absence of symptoms. Once initial relief is obtained, the dose should be reduced to the minimal effective dosage.

Local side effects of intranasal steroids include nasal irritation, bleeding, dryness, and sneezing.[2] Nasal irritation, characterized by burning and stinging, may be associated with mild epistaxis. Rarely, nasal septal perforation has been reported with long-term use of high-dose intranasal corticosteroids.[1] Oral candidiasis may occur if the corticosteroid is swallowed.

Systemic side effects from intranasal steroids (i.e., growth retardation, hypothalamic-pituitary-

Table 15-9

Comparison of Intranasal Corticosteroids

DRUG NAME		DOSE/ ACTUATION	DOSAGE (PER NOSTRIL)	
GENERIC	TRADE		PEDIATRIC	ADULT
Beclomethasone dipropionate	Beconase Vancenase Vancenase Pockethaler	42 µg	6–12 years: 1 spray TID	1 spray B-QID
	Beconase AQ		6–12 years: 1 spray BID	1–2 sprays BID
	Vancenase AQ	84 µg	6–12 years: 1 spray QD	1–2 sprays QD
Budesonide	Rhinocort	32 µg	6–12 years: 2 sprays BID or 4 sprays QD	2 sprays BID or 4 sprays QD
Flunisolide	Nasarel Nasolide	25 µg	6–14 years: 1 spray TID or 2 sprays BID	2 sprays B-TID
Fluticasone	Flonase	50 µg	4–12 years: 1 spray QD increased to 2 sprays BID or 4 sprays QD	2 sprays BID or 4 sprays QD
Mometasone	Nasonex	50 µg	3–12 years: 1 spray QD	2 sprays QD
Triamcinolone	Nasocort Nasocort AQ	55 µg	6–12 years: 2 sprays QD	2 sprays Q-BID

SOURCE: Adapted from American Academy of Allergy, Asthma, and Immunology[2] and Cada,[26] with permission.

adrenal suppression, cataracts, and glaucoma) are extremely rare.[1] Mometasone and fluticasone are less likely to cause systemic side effects because of their poor gastrointestinal absorption. These agents may be preferred in adults with contraindications to systemic corticosteroids, adults with asthma using inhaled oral corticosteroids, and growing children.[31,34] Clinical trials of low doses of intranasal corticosteroids for children with allergic rhinitis have not demonstrated sustained effects on growth or adrenal suppression.[2,31,35] While oral antihistamines and intranasal cromolyn sodium remain first-line agents in children, corticosteroids are used in conjunction with other therapies in children with severe symptoms that are not resolved with other therapies. In children, fluticasone or mometasone are preferred because of their low systemic bioavailability and because they have been approved for use in younger children (Table 15-9).[2,26]

Although systemic steroids are not appropriate for chronic use in allergic rhinitis, short bursts of therapy are appropriate for severe cases that are unresponsive to intranasal corticosteroids, oral antihistamines, or other products. If used, a short course (3 to 7 days) of short-acting oral corticosteroids (e.g., prednisone 40 mg daily) should be chosen.[1] Intranasal corticosteroid use should be continued during this period. Intramuscular and intraturbinate injections of corticosteroids are not recommended.[1,2]

MAST CELL STABILIZERS

Intranasal cromolyn inhibits the degranulation of mast cells, preventing the release of histamine and other allergic mediators of inflammation.

Effective in preventing both the early- and late-phase allergic reaction, cromolyn minimizes sneezing, itching, congestion, and rhinorrhea (Table 15-7).[2] Intranasal cromolyn is available as an over-the-counter product.

Cromolyn must be administered as one spray in each nostril 3 to 4 times daily. The protective effect after inhalation lasts between 4 and 8 h, and maximum efficacy is usually reached after 7 days of use.[1] The frequency of administration and prolonged period prior to achieving maximum effect may significantly inhibit compliance.

Cromolyn is generally considered to be less effective than intranasal corticosteroids. Therefore, this agent should be used for pretreatment of patients with predictable periods of exposure to allergens who do not tolerate oral antihistamines or corticosteroids.[1,28] Cromolyn is not very effective once symptoms have started.[2]

Cromolyn has an excellent safety profile and can be used in children and pregnant women.[1,31] Side effects include sneezing, nasal stinging, burning, irritation, and bad taste.[1,2]

ANTICHOLINERGIC AGENTS

Ipratropium bromide is the only intranasal anticholinergic drug that is approved for allergic rhinitis. Cholinergic hyperreactivity has been demonstrated in patients with allergic rhinitis, and a significant portion of histamine release appears to be cholinergically mediated. Ipratropium blocks receptors on cholinergic neurons, resulting in decreased stimulation of mucus glands.[1]

Anticholinergic agents are primarily effective in reducing rhinorrhea; they have little effect on sneezing, itching, congestion, or eye symptoms (Table 15-7).[1,2,28] Therefore, ipratropium is most appropriate when rhinorrhea is refractory to the effects of intranasal corticosteroids and/or oral antihistamines. The most common side effects are nasal irritation, crusting, and occasional mild epistaxis.

CONSIDERATIONS IN THE PHARMACOTHERAPEUTIC MANAGEMENT OF ALLERGIC RHINITIS

Management of allergic rhinitis should be individualized based on the severity of symptoms (Table 15-10).[2] Patients with intermittent symptoms should take rapid-onset, nonsedating oral antihistamines or intranasal antihistamines on an as-needed basis. When the period of exposure to allergens is anticipated, nasal cromolyn may be used as a preventive measure.

For patients with mild to moderate symptoms that are persistent, initial therapy should be an oral nonsedating antihistamine or an intranasal corticosteroid on a regular basis. An oral decongestant may be added to the antihistamine either separately or as part of a combination product. If patients do not tolerate oral antihistamines, intranasal products can be used. Children should receive intranasal cromolyn sodium as first-line therapy. Clinicians should consider referral to an allergy specialist for co-management or consultation.

Patients with severe allergic rhinitis should use a combination of intranasal corticosteroids and antihistamines (oral or topical). Short bursts of oral corticosteroids also may be used. If rhinorrhea is particularly bothersome, intranasal ipratropium should be added. Patients with eye symptoms can receive topical ophthalmic antihistamines, vasoconstrictors, mast cell stabilizers, or topical nonsteroidal anti-inflammatory agents. Children should still be treated initially with cromolyn sodium. If this agent is ineffective or is impractical for the family, a second-generation oral antihistamine or low-dose intranasal corticosteroid should be recommended.

Immunotherapy

Immunotherapy with allergens that induce the formation of protective blocking IgG antibodies should be considered for patients who cannot control their symptoms with the usual methods of avoidance and pharmacotherapy.[36] Well-controlled clinical studies have demonstrated

Table 15-10

Stepwise Approach to Pharmacotherapy for Allergic Rhinitis

SEVERITY	DAILY MEDICATION	QUICK-RELIEF MEDICATION
SEASONAL ALLERGIC RHINITIS		
Intermittent symptoms	None	Rapid onset, oral, nonsedating antihistamine
Persistent mild to moderate symptoms	Oral nonsedating antihistamine (alone or with decongestant) **OR** Topical intranasal corticosteroid **CONSIDER** Topical intranasal antihistamine Nasal cromolyn sodium for children If prominent eye symptoms, consider topical ophthalmic antihistamine +/− vasoconstrictor, topical ocular mast cell stabilizer, +/− topical ocular nonsteroidal anti-inflammatory drug	**OR** Topical nasal antihistamine
Severe symptoms (referral to specialist for consultation/ co-management recommended)	Topical intranasal corticosteroid **AND** Oral nonsedating antihistamine (alone or with decongestant) **CONSIDER** Topical intranasal antihistamine Nasal cromolyn sodium for children **AND, IF NEEDED,** A short course (3–7 days) of oral corticosteroids If prominent eye symptoms, consider topical ophthalmic antihistamine +/− vasoconstrictor, topical ocular mast cell stabilizer, +/− topical ocular nonsteroidal anti-inflammatory drug	
PERENNIAL ALLERGIC RHINITIS		
Intermittent symptoms	None	Rapid onset, oral, nonsedating antihistamine
Persistent mild to moderate symptoms	Oral nonsedating antihistamine (alone or with decongestant) **AND/OR** Topical intranasal corticosteroid **CONSIDER** Topical intranasal antihistamine Nasal cromolyn or oral nonsedating antihistamine for children	**OR** Topical nasal antihistamine
Severe symptoms (referral to specialist for consultation/ co-management recommended)	Topical intranasal corticosteroid **AND** Oral nonsedating antihistamine (alone or with decongestant) **AND, IF NEEDED,** A short course (3–7 days) of oral corticosteroids If copious watery discharge, consider intranasal anticholinergic	

SOURCE: Adapted from American Academy of Allergy, Asthma, and Immunology,[2] with permission.

that allergen immunotherapy is beneficial in the treatment of allergic rhinitis caused by tree pollens, grass pollens, weed pollens, mold spores, dust mites, and animal dander.[9] Considerations favoring the use of immunotherapy include long allergen seasons; perennial symptoms; poor response to, poor tolerance of, or unwillingness to use symptomatic medications; presence of chronic or recurrent rhinosinusitis; or the presence of chronic or recurrent middle ear disease.[2] Immunotherapy also may be beneficial in patients with coexisting asthma, since treatment of the allergic problems may reduce the severity of asthma symptoms.

To start immunotherapy, the patient undergoes administration of increasing amounts of allergen every 5 to 7 days until either a symptom-relieving dose is obtained or a maximal tolerance dose is achieved.[36] Once maintenance is reached, the patient receives allergy shots for approximately 3 to 5 years. About 75 percent of patients develop a permanently diminished allergen response and can discontinue injections; the remainder may required lifelong immunotherapy.

References

1. Joint Task Force on Practice Parameters in Allergy, Asthma and Immunology: Diagnosis and management of rhinitis: complete guidelines of the Joint Task Force on Practice Parameters in Allergy, Asthma and Immunology. *Ann Allergy Asthma Immunol* 81:478–518, 1998.
2. American Academy of Allergy, Asthma, and Immunology: *The Allergy Report*, vol. 2, *Diseases of the Atopic Diathesis*. Milwaukee, WI, American Academy of Allergy, Asthma, and Immunology; 2000.
3. Linneberg A, Nielsen NH, Madsen F, et al: Increasing prevalence of allergic rhinitis symptoms in an adult Danish population. *Allergy* 54:1194–1198, 1999.
4. Sly RM: Changing prevalence of allergic rhinitis and asthma. *Ann Allergy Asthma Immunol* 82:233–248, 1999.
5. Juniper EF: Rhinitis management: the patient's perspective. *Clin Exp Allergy* 28(suppl 6):34–38, 1998.
6. Weiss KB, Sullivan SD: The health economics of asthma and rhinitis. *J Allergy Clin Immunol* 107:3–8, 2001.
7. Malone DC, Lawson KA, Smith DH, et al: A cost of illness study of allergic rhinitis in the United States. *J Allergy Clin Immunol* 99:22–27, 1997.
8. Ross RN: The costs of allergic rhinitis. *Am J Managed Care* 2:285–290, 1996.
9. American Academy of Allergy, Asthma, and Immunology: *The Allergy Report*, vol. 1, *Diseases of the Atopic Diathesis*. Milwaukee, WI, American Academy of Allergy, Asthma, and Immunology; 2000.
10. Eggleston PA, Bush RK: Environmental allergen avoidance: an overview. *J Allergy Clin Immunol* 107:S403–S405, 2001.
11. Kaliner M, Lemanske R: Rhinitis and asthma. *JAMA* 268:2807–2829, 1992.
12. Togias A: Unique mechanistic features of allergic rhinitis. *J Allergy Clin Immunol* 105:S599–S604, 2000.
13. Baraniuk JN: New insights into allergic rhinitis: quality of life, associated airway diseases, and antihistamine potency. *J Allergy Clin Immunol* 99:763–772, 1997.
14. Naclerio RM: Pathophysiology of perennial allergic rhinitis. *Allergy* 52(36 suppl):7–13, 1997.
15. Pearlman DS: Pathophysiology of the inflammatory response. *J Allergy Clin Immunol* 104:S132–S137, 1999.
16. Urval KR: Overview of diagnosis and management of allergic rhinitis. *Primary Care Clin* 25:649–662, 1998.
17. Variant FS: Allergic rhinitis. *Immunol Allergy Clin North Am* 20:265–282, 2000.
18. Smart BS: Allergy testing using in vivo and in vitro techniques. *Immunol Allergy Clin North Am* 19:35–45, 1999.
19. Droste JH, Kerhoff M, de Monchy JG, et al: Association of skin test reactivity, specific IgE, total IgE, and eosinophils with nasal symptoms in a community-based population: the Dutch ECRHS Group. *J Allergy Clin Immunol* 97:922–932, 1996.
20. Sampson HA. Food allergy. Immunopathogenesis and clinical disorders. *J Allergy Clin Immunol* 103:717–728, 1999.
21. Kelso JM, Sodhi N, Gosselin VA, et al: Diagnostic performance characteristics of the standard

Phadebas RAST, modified RAST, and Pharmacia CAP system versus skin testing. *Ann Allergy* 67: 511–514, 1991.

22. Crobach MJ, Hermans J: Diagnosis of allergic rhinitis. *Br J Gen Pract* 46:437, 1996.

23. Dolen WK, Selner JC: Endoscopy of the upper airway, in Middleton E, Reed CE, Ellis EF (eds): *Allergy Principles and Practice*, 5th ed. St. Louis, Mosby-Year Book; 1998: pp 1017–1023.

24. Matthews KP: Allergic and non-allergic rhinitis, nasal polyposis, and sinusitis, in Kaplan AP (ed): *Allergy*. New York, Churchill Livingstone; 1985: pp 331–366.

25. Graf P: Rhinitis medicamentosa: aspects of pathophysiology and treatment. *Allergy* 52:28–34, 1997.

26. Cada DJ (ed): Respiratory agents, in *Drug Facts and Comparisons*. St. Louis, Wolters Kluwer; 2001: pp 698–707.

27. Newer antihistamines. *Med Lett* 43(1103):35, 2001.

28. Corren J: Allergic rhinitis: treating the adult. *J Allergy Clin Immunol* 105(6 pt 2):S610–615, 2000.

29. Walsh JK, Muehlbach MJ, Schweitzer PK: Simulated assembly line performance following ingestion of cetirizine or hydroxyzine. *Ann Allergy* 69:195–200, 1992.

30. Gilmore TM, Alexander BH, Mueller BA, Rivera FP: Occupational injuries and medical use. *Am J Ind Med* 30:234–239, 1996.

31. Fireman P: Therapeutic approaches to allergic rhinitis: treating the child. *J Allergy Clin Immunol* 105(6 pt 2):S616–S621, 2000.

32. Kernan WN, Viscoli CM, Brass LM, et al: Phenylpropanolamine and the risk of hemorrhagic stroke. *N Engl J Med* 343(25):1826–1832, 2000.

33. Weiner JM, Abramson MJ, Puy RM: Intranasal corticosteroids versus oral H_1 receptor antagonists in allergic rhinitis: systematic review of randomised controlled trials. *Br Med J* 317:1624–1629, 1998.

34. Corren J, Adinoff AD, Buchmeier AD, et al: Nasal beclomethasone prevents the seasonal increase in bronchial responsiveness in patients with allergic rhinitis and asthma. *J Allergy Clin Immunol* 90: 250–256, 1992.

35. Rachelefsky GS: An approach to intranasal corticosteroid use in the pediatric patient with allergic rhinitis: friend or foe? *Fam Pract Recert* 22(13): 16–22, 2000.

36. Hadley JA: Evaluation and management of allergic rhinitis. *Med Clin North Am* 83:13–25, 1999.

Barbara P. Yawn

Chapter

16

Asthma

Asthma is a complex inflammatory syndrome with many clinical presentations. Not all wheezing is asthma, and not all asthma presents with wheezing. A definitive diagnosis of asthma is based on the demonstration of reversible airway obstruction using spirometry. The clinical spectrum of asthma varies from severe persistent disease with daily symptoms to intermittent disease with two or three short episodes each year. Few clinicians see the entire spectrum, and so they often believe that all asthma is similar to the type seen in their office or hospital. This limited perspective may lead generalists and specialists to wonder if they are even treating the same condition.[1]

Clinical, research, and epidemiologic information related to the mildest and intermittent forms of asthma is scant, but, overall, 60 to 70 percent of patients with asthma fall into the categories of "mild persistent" or "intermittent" asthma.[2] The relative frequency of mild persistent and intermittent asthma is not known. Nevertheless, a substantial percentage of people with asthma appear to have only two to four episodes of recognized asthma symptoms each year, separated by long periods without any recognized symptoms of bronchospasm. However, significant concern exists that many of the people labeled as having "intermittent" asthma may have unrecognized and untreated chronic and persistent symptoms.

The emphasis of this chapter will be on the recognition and treatment of persistent asthma. Intermittent asthma will be considered a diagnosis of exclusion, made only after assuring that no persistent and previously unrecognized ongoing symptoms exist. Recommendations for evaluation and treatment are based on our current understanding of the inflammatory and allergic pathophysiology of asthma.

Epidemiology

Asthma is common, affecting more than 25 percent of children at some time before age 18[3,4] and 3 to 5 percent of adults.[4–7] Exercise-induced bronchospasm (EIB), also called exercise-induced asthma, may coexist with asthma, but also occurs in another 3 to 5 percent of children and adults[3,8–10] with no other recognized asthma episodes. Other than myopia, asthma is the most common chronic condition in children, and asthma-related problems are among the most common causes of missed school and workdays. Asthma also is a frequent reason for visits to emergency departments and potentially preventable hospitalizations.[3,11,12]

By age 6 almost half (48 percent) of children have had a recognized episode of wheezing illness.[13] Before the age of 2 years, however, asthma is difficult to diagnose, primarily because of the overlap with bronchiolitis due to respiratory syncytial virus (RSV) infections, the small lungs of premature infants, and the difficulty in confirming reversible airway obstruction. After age 2, asthma is more commonly diagnosed in boys until puberty, when girls have an accelerated rate of new asthma diagnoses.[4]

Among all school-age children (K–12th grades), almost 1 in 4 (24 percent) report having at some time had a physician diagnosis of asthma, and over 1 in 6 (17 percent) report having made a medical visit for asthma in the past 2 years.[4] Between 1 in 10 and 1 in 20 adults report making asthma-related visits after age 20. In adults, asthma appears to be more common in women. After age 45 to 50 new-onset asthma is not common, and the increasing occurrence of chronic obstructive lung disease (COPD) complicated with intermittent wheezing can make identification of asthma difficult.

Asthma appears to be more common in all nonwhite ethnic groups.[3] Some of the ethnic differences may be confounded by socioeconomic differences among racial groups. However, when only middle-class children living in suburban areas are considered, asthma is still most common among African Americans, then Hispanics, and least common in white non-Hispanic children.[14] Causes for ethnic or racial differences after controlling for socioeconomic status are unknown; environmental or genetic factors may account for the difference.

Children and adults living in poverty are at significantly higher risk for asthma. Environmental exposure, including molds, dust mites, cigarette smoke, and cockroaches, may explain this difference. Ethnic and economic differences in mortality rates may be due to differences in access to medical care and medications.[15]

The majority of the 11.9 million asthma-related medical visits made to U.S. health care clinicians are made to primary care physicians.[16] Although the majority of asthma exacerbations are mild to moderate, 5000 Americans die each year as a direct result of their asthma. Both the number of new diagnoses of asthma and the number of deaths from asthma have increased since 1980.[3,4,17] While part of the increase is undoubtedly due to increased recognition and labeling of disease as asthma, the increase in the prevalence of and mortality from asthma appears to be real.

Pathophysiology

Asthma can be viewed as similar to other chronic inflammatory conditions such as rheumatoid arthritis, with some level of persistent underlying disease punctuated by recurrent "flares," exacerbations, or "attacks." Focusing only on exacerbations may lead patients, parents, and clinicians to view asthma as an episodic rather than a chronic illness. Yet the subacute inflammatory process continues during the period of relative quiescence. Patients and families may fail to recognize mild persistent or recurrent symptoms or may dismiss them as normal limitations of asthma, thus disguising the chronic nature of the illness. When asthma is treated as an episodic illness, important aspects of therapy such as control of the inflammatory process and investigation and management of allergic disease may be ignored.

The anatomic hallmarks of asthma are reduced diameter of the airways from bronchial smooth muscle contraction, along with vascular congestion and edema of the bronchial walls and thickening of bronchial secretions. The net result is increased airway resistance. Decreased forced expiratory volumes and flow rates may leave the lungs hyperinflated, with an imbalance of the ventilation/blood flow distribution within the lungs and ineffective elastic recoil in the bronchi and bronchioles. These changes result in increased work of breathing.

Lung Changes in Asthma

The anatomic changes in asthma include both acute and chronic reversible changes and possibly permanent airway remodeling. Acute changes can be divided into early-phase and late-phase reactions as well as bronchial hyperresponsiveness. The normal inflammatory response is aimed at removing or neutralizing toxic agents and healing areas of tissue damage. In asthma, exposure to allergens or other stimuli triggers the inflammatory cascade, bringing mast cells, neutrophils, and eosinophils to the bronchi and alveoli. The early-phase reaction occurs as inflammatory cells release histamines and other chemicals that produce acute bronchial constriction, usually within minutes to a few hours. The process continues with recruitment of other inflammatory cells such as macrophages, basophils, and neutrophils that release the cytokines, tissue necrosing factors, and leukotrienes that result in the late-phase reaction. In intermittent asthma this process appears to be self-regulating and will shut down if the stimuli (allergic or other) are removed.[18]

In persistent asthma the down regulation of the inflammation appears to be faulty, with continuation of the inflammatory process into a chronic phase. Untreated, the chronic inflammation results in symptoms that are clinically evident on a weekly or even daily basis. The normal balance of the immune system may shift to increased production of T cells (specifically Th2 cells) that produce activated B cells—cells that are hyperresponsive to allergic and inflammatory stimulation. The result is a spiral of chronic inflammation with airway narrowing, continued recruitment of inflammatory cells, and hyperresponsiveness to allergens and other stimuli that feed the inflammatory cycle.

In some people with asthma, the chronic ongoing inflammatory response may result in structural changes in the walls of the bronchi. In a subset of children and adults with asthma, the chronic damage to the epithelial cells from mast cells, eosinophils, and the inflammatory mediators leads to increases in the bronchial smooth muscle mass, sub-basement membrane collagen deposition, and vascular hypertrophy. The epithelial cells become denuded and scarred with fibroblasts, thus decreasing the transfer of oxygen across the basement membranes. Eventually the airway remodeling is permanent and not reversible with therapy.[19] While control of the inflammatory and allergic processes seems a reasonable first step, it is not clear that controlling the inflammatory reaction is effective in preventing airway remodeling at all ages and stages of the asthma continuum.[20]

For children, both the inflammatory nature of asthma and the strong association with allergies are important in designing the evaluation and management of the condition. In children, 80 percent of asthma is believed to be allergic asthma, i.e., asthma that is triggered by the exposure and processing of allergens that result in allergic inflammation. A continuum of allergic conditions has been hypothesized and supported by some observations, including the apparent progression of symptoms from food sensitivity and gastrointestinal (GI) distress in infants to allergic rhinitis in toddlers and preschoolers to asthma in young school-age children.[21] In addition, preliminary research suggests that identification and management of allergies early in the progression from GI-based symptoms to asthma may blunt this progression and the expression of future symptoms.[16]

Genetics

Little doubt remains that there is a very strong familial component of asthma. However, the specific genetic mechanisms and the identification of a gene or genes linked to asthma remain elusive. Several candidate genes have been identified that correlate well with the high levels of serum IgE and atopy seen in young children destined to develop asthma.[19] Some of these genes are also linked to hyperresponsiveness of the bronchial airways as well as to receptors associated with the inflammatory and allergic cascade known to be of importance in asthma, including interleukin-4 (IL-4), IL-5, beta-adrenergic, and glucocorticoid receptors. Sorting out the number of candidate genes and the complex nature of asthma and its relationship to early allergen and other antigen exposure may require many years.

Asthma in Children

Diagnosis

DIFFERENTIAL DIAGNOSIS

The first step in diagnosis is to consider asthma in the differential diagnosis of respiratory symptoms. This is facilitated by including an asthma focus in the child presenting for recurrent coughing, recurrent and prolonged "colds," trouble sleeping, or difficulty exercising. A series of questions such as those in Table 16-1[18] has been shown to identify children at high risk of asthma[5,6,22] and could be the basis for questions used in the physician's office. Questions about exercise-related symptoms should also be included on all well child visits and sports preparticipation examinations.

Other causes of asthma-like symptoms in children are shown in Table 16-2.[18] Most of these may be ruled out by history, but others may require additional testing. These etiologies should be considered in the child presenting with the first episode of wheezing, with incomplete response to bronchodilator therapy, or

Table 16-1

An Asthma-Focused History: Questions to Ask

Sample Questions for the Diagnosis and Initial Assessment of Asthma

A "yes" answer to any question suggests that an asthma diagnosis is likely.

In the past 12 months,

- Have you had a sudden severe episode or recurrent episodes of coughing, wheezing (high-pitched whistling sounds when breathing out), or shortness of breath?
- Have you had colds that "go to the chest" or take more than 10 days to get over?
- Have you had coughing, wheezing, or shortness of breath during a particular season or time of the year?
- Have you had coughing, wheezing, or shortness of breath in certain places or when exposed to certain things (e.g., animals, tobacco smoke, perfumes)?
- Have you used any medications that help you breathe better? How often?
- Are your symptoms relieved when the medications are used?
- In the past 4 weeks, have you had coughing, wheezing, or shortness of breath:
  - At night that has awakened you?
  - In the early morning?
  - After running, moderate exercise, or other physical activity?

These questions are examples and do not represent a standardized assessment or diagnostic instrument. The validity and reliability of these questions have not been assessed.

SOURCE: Adapted from NIH,[18] with permission.

with concomitant problems such as failure to thrive.

For children presenting to the emergency department with a recurrent episode of wheezing, the diagnosis is usually clear. However, a significant portion of children with asthma remain unrecognized, undiagnosed, and therefore inadequately treated.[4,5,7] Asthma symptoms may be labeled recurrent colds, nocturnal symptoms may be ignored, and exercise-induced symptoms may be accepted as normal or due to poor fitness levels. In addition, it is not clear how many children currently being treated for intermittent asthma actually have chronic asthma.

The diagnosis of asthma in children less than age 7 is based on relief or diminution of symptoms following inhalation of a short-acting beta-agonist. In practice, many diagnoses of asthma in older children and adults are presumptive,

based on observed or patient-reported response to therapy or changes in peak flow measurements. When in doubt, asthma is diagnosed using spirometry. A 12 percent increase in forced expiratory volume in 1 s (FEV_1) following 2 puffs of a beta-agonist is considered diagnostic. If the pretreatment FEV_1 is normal, the diagnosis can be made by heightened bronchial responsiveness (bronchial hyperresponsiveness) to histamine, methacholine, or cold air during a challenge test. Children as young as age 7 can usually participate in spirometry assessment.

HISTORY

The presenting symptoms of asthma may vary by age. The infant or young child may have a history of recurrent bronchitis or pneumonia, persistent coughing with colds, recurrent croup, or just a chronic chest rattle. Older children may

Table 16-2

Differential Diagnostic Possibilities for Asthma in Infants and Children

Upper airway diseases
- Allergic rhinitis and sinusitis

Obstructions involving large airways
- Foreign body in trachea or bronchus
- Vocal cord dysfunction
- Vascular rings or laryngeal webs
- Laryngotracheomalacia, tracheal stenosis, or bronchostenosis
- Enlarged lymph nodes or tumor

Obstructions involving small airways
- Viral bronchiolitis or obliterative bronchiolitis
- Cystic fibrosis
- Bronchopulmonary dysplasia
- Heart disease

Other Causes
- Recurrent cough not due to asthma
- Aspiration from swallowing mechanism dysfunction or gastroesophageal reflux

report recurrent chest congestion, bronchitis, or persistent coughing with upper respiratory tract infections (URIs). The respiratory symptoms may be precipitated or aggravated by common allergens or irritants such as pollens, cats, dogs, cold air, or tobacco smoke. Recurrent episodes of coughing are especially likely to be labeled recurrent URIs or allergies without recognition or diagnosis of the airflow obstruction component. Cough-variant asthma may not be associated with any audible wheezing and can be diagnosed only with careful history, spirometry, or appropriate challenge tests. Special attention should be paid to the diurnal variation of symptoms, since asthma-related symptoms are more commonly noticed during the night and in the early morning.

A personal history of atopy is the strongest predisposing genetic factor for childhood asthma. Atopy is the predisposition to develop an IgE-mediated response to allergens and is most commonly manifest as eczema in infants. A family history of asthma is also suggestive in a child with the other key indicators of asthma. While not diagnostic, both a personal history of atopy and a family history of asthma may be important in developing an evaluation and treatment plan. For example, a history of atopy strongly suggests an allergic component to the asthma. This requires evaluation of allergen exposure and sensitivity and highlights the need for the physician or asthma educator to discuss allergen avoidance. Recognition, specific evaluation, and treatment of the allergic component of asthma is often overlooked and can adversely affect the ability to achieve optimal therapeutic outcomes.

In addition, the exposure to airway irritants should be assessed. Tobacco smoke is the most common irritant. Exposure to tobacco smoke in all sites where the child spends time should be considered. To include all potential tobacco smoke exposure, the history should include smoking by friends and older siblings, not just parents. Smoking in another room within the house will not remove the smoke from the ventilation system of the house or other building. Air pollution is an important consideration in large cities and industrial centers. Strong odors or perfumes can also be irritants for hyperreactive airways.

The evaluation of the child with asthma must include evaluation of the persistent versus intermittent nature of the child's disease. Studies of asthma treatment suggest that primary care physicians consider or at least treat > 70 percent of asthma as intermittent. However, the exact proportion of intermittent asthma is unknown. Children may be treated with intermittent therapy without evaluation for the presence of persistent airflow obstruction. To detect symptoms of persistent airflow obstruction, each child and parent should be asked about daily or weekly problems with nocturnal cough, restless sleep, chronic cough, shortness of breath, chest tightness, or breathing problems with exercise or playing. A symptoms diary that records symptoms, changes in activity level, or sleep problems may be helpful. Recurrent cough is the most common unrecognized asthma symptom and may be present during sleep, at rest, or during or shortly after exercise.

PHYSICAL EXAMINATION

Depending on the timing, the examination of a child with asthma can range from very dramatic to completely unrevealing. Wheezing is the most common symptom observed in asthma. Wheezing may be heard during inspiration, expiration, or both. The pitch of the wheezing can vary from low to high as the airways get tighter. With severe airflow obstruction, insufficient air may be moving to generate audible wheezes. However, the degree of airway obstruction correlates poorly with the type and pitch of wheezing. Therefore, auscultation alone is insufficient to assess the severity of the asthma or the bronchospasm.

In those without wheezing, a prolonged forced expiratory phase may be observed. The expiratory phase can be compared to that of the physician or a sibling in the room. The presence or absence of wheezing during forced expiration is not a reliable indicator of airflow limitation and should not be used as the sole criterion to assess asthma.

During an acute episode, signs of hyperexpansion of the chest, such as an increased front-to-back diameter, may be present. Use of the accessory respiratory muscles can result in retraction of the spaces between the ribs on inspiration, and many children find a hunched position more comfortable during an asthma "attack." More severe exacerbations are often associated with anxiety, apparent dyspnea, and tachypnea.

Examining the head and neck can provide important findings that relate to other allergic phenomena, and some of these may precipitate or prolong an asthma exacerbation and interfere with treatment results. The ears can show signs of middle ear disease. Conjunctival edema and slight erythema can suggest ocular allergies. Allergic shiners (periorbital edema and discoloration due to venous and lymphatic stasis) point to the allergic basis of the child's disease. The nasal salute (a crease across the end of the nose from constant wiping of a runny nose) further confirms allergies. In young children, the presence of eczema or lichenification and a forearm flexor crease rash frequently precedes and then accompanies asthma. The child's general demeanor can suggest agitation or anxiety associated with hypoxia.

PULMONARY FUNCTION TESTING

Spirometry is an essential diagnostic tool in confirming the diagnosis of asthma. Both the FEV_1 and the ratio of FEV_1 to forced vital capacity (FVC) are important in diagnosing airflow obstruction. Most children over the age of 5 years and some as young as 4 years can successfully complete spirometry testing.

Since maximal patient effort is required when performing spirometry, one of the most important roles of the individual conducting the test is effective coaching. Repeated and enthusiastic encouragement during exhalation is usually required. Children who have trouble understanding forced exhalation may be taught to perform the maneuver using blowout party favors that whistle. The child needs to blow hard enough to snap the blowout to full extension.

Spirometry should be performed both before and after 2 puffs of a beta-agonist in a child who has not used a short-acting beta-agonist for at least 6 h or a long-duration beta-agonist for at least 24 h. Recent beta-agonist use will blunt the response, making the diagnosis more difficult. Significant reversibility of the airflow obstruction is indicated by an increase in FEV_1 of ≥ 12 percent. Peak flow meters can be used to follow a child's course but are not recommended as a substitute for spirometry, since they are not as accurate as FEV_1 and are primarily a measure of large airway function, whereas asthma affects all of the airways

In children with a normal baseline FEV_1, it may be necessary to use a challenge test to demonstrate bronchial hyperreactivity and reversible airway obstruction. In children believed to have only mild intermittent episodes, it may be acceptable to inform parents of your suspicion regarding asthma and wait until the next exacerbation. However, in children with a history of recurrent prolonged coughs with colds, sleep disturbances, or exercise-induced symptoms, delaying diagnosis until the next recognized acute attack may be inappropriate and result in unnecessary morbidity.

ALLERGY TESTING

Greater understanding of the association between allergy and asthma has occurred, with clearer elucidation of the role of eosinophils, mast cells, histamines, and leukotrienes in producing acute asthma symptoms. The allergic response has also been traced through the more prolonged late-phase reaction (4 to 6 h after allergen exposure) of airway obstruction due to cytokines and chemokines from inflammatory cells such as macrophages, epithelial cells, lymphocytes, and eosinophils. These observations clearly link the allergy and inflammatory cascades, now referred to as allergic inflammation in asthma.[18]

If the patient's history provides evidence of responses to indoor and outdoor allergens, additional testing may be indicated. For some allergens, such as dust mites and mold, effective avoidance strategies may be all that is necessary. Additional testing for these allergens may not be necessary, but when done it can reinforce the need to implement avoidance strategies. For other allergens, the history of exposure may be unclear or insufficient. For these cases and for any child for whom allergy desensitization is being considered, further testing is indicated. Suspected pet allergies can result in great angst. Objective test results may help assure the imple-

mentation of at least minimal avoidance strategies involving the family dog, cat, or hamster.

Both in vitro and in vivo allergy testing quantify allergen-specific IgE. Neither type of testing should be used without some other confirmation that the allergen being tested is actually causing symptoms. For example, it makes no sense to test for ragweed-specific IgE in a child with no seasonal component to the asthma or one whose parents say he or she actually has fewest symptoms during the fall.

IN VITRO ALLERGY TESTING   In vitro blood testing for allergen-specific IgE can be accomplished on any patient at any time, regardless of atopic disease, current symptoms, and current medications. There is no risk of anaphylaxis, and the testing can be performed in any office setting where phlebotomy is possible. The original in vitro tests [Phadebas and Phadezym radioallergosorbent (PhRAST)] were specific but not sensitive, giving many false negative results. Newer technology [modified radioallergosorbent (modified RAST)] has significantly improved both the specificity and the sensitivity, making accuracy comparable to that of skin testing.

The major drawback of in vitro testing has been the expense in children who require assessment for multiple individual allergens. Alternative methods of testing that use screening batteries of allergens are available using Immuno Cap radioallergosorbent (CAP-RAST) technology (www.ImmunoCap.com). This quantitative mini-panel test includes the most common allergen in each of the major inhalant groups of allergens, tailored to the patient's region of the country, and is about 95 percent sensitive. It is used to confirm sensitivity to specific allergens in a child who has a history consistent with reactions to multiple allergens such as dust mites, cats, and ragweed. The panel is less expensive than ordering multiple single allergen-specific blood tests. However, it may miss some allergens. If the presence of atopy is unclear, a qualitative multiallergen assay can be used. The results will simply identify the presence or absence of any IgE reaction to any of the included allergens. This is seldom necessary in children, since 80 percent have some allergic basis for their asthma. Testing for food allergies is not appropriate, since only inhalant allergies have been shown to be related to asthma.

IN VIVO ALLERGY TESTING In vivo testing can be skin prick (epicutaneous) or intradermal. Test results can be affected by certain medications, including antihistamines and corticosteroids, and both classes of drugs should be discontinued for 4 to 7 days prior to testing. Young children and those with widespread eczema are not appropriate for skin testing. As with in vitro testing, allergen selection should be based on careful history, and multiple tests should not be applied to a larger patient simply because the patient has room for them. Few primary care physicians do in vivo testing in their offices. The use of skin prick testing in general practice offices is being studied in the United Kingdom.

OTHER TESTS

Other testing for the diagnosis of asthma in a child with spirometry-proven reversible airflow obstruction and typical recurrent episodes of bronchospasm is usually not required but may be important in developing the plan of therapy. In infants less than 1 year of age, the salty kiss test (ask the mother if the child tastes salty when kissed) or a sweat test should be considered when eating, digestion, or growth problems suggest that cystic fibrosis may be possible. Blood smears for eosinophilia, total serum IgE counts, and nasal smears for eosinophils have been used to diagnose allergic disease in a child with asthma but are imperfect allergy screening tests. Chest x-rays are not useful unless they are needed to rule out other diagnoses such as foreign body aspiration or bronchopulmonary dysplasia in children who were markedly premature. During hospitalization, however, chest radiography may be appropriate to rule out coexisting infiltrates, pneumonia, or atelectasis.

Management

The National Asthma Education and Prevention Program[18] (NAEPP) has established goals for asthma management. Meeting these goals requires a coordinated disease management strategy that can be separated into four components: (1) measures of assessment and monitoring, (2) control of factors contributing to asthma severity, (3) pharmacologic therapy, and (4) education for a partnership in asthma care. In addition, allergic triggers should be avoided, if possible. The role of immunotherapy in asthma management in children remains controversial.

MEASURES OF ASSESSMENT AND MONITORING

Asthma should be viewed as having a chronic or baseline severity ranging from no chronic symptoms in intermittent asthma to the almost continuous symptoms of severe asthma. Asthma severity is a continuum, and the child may move up and down the scale depending on his or her extrinsic and intrinsic environment. Therefore, a single assessment of severity is inadequate to classify a child for months or years into the future. As in management of other chronic conditions, comprehensive asthma care for persistent disease requires routine follow-up visits or education and assessment visits not devoted to the care of an urgent episode.

Asthma is categorized as intermittent or persistent with levels of mild, moderate, and severe asthma (Table 16-3).[18] The severity of asthma refers to baseline asthma symptoms in an untreated child, not to the symptoms that occur during an exacerbation. Severity is assessed by the frequency, intensity, and duration of baseline symptoms; the level of airflow obstruction; and the extent to which asthma interferes with daily activities. The presence of any single element from a higher category places the child in that

Table 16-3

Classification of Asthma Severity*

	SYMPTOMS[†]	NIGHTTIME SYMPTOMS	LUNG FUNCTION
Step 4, severe persistent	• Continual symptoms • Limited physical activity • Frequent exacerbations	Frequent	• FEV_1 or PEF ≤ 60% predicted • PEF variability > 30%
Step 3, moderate persistent	• Daily symptoms • Daily use of inhaled short-acting beta$_2$-agonist • Exacerbations affect activity • Exacerbations ≥ 2 times a week; may last days	> 1 time a week	• FEV_1 or PEF > 60% but < 80% predicted • PEF variability > 30%
Step 2, mild persistent	• Symptoms > 2 times a week but < 1 time a day • Exacerbations may affect activity	> 2 times a month	• FEV_1 or PEF ≥ 80% predicted • PEF variability 20–30%
Step 1, mild inter-mittent	• Symptoms < 2 times a week • Asymptomatic and normal PEF between exacerbations • Exacerbations brief (from a few hours to a few days); intensity may vary	≤ 2 times a month	• FEV_1 or PEF ≥ 80% predicted • PEF variability < 20%

*The presence of one of the features of severity is sufficient to place a patient in that category. An individual should be assigned to the most severe grade in which any feature occurs. The characteristics noted in this figure are general and may overlap because asthma is highly variable. Furthermore, an individual's classification may change over time.

†Patients at any level of severity can have mild, moderate, or severe exacerbations. Some patients with intermittent asthma experience severe and life-threatening exacerbations separated by long periods of normal lung function and no symptoms.

ABBREVIATIONS: FEV_1, forced expiratory volume in 1 s; PEF, peak expiratory flow.

category. For example, a child with daytime symptoms three or four times a year, normal spirometry FEV_1, and brief exacerbations but who wakes up at least once a week with a "coughing" spell would be classified as mild persistent because of the frequency of nighttime symptoms.

Since many symptoms of asthma are unrecognized by the parent or the child, it is important to ascertain whether the patient is experiencing unrecognized symptoms between recognized exacerbations. Clues to ongoing symptoms include frequent visits to the office, urgent care center, or emergency department for severe or lingering colds, bronchitis, or coughing spells; frequent sleep disturbances; and missed school days. The use of daily home peak flow monitoring for a period of 2 or 3 weeks may provide objective evidence of unrecognized problems. For example, monitoring may repeatedly show peak flow rates that are less than 80 percent of the child's "best" or that demonstrate 20 percent variation between morning and evening peak flow measurements (morning is usually lower in these cases). The "best" peak flow level should be assessed during periods of chronic daily therapy or during a period of treatment for an exacerbation once the symptoms are fully under control—usually 5 to 7 days after beginning therapy.

Chronic diseases are uncommon in children. When treating asthma, chronic disease management strategy may be overlooked, and asthma management becomes a series of acute care visits, with little time available for a comprehensive history, patient education or monitoring, and evaluation of the long-term course of the asthma. In addition to carefully elucidating the description of symptoms and allergen and irritant exposure, it is important to understand what asthma means to the child and family and how it affects their lives. During routine asthma rechecks it is important to discuss

- The impact of asthma on the child and family (unscheduled care visits, limitation of activities, number of missed school or play days, nocturnal effects)
- The child's and parents' perception of asthma (knowledge and beliefs about etiology, allergies, treatment—especially long-term medications, economic resources, and insurance concerns)
- History of asthma in the family (severity of disease in others, health beliefs about asthma)
- Social history (living situation and conditions, pets, day care, school, tobacco smoke, parents' level of education, child's level of maturity)

CONTROL OF FACTORS CONTRIBUTING TO EXACERBATIONS

One of the most important steps in controlling asthma is the reduction of exposure to factors that exacerbate symptoms and inflammation. Many common activities, such as exercise, can trigger an acute attack. However, exercise should not be avoided but encouraged, and pre-exercise treatment with a bronchodilator or cromolyn should be used prior to any sustained exercise. Exercise-induced bronchospasm usually occurs in conjunction with asthma and may clear when asthma is under good control.

Cold air may worsen asthma symptoms, especially during exercise. Cold air cannot be avoided, but children with asthma should be encouraged to wear a muffler or scarf over their mouth when temperatures dip to below freezing to warm the air before it is breathed. In cold climates, finding indoor sites for exercise is important in order to allow children to continue to play and be active but avoid exposure to cold air.

When viral infections are recognized as a recurrent trigger, it may be necessary to increase asthma medications at the start of the URI. In some cases it is necessary to begin a short course (usually 3 to 5 days) of oral steroids at the beginning of the viral infection. Antibiotics are not helpful in either treating the viral infection or preventing an asthma exacerbation.

Avoidance is the best strategy for wood and cigarette smoke and for perfumes and other strong odors. Parents who smoke should be repeatedly offered either smoking cessation help in your office or referral for smoking cessation. Children need early and repeated advice to avoid smoking. This should begin with the first diagnosis of asthma. Remember that many children begin smoking at ages as young as 8 to 12 years. Smoking cessation programs and nicotine replacement support are appropriate for teens as well as adults. Special programs that address preteen and adolescent concerns may be more successful than mixing adults and teens in one program.

Allergy management is one of the most important aspects of asthma treatment. Avoidance of allergens, especially indoor allergens, is the first step in managing allergy-related asthma. Many families do not recognize potential sources of allergens, so providing a list for them to consider is useful.

Removing the patient from the allergen source, however, is not always practical, and suggested interventions must be sensitive to the lifestyle and resources of the family. For example, suggestions such as purchasing high-energy particulate air (HEPA) filters and replacing carpets or a heating system are not acceptable or possible for many families. Suggesting a series of low-cost steps is more likely to engage the family's support.

PHARMACOLOGIC THERAPY

The drug therapy choices for asthma should be based on the child's age and maturity level and the severity of the asthma. For example, drug delivery systems such as the metered-dose inhaler (MDI) cannot be used by most children before the age of 4 to 6 years. However, for almost all classes of asthma medications, there is some drug within that class that is available for young children and has a delivery system designed to allow its use in infants or preschoolers. Therefore, the main basis on which therapy should be selected is the severity of the child's asthma.

A stepwise approach to asthma management provides a guideline for beginning therapy. Therapy should be based on the underlying frequency and severity of daytime and nocturnal symptoms, not on the level of symptoms during an exacerbation. For persistent asthma, it may be helpful to begin therapy one step above the assessed level of severity to provide the child with good control more quickly. Rapid control of the child's symptoms may encourage both the child and especially the adolescent and parent to continue asthma care with you. Many patients stop their medications soon after they are begun, and a follow-up visit in 2 to 4 weeks can be useful to emphasize the need for continued therapy.

Only persistent asthma requires regular therapy. Again, the selection of daily medications should be based on the usual level of symptoms, not on the severity of symptoms during an exacerbation. The stepwise approach to drug therapy is different for children ≤ 5 years of age (Table 16-4)[18] and those 6 years of age (Table 16-5)[18] and older.

For a child using any type of inhaler, it is important to observe inhaler technique at each visit, since many children (and adults) fail to properly initialize, prime, and use the inhalers. For children, a spacer device can overcome some of the problems with lack of coordination of inhaler initiation and inspiration.

TYPES OF MEDICATIONS USED IN ASTHMA

The following sections will review each of the groups of asthma medications. In general, asthma drugs are divided into two broad groups: medications that address the inflammation of asthma (such as corticosteroids, cromoglycates, and leukotriene antagonists) and those that primarily control symptoms by direct bronchodilation (such as beta-agonists, anticholinergics, and methylxanthines). Not all drugs fit nicely into one class, however, since evidence suggests that some drugs thought of as bronchodilators also have some anti-inflammatory activity.

CORTICOSTEROIDS Oral and inhaled steroids are the most potent and effective anti-inflammatory drugs currently available. The inhaled steroids are used for long-term asthma management to break the inflammatory cycle (Table 16-6). Short-term bursts of oral steroids may be necessary during moderate or severe acute exacerbations. The full therapeutic effect of inhaled steroids may require up to 2 weeks, although some impact is noted within days. Systemic steroids have an effect within hours to a day.

The most common side effects from inhaled steroids include cough, hoarseness, and oral thrush, but the risk of these can be reduced by the use of a spacer or holding chamber in conjunction with the inhaler. The most severe side effects of glucocorticoids include adrenal suppression, osteoporosis, thinning of the skin, and easy bruising. Of great concern to parents has been the potential for growth suppression with chronic use of inhaled steroids. Daily corticosteroid use does slow linear growth in children and adolescents. The greatest growth reduction appears to occur in the first year, with about 1 in

Table 16-4

Asthma Drug Therapy Based on Severity (Age Birth to 6 Years)

	DAILY ANTI-INFLAMMATORY MEDICATIONS	QUICK RELIEF
Step 4, severe persistent	• High-dose inhaled corticosteroid with spacer/holding chamber and face mask **AND** • If needed, add systemic corticosteroids 2 mg/kg/day and reduce to lowest daily or alternate-day dose that stabilizes symptoms	• Short-acting bronchodilator as needed for symptoms by nebulizer or MDI with spacer/holding chamber and face mask **OR** • oral beta$_2$-agonist *Daily or increasing use of short-acting inhaled beta$_2$-agonist indicates need for additional long-term control therapy.*
Step 3, moderate persistent	• Either medium-dose inhaled corticosteroid with spacer/holding chamber and face mask **OR** • low- to medium-dose inhaled corticosteroid and long-acting bronchodilator (theophylline)	• Short-acting bronchodilator as needed for symptoms by nebulizer or MDI with spacer/holding chamber and face mask **OR** • oral beta$_2$-agonist *Daily or increasing use of short-acting inhaled beta$_2$-agonist indicates need for additional long-term control therapy.*
Step 2, mild persistent	• Infants and young children usually begin with a trial of cromolyn **OR** • low-dose inhaled corticosteroid with spacer/holding chamber and face mask	• Short-acting bronchodilator as needed for symptoms by nebulizer or MDI with spacer/holding chamber and face mask **OR** • oral beta$_2$-agonist *Daily or increasing use of short-acting inhaled beta$_2$-agonist indicates need for additional long-term control therapy.*
Step 1, intermittent	• No daily medication	• Short-acting bronchodilator as needed for symptoms < 2 times/week by nebulizer or MDI with spacer/holding chamber and face mask **OR** • oral beta$_2$-agonist *Two times weekly or increasing use of short-acting inhaled beta$_2$-agonist indicates need for additional long-term control therapy.*
STEP DOWN	**STEP UP**	
Review treatment every 1 to 6 months; a gradual stepwise reduction in treatment may be possible.	If control is not maintained, consider stepping up. First, review patient medication technique, adherence, and environmental control (avoidance of allergens and/or other factors that contribute to asthma severity).	

ABBREVIATION: MDI, metered-dose inhaler.
SOURCE: Reprinted as modified from NIH,[18] with permission.

Table 16-5

Asthma Drug Therapy Based on Severity (Ages 6 Years through Adulthood)

	DAILY MEDICATIONS (CHOOSE ALL NEEDED)	QUICK RELIEF
Step 4, severe persistent	• High-dose inhaled corticosteroid • Long-acting bronchodilator • A leukotriene modifier • Oral corticosteroid	• Short-acting bronchodilator *Daily or increasing use of short-acting inhaled beta$_2$-agonist indicates need for additional long-term control therapy.*
Step 3, moderate persistent	*Daily medication (usually need two):* • Either low- or medium-dose inhaled corticosteroid • Long-acting bronchodilator • A leukotriene modifier	• Short-acting bronchodilator *Daily or increasing use of short-acting inhaled beta$_2$-agonist indicates need for additional long-term control therapy.*
Step 2, mild persistent	*One daily medication (choose one):* • Low-dose inhaled corticosteroid • Cromolyn • Sustained-release theophylline (to serum concentration of 5–15 µg/mL) • A leukotriene modifier	• Short-acting bronchodilator *Daily or increasing use of short-acting inhaled beta$_2$-agonist indicates need for additional long-term control therapy.*
Step 1, intermittent	• No daily medication needed	• Short-acting bronchodilator *Use of short-acting inhaled beta$_2$-agonist > 2 times per week indicates need for additional long-term control therapy.*

STEP DOWN	STEP UP
Review treatment every 1 to 6 months; a gradual stepwise reduction in treatment may be possible.	If control is not maintained, consider stepping up. First, review patient medication technique, adherence, and environmental control (avoidance of allergens and/or other factors that contribute to asthma severity).

SOURCE: Reprinted as modified from NIH,[18] with permission.

of reduction in overall adult height as a result of long-term steroid use. Whether this is a larger, smaller, or similar height reduction than would occur in patients with chronic untreated asthma is unknown.[23–26]

CROMOGLYCATES The cromoglycates, which include cromolyn and nedocromil, produce anti-inflammatory effects by stabilizing mast cells, eosinophils, and epithelial cells and consequently blocking both early and late reaction to

Table 16-6

Anti-inflammatory Medications: Inhaled Corticosteroids

Generic Name	Brand Name	Dosage Form(s)	Cost per Day, $	Low	Medium	High	Potential Adverse Effects and Therapeutic Issues
Beclomethasone dipropionate	Beclovent, Vanceril, Vanceril-DS	MDI: 42 µg/puff MDI: 84 µg/puff	2.84 2.64	2–8 puffs/day 1–4 puffs/day	8–16 puffs/day 4–8 puffs/day	>16 puffs/day >8 puffs/day Max: 0.84 mg/day adults, 0.42 mg/day children	**FOR ALL INHALED CORTICOSTEROIDS:** • Cough, dysphonia, moniliasis; high doses may have systemic effects, although studies are not conclusive and clinical significance is not clear. • Monitoring of growth is recommended when used in children. • The potential risks of inhaled corticosteroids are well balanced by their benefits. • To minimize local and systemic adverse events, use MDI with a spacer/holding chamber.
	QVAR CFC free§	MDI: 40–80 µg/puff	1.04–1.64	1–2 puffs/day	2–4 puffs/day	Max: 0.64 mg/day children	
Budesonide	Pulmicort Turbuhaler	DPI: 200 µg/puff	1.24	2 puffs/day	4 puffs/day	8 puffs/day Max: 1.6 mg/day adults, 0.8 mg/day children	
Flunisolide	AeroBid, AeroBid-M	MDI: 250 µg/puff	2.68 2.68	2–3 puffs/day 2–3 puffs/day	4–5 puffs/day 4–5 puffs/day	>5 puffs/day Max: 2 mg/day adults, 1 mg/day children	
Fluticasone propionate	Flovent	MDI: 44 µg/puff 110 µg/puff 220 µg/puff	NA 2.28 1.74	2–4 puffs/day — —	4–10 puffs/day 2–4 puffs/day 1–2 puffs/day	— >4 puffs/day >2 puffs/day Max: 1 mg/day adults, 0.2 mg/day children	
	Flovent Rotadisk	DPI: 50 µg/puff 100 µg/puff 250 µg/puff	NA 2.28 1.74	2–4 puffs/day 1–2 puffs/day —	— 2–4 puffs/day 1–2 puffs/day	— >4 puffs/day >2 puffs/day Max: 1 mg/day adults, 0.2 mg/day children	
Triamcinolone acetonide	Azmacort	MDI: 100 µg/puff	2.50	4–8 puffs/day	8–12 puffs/day	>12 puffs/day Max: 1.6 mg/day adults, 1.2 mg/day children	
Budesonide	Pulmicort Respules	Nebulizing suspension: 0.125 mg/mL 0.25 mg/mL 0.50 mg/mL per 2-mL respule	8.40 4.20 2.10	0.50 mg/day 0.50 mg/day 0.50 mg/day	1.0 mg/day 1.0 mg/day 1.0 mg/day	2.0 mg/day 2.0 mg/day 2.0 mg/day	
Mometasone furoate	Asmanex	DPI: 200 µg/puff DPI: 400 µg/puff	NA NA	200 mg, QD 200 mg, QD	400 mg, QD 400 mg, QD	400 mg, BID 400 mg, BID	

†These doses are suggested as guides for making clinical decisions. The clinician must use his/her judgment to tailor treatment to the specific needs and circumstances of the patient.

§CFC refers to chlorofluorocarbons

ABBREVIATIONS: CFC, chlorofluorocarbon; DPI, dry powder inhaler; MDI, metered-dose inhaler.

allergens (Table 16-7). These drugs have also been shown to block the acute response to irritants or symptom enhancers such as exercise and cold air.

Cromoglycates may be used as first-line medications (instead of inhaled corticosteroids) in children where growth is a special concern and for exercise-induced symptoms. It is important to remember that 2 to 4 weeks may be required to see the full therapeutic effect. Conversely, when these drugs are used for exercise-induced asthma, the effect is almost immediate.

The most common complaint associated with these inhaled medications is the unpleasant taste. In one study, up to 13 percent of children refused to use nedocromil, while another larger percentage found it unpleasant but tolerable.

LEUKOTRIENE MODIFIERS   Zafirlukast and zileuton are oral medications that suppress the inflammatory cascade associated with asthma (Table 16-8). They have few reported side effects except for rare instances of reversible hepatitis. Although not initially approved for use in children, experience with using these drugs in children is growing, and some formulations are now approved for use in children as young as 4.

Controversy continues to surround whether to use leukotriene modifiers as first-line asthma drugs or as monotherapy. The usual indication is as a concurrent medication in children using daily inhaled or oral corticosteroids to allow reduction in the dose of required steroids.

BETA-AGONISTS   This class can be subdivided into short-acting (albuterol, biotolterol, pirbuterol, and terbutaline) and long-acting agents (salmeterol and fomeral) (Table 16-9). Both types of agents act as direct bronchodilators. They are the most effective therapy for acute bronchospasm. The longer-acting drugs may also have some effect on stabilizing inflammatory cells.

Short-acting beta-agonists should be used to treat acute symptoms and exacerbations. Daily use or use of more than 1 canister per month of a beta-agonist suggests that additional therapy may be needed for adequate control. Since the short-acting beta-agonists do not affect the chronic inflammation of asthma, they may also not prevent long-term complications such as basement membrane remodeling. However, in mild persistent asthma, daily and regular use of beta-agonists (as opposed to use as needed) has been found to adequately control symptoms in those with few nocturnal problems.[27]

Long-acting beta-agonists should never be used for treatment of acute symptoms or exacerbations. Salmeterol, in particular, has a slow onset of action and may lead the patient or parents to believe that the drug has not been effective and give another dose, leading to acute overdosing and failure to seek other appropriate therapy. Long-acting beta-agonists are effective for control of nocturnal symptoms and exercise-induced symptoms over an extended period. They may be especially useful to prevent the need to use medication during school hours and repeated dosing for children and young athletes competing in sporting events. Long-acting beta-agonists also can be added to inhaled corticosteroids to help maintain steroid doses at the lowest possible level. Asking parents to put a red glow-in-the-dark sticker on the long-acting drug canister may help prevent improper use of long-acting beta-agonists during an acute exacerbation.

ANTICHOLINERGICS   Ipratropium bromide is an anticholinergic agent that can be used for treatment of acute symptoms and may be useful when large amounts of mucus are being produced. The drug is delivered via an inhaler, and bronchodilation is the main mechanism of action, with an adjunct increase in vagal tone. Anticholinergics also appear to block bronchoconstriction due to irritants such as cigarette smoke or the reflux of gastric contents. These drugs have very limited use in children, since they have no or limited effect on

Table 16-7

Anti-inflammatory Medications: Cromolyn Sodium/Nedocromil Sodium

Generic Name	Brand Name(s)	Dosage Form(s)	Cost per Day, $	Dose*	Potential Adverse Effects and Therapeutic Issues
Cromolyn sodium	Intal	MDI: 1 mg/puff Nebulizer solution: 20 mg/ampule	1.88	1–2 puffs, 10–15 min before exercise 1–2 puffs, TID–QID 1 ampule, TID–QID	• Therapeutic response to cromolyn and nedocromil often occurs within 2 weeks, but a 4- to 6-week trial may be needed to determine maximum benefit. • Dose of cromolyn MDI (1 mg/puff) may be inadequate to affect airway hyperresponsiveness. Nebulizer delivery (20 mg/ampule) may be preferred for some patients. • Safety is the primary advantage of these agents.
Nedocromil sodium	Tilade	MDI: 1.75 mg/puff	1.44	1–2 puffs, 30 min before exercise 1–2 puffs, BID–QID	• Unpleasant taste for some patients.

*These doses are suggested as guides for making clinical decisions. The clinician must use his/her judgment to tailor treatment to the specific needs and circumstances of the patient.

Abbreviation: MDI, metered-dose inhaler.

Table 16-8

Leukotriene Modifiers

GENERIC NAME	BRAND NAME(s)	COST PER DAY, $	DOSAGE FORM(s)	DOSE*	POTENTIAL ADVERSE EFFECTS AND THERAPEUTIC ISSUES
Montelukast	Singulair	2.43	Tablet: 5 mg, chewable, for ages 6 through 14 years	1 tablet in evening	
		2.37	10 mg for ages 15 years and older	1 tablet in evening	
Zafirlukast	Accolate	1.24	Tablet: 20 mg, for ages 12 years and older 10 mg, for ages 7 through 11 years	1 tablet BID; take 1 h before or 2 h after meals	• Drug interactions (warfarin); increases prothrombin time[†]
Zileuton	Zyflo	3.03	Tablet: 600 mg, for ages 12 years and older	1 tablet QID	• Possible elevation of liver enzymes requires monitoring; drug interactions (warfarin, theo- phylline)[†]

*These doses are suggested as guides for making clinical decisions. The clinician must use his/her judgment to tailor treatment to the specific needs and circumstances of the patient.

[†]Data about adverse effects in patients are limited. Increased clinical experience and further study in a wide range of patients are needed to determine those patients most likely to benefit from leukotriene modifiers and to establish a more specific role for these medications in asthma therapy.

bronchoconstriction due to allergens and exercise. Side effects include drying of the mouth.

METHYLXANTHINES Theophylline products can be used for long-term control and may be helpful for nocturnal symptoms. These drugs are primarily bronchodilators, but they have some anti-inflammatory effect on eosinophils and T-lymphocytes and increase diaphragmatic contractility. Side effects of this class include vomiting, nausea, central nervous system stimulation, and tachyarrhythmias.

The major drawback to the use of methylxanthines is the need to monitor blood levels, which may vary significantly depending on diet and other medications, especially drugs that affect the P-450 cytochrome system. Furthermore, febrile illnesses such as influenza can markedly elevate serum theophylline levels. Serum the-

ophylline levels should be kept between 5 and 15 µg/mL to prevent toxicity. The indications for use of methylxanthines have decreased as experience with other medications in young children has grown.

THE USE OF INHALERS IN ASTHMA

When inhaled drugs are used, variations in delivery systems may enhance the amount of drug deposited in the airways. These include the use of powder delivery systems, chlorofluorocarbon (CFC)-free inhalers, and breath-activated metered-dose inhalers (MDIs) (Table 16-10). Newer delivery systems such as the CFC-free inhalers deliver a greater portion of the dosage to the lungs and therefore provide greater levels of active drug with the same dosage of drug per puff. When changing from a CFC MDI to a CFC-free unit, patients should be cautioned to reduce their dose of inhaled corticosteroids so that they do not exceed maximal recommended doses.

Spacers or holding chambers are suggested for any child or adult having difficulty coordinating actuation and inhalation with any MDI. The spacer or holding chamber increases the dose of drug delivered to the lungs and may reduce the amount of drug deposited in the mouth and absorbed into the bloodstream. They should be used at home for all inhalations with CFC MDIs, although the need for their use with the new CFC-free reengineered inhalers is controversial. Spacers also are recommended for use in all children on daily inhaled corticosteroids to reduce the risks of adrenal suppression and inhibition of linear growth.

Dry powder inhalers are available for beta-agonists and corticosteroids. These devices require a specific minimal strength of inhalation and may not work as well in moderate to severe asthma episodes as nebulizers or self-actuated MDIs. The mouth should be rinsed out after each use of the dry powder MDI to decrease systemic drug absorption. Dry powder inhalers do not require spacers or holding chambers.

Nebulizers can be used to deliver beta-agonists, cromolyn, anticholinergics, and corticosteroids. They are also very useful in treating moderate and severe exacerbations in the office or emergency department. Face masks allow nebulizer use without the need to hold a mouthpiece in place. For infants and young children, a nebulizer can be used by parents at home, and they are available now in many elementary schools.

MANAGING AN EXACERBATION

Managing an exacerbation or asthma attack may begin at home or at school. If treatment there is not successful or if the attack is severe, the child may need to come to the office, to an urgent care center, or to the emergency department (ED). It is useful for parents and schools to have a written plan of action that provides step-by-step measures to deal with an asthma exacerbation, including when to call the physician, call 911, or transfer the child to a care center.

Treatment of the exacerbation must begin with assessment of the exacerbation's intensity (Table 16-11). This is best done by peak flow assessment or spirometry in a child with more than minimal symptoms. A severe attack, one associated with a 50 percent decrease in FEV_1 or peak flow or one in which a child is unable to talk or walk because of shortness of breath or severe coughing, is best treated in an ED. If the exacerbation is severe, the ability to assess oxygen saturation and provide supplemental O_2 is important.

If the exacerbation is less severe, it can be treated at home or in a medical office. Treatment should begin with 2 to 4 puffs of a short-acting beta-agonist by MDI or equivalent dose by nebulizer. Follow-up treatment is based on response to the beta-agonist (Table 16-12).[28] When home or school management fails, the child should be brought to a care site where spirometry or peak flow assessment is available. An algorithm for dealing with the asthmatic child can be useful for both the busy urban ED and the small rural ED with infrequent experience with children with asthma (Fig. 16-1).

A child with underlying mild asthma may have a severe exacerbation, including life-threatening episodes. Therefore, all children and their parents need to understand the possibility of an exacerbation of greater intensity than previous exacerbations or "attacks." Attacks are layered on top of the baseline severity and are classified during the acute episode regardless of baseline medications.

ESTABLISHING A PARTNERSHIP

Education is essential for the adequate management of asthma. When children are involved, it is important to educate the parents, but the child must remain the focus of the visit. Even very young children can be included in the educational process. Education must begin at the

Table 16-9

Bronchodilators

GENERIC NAME	BRAND NAME(S)	COST PER DAY, $	DOSAGE FORM(S)	DOSE[a]	POTENTIAL ADVERSE EFFECTS AND THERAPEUTIC ISSUES
			LONG-ACTING BRONCHODILATORS		
Salmeterol	Serevent	1.45	MDI: 21 μg/puff DPI: 50 μg/blister	2 puffs, 30–60 min before exercise 1–2 puffs, q12h 1 blister, q12h	• Tachycardia, tremor. The clinical relevance of potential diminished bronchoprotective effect is uncertain. **DO NOT USE** in place of anti-inflammatory therapy.
Sustained-release albuterol	Volmax Proventil Repetabs	0.83 0.78	Tablet: 4, 8 mg Tablet: 4 mg	0.3–0.6 mg/kg/day, not to exceed 4–8 mg/day, q12h	• Tachycardia, tremor, irritability.
Theophylline[b]	Aerolate-III Aerolate-JR Aerolate-SR Choledyl-SA Elixophyllin Quibron-T QuibronOT/SR Slo-b.i.d. Slo-phyllin Theo-24 Theochron Theo-Dur Theolair Theolair-SR T-Phyll Uni-Dur Uniphyl	NA NA 0.41 0.40 NA 0.35 0.28 0.50 0.35 0.28 NA 0.25 0.40 0.25 NA NA NA	Capsules, tablets	Starting dose: 10 mg/kg/day Maximal dose: <1 year[c]: (0.2 × age in weeks) + 5 mg/kg/day Maximal dose: ≥ 1 year: 16 mg/kg/day, not to exceed the adult maximum (800 mg/day)	• Tachycardia, nausea, vomiting, headache, CNS stimulation. • Monitoring serum levels (5–15 μg/mL) is essential to ensure that therapeutic, but not toxic, doses are achieved. • Serum levels may be affected by numerous factors (diet, febrile illness, other medications).
Formoterol	Foradil	NA	DPI (12 μg)	1 puff BID	Tachycardia, tremor. The clinical relevance of potential diminished bronchoprotective effect is uncertain. **DO NOT USE** in place of anti-inflammatory therapy.
			SHORT-ACTING BETA₂-AGONISTS		
Albuterol	Airet Proventil Ventolin	NA NA NA	MDI: 90 μg/puff Nebulizer solution: 5 mg/mL (0.5%); 0.083% (unit dose[d]) containing 2.5 mg	1–2 puffs, 15 min before exercise 2 puffs, TID-QID PRN 0.05 mg/kg (minimum: 1.25 mg; maximum: 2.5 mg)	For all short-acting beta₂-agonists: • Tremor, tachycardia, headache.
	Proventil-HFA CFC-free	0.82	MDI: 90 μg/puff	1–2 puffs, 15 min before exercise 2 puffs, TID-QID PRN	Note: Increasing use of short-acting beta₂-agonists, use of > 1 canister/ month, or lack of expected effect indicates

Drug		Ratio	Dosage Form/Strength	Dosing	Comments
	Ventolin Rotacaps	1.28	DPI: 200 µg/capsule	1 capsule, 15 min before exercise; 1 capsule, TID-QID PRN; 2–6 years, 0.1 mg/kg TID-QID; 6–14 years, 2 mg TID-QID; > 14 years, 2–4 mg TID-QID	inadequate asthma control. See doctor to increase or add long-term control medication(s).
	Proventil Syrup	NA	2 mg/5 mL		
	Ventolin Syrup	NA	2 mg/5 mL		
Bitolterol	Tornalate	NA	MDI[e]: 370 µg/puff; Nebulizer solution: 2 mg/1 mL (0.2%)	1–2 puffs, 15 min before exercise; 2 puffs, TID-QID PRN; 10–15 min administration; 8 mg max intermittent; 14 mg max continuous	
Levalbuterol	Xopenex	NA	Nebulizer solution: Unit dose vials: 0.63 mg/3 mL; 1.25 mg/3 mL	0.63 mg q4–6h for maintenance; 1.25 mg q4–6h for acute bronchospasm and for patients unresponsive to lower dose	
Metaproterenol	Alupent	NA	Tablets: 10, 20 mg; Syrup: 10 mg/5 mL; Nebulizer: Unit dose vial 5% nebulizer solution	Under 6 years, 10 mg TID-QID; Over 6 years, 20 mg TID-QID; Age 12 and over 0.2 mL in 2.5 mL saline	
	Alupent inhaler	NA			
Pirbuterol	Maxair	1.15	MDI: 200 mg/puff	1–2 puffs, TID-QID PRN	
Terbutaline	Brethaire	NA	MDI: 200 µg/puff	1–2 puffs, TID-QID PRN	
	Brethine	NA	Tablets: 2.5, 5 mg	Over age 12: 2.5 to 5 mg TID	
ANTICHOLINERGICS					
Ipratropium bromide	Atrovent	NA	MDI: 18 µg/puff; Nebulizer solution: 0.5 mg/2.5 mL (0.02%)	1–2 puffs every 6 h; 0.5 mg every 6 h	Dry mouth; avoid contact with eyes. May provide additive effect(s) to short-acting beta$_2$-agonist.
COMBINATION INHALERS					
Salmeterol/Fluticasone	Advair 110/50	3.46	DPI: 100 µg/50 µg	1 puff QD	
	Advair 250/50	3.46	250 µg/50 µg	1 puff QD	
	Advair 500/50	3.46	500 µg/50 µg	1 puff QD	

[a] These doses are suggested as guides for making clinical decisions. The clinician must use his/her judgment to tailor treatment to the specific needs and circumstances of the patient.

[b] Sustained-release theophylline may be considered an alternative, but not preferred, long-term control medication when issues arise related to cost, adherence, or ability to use inhaled medications.

[c] Sustained-release theophylline may have particular risks of adverse effects in infants, who frequently have febrile illnesses that increase theophylline levels. Consider theophylline for infants only if serum levels will be carefully monitored.

[d] Do not use partial unit dose.

[e] Also available as a nebulizer solution (2 mg/mL = 0.2%), but a children's dose has not been established.

[f] A course of 7 days or less is usually sufficient. In some cases, the exacerbation may require up to 10 days of treatment.

ABBREVIATIONS: MDI, metered-dose inhaler; DPI, dry powder inhaler; CNS, central nervous system.

Table 16-10

Inhaler Types and Use

DEVICE/MEDICATIONS	AGE	COMMENTS
Metered-dose inhaler (MDI) Beta$_2$-agonists Corticosteroids Cromolyn sodium Nedocromil sodium Anticholinergics	Adults: Spacer/holding chamber recommended for patients having difficult with inhalation technique. Recommended routinely for patients on corticosteroids. Children: ≥ 5 years: spacer/holding chamber recommended. < 5 years: spacer/holding chamber with face mask recommended.	• A spacer/holding chamber may be helpful if patient has difficulty coordinating inhalation and triggering a puff.
Breath-actuated MDI Beta$_2$-agonists	Children > 12 years and adults	• Some patients have difficulty triggering a puff while inhaling.
Dry powder inhaler (DPI) Beta$_2$-agonists Corticosteroids	Children ≥ 4 years and adults	• Dose delivered may differ from the MDI for some medications. • Can be effort-dependent.
Nebulizer Beta$_2$-agonists Cromolyn sodium Anticholinergics	Patients of any age who cannot use an MDI with spacer/holding chamber with or without face mask	• Useful for infants, very young children, elderly patients, and any patient with a moderate to severe asthma episode (although MDI with spacer/holding chamber may be as effective).

first asthma visit and be included as a routine part of every visit, whether that visit is to the office, the urgent care center, or the ED. Recent studies have shown that children who received asthma education and referral to a personal physician during ED visits made fewer urgent care and ED visits in the future.

Asthma education is similar to education for other chronic conditions. Developing a list of key messages can guide the educational process, assure that the child and family are hearing consistent messages, and allow tracking of the education over time. These topics should include education about the chronic nature of the disease and how medications work, assuring that

inhaler technique is appropriate, reviewing environmental control measures and avoiding triggers, education about long-term management goals, and information on how to manage an exacerbation. A copy of the key messages can be kept in the child's medical record and used as a checklist to guide education over several visits. Asking the child's and parent's goals for asthma management and sharing your goals sets the stage for negotiating a set of mutual goals.

Understanding the child's and parents' most pressing concerns allows you to prioritize the educational messages and reaffirm the importance of a partnership in controlling asthma. For children with moderate, severe, or difficult to

Table 16-11

Assessing Intensity of an Exacerbation (Attack)

PARAMETER*	MILD	MODERATE	SEVERE	RESPIRATORY ARREST IMMINENT
Breathless	Walking	Talking Infant: softer, shorter cry; difficulty feeding	At rest Infant: stops feeding	
	Can lie down	Prefers sitting	Hunched forward	
Talks in	Sentences	Phrases	Words	
Alertness	May be agitated	Usually agitated	Usually agitated	Drowsy or confused
Respiratory rate	Increased	Increased	Often ≥ 30/min	

Guide to rates of breathing associated with respiratory distress in awake children:

Age	Normal rate
<2 months	<60/min
2–12 months	<50/min
1–5 years	<40/min
6–8 years	<30/min

PARAMETER*	MILD	MODERATE	SEVERE	RESPIRATORY ARREST IMMINENT
Accessory muscles and suprasternal retractions	Usually not	Usually	Usually	Paradoxical thoraco-abdominal movement
Wheeze	Moderate, often only end expiratory	Loud	Usually loud	Absence of wheeze
Pulse (beats/min)	<100	100–120	>120	Bradycardia

Guide to limits of normal pulse rate in children:

Infants	2–12 months	Normal rate < 160/min
Preschool	1–2 years	Normal rate < 120/min
School age	2–8 years	Normal rate < 110/min

PARAMETER*	MILD	MODERATE	SEVERE	RESPIRATORY ARREST IMMINENT
Pulsus paradoxus	Absent <10 mmHg	May be present 10–25 mmHg	Often present >25 mmHg (adult), 20–40 mmHg (child)	Absence suggests respiratory muscle fatigue
PEF after initial bronchodilator, % predicted or % personal best	Over 80%	Approximately 60–80%	<60% predicted or personal best (<100 L/min adults) or response last <2 h	
PaO$_2$ (on air)† and/or	Normal Test not usually necessary	>60 mmHg	<60 mmHg Possible cyanosis	
PaCO$_2$†	<45 mmHg	<45 mmHg	>45 mmHg: Possible respiratory failure (see text)	
SaO$_2$% (on air)†	>95%	91–95%	<90%	

Hypercapnia (hypoventilation) develops more readily in young children than in adults and adolescents.

*Note: The presence of several parameters, but not necessarily all, indicates the general classification of the attack.

†Kilopascals are also used internationally; conversion would be appropriate in this regard.

ABBREVIATION: PEF, peak expiratory flow.

Table 16-12

Home Treatment Response to Initial Treatment Assessment

Good If . . .	Incomplete If . . .	Poor If . . .
Symptoms subside after initial beta$_2$-agonist and relief is sustained for 4 h.	Symptoms decrease but return in less than 3 h after initial beta$_2$-agonist treatment.	Symptoms persist or worsen despite initial beta$_2$-agonist treatment.
PEF is greater than 80% predicted or personal best.	PEF is 60–80% predicted or personal best.	PEF is less than 60% predicted or personal best.
ACTIONS: • May continue beta$_2$-agonist every 3–4 h for 1–2 days. • Contact physician for follow-up instructions.	**ACTIONS:** • Add corticosteroid tablets or syrup. • Continue beta$_2$-agonist. • Consult physician urgently for instructions.	**ACTIONS:** • Add corticosteroid tablets or syrup. • Repeat beta$_2$-agonist immediately. • Immediately transport to hospital emergency department (see Fig. 16-1).

ABBREVIATION: PEF, peak expiratory flow.
SOURCE: Adapted from NIH.[28]

control asthma, the partnership may extend to an asthma specialist for co-management, consultation, or referral. It is important to establish the role of each physician early in the course of co-management. If this is not established, the family can be confused about whom to contact for what type of problem.

The asthma messages also need to be the same whether they are coming from the child's primary care clinician or from the specialist's office. This process can be enhanced when the primary care clinician selects (in consultation with the family) the specialist to be included in care. Developing a working relationship with one or two specialists, asking to have copies of their patient and family education materials, and negotiating roles can facilitate care.

For children in day care, the caregivers and owners of the day care center will require asthma information. Although many schools have plans for administering asthma medications in school, few have any type of asthma management strategy. An action plan should be developed with the parents and the school to deal with current management decisions and re-

sponses to an exacerbation. Action plans should include the list of usual medications and maximum usage in a day, a list of common triggers and allergens, signs and symptoms indicating when additional treatment is needed, medications to take during an exacerbation, warning signs for a severe attack, when to call parents, and when to call 911 for emergency assistance. Family members should be instructed where to find these action plans in the event of an emergency.

COMPLICATIONS

The most severe complication of asthma in children is death. Indicators of increased risk of death should be evaluated in each child (Table 16-13). In addition, during an acute attack, respiratory distress (shortness of breath or tachypnea), inability to speak, use of accessory muscles (retractions), disappearance of wheezing in a silent chest, decreased peak expiratory flow (PEF) (<50 percent of child's normal), agitation, and cyanosis all suggest a severe exacerbation that requires immediate and emergent action.

Figure 16-1　Emergency Department or Office Treatment of Acute Exacerbation

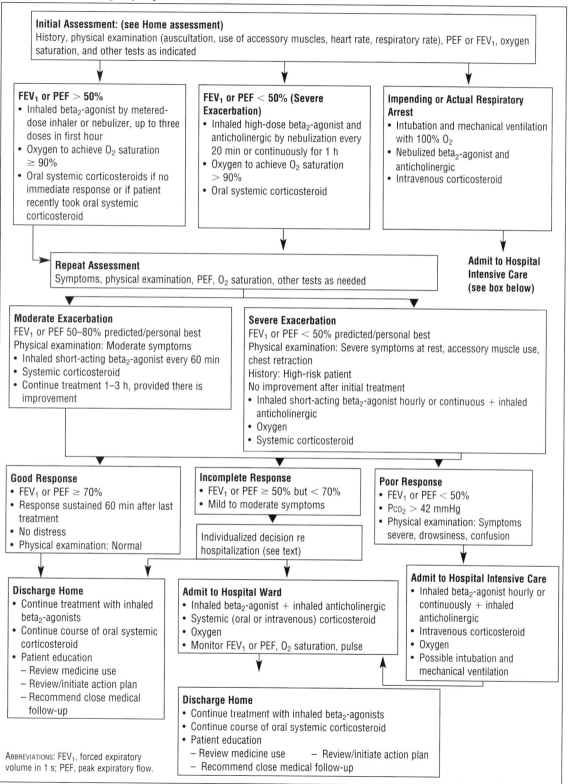

Initial Assessment: (see Home assessment)
History, physical examination (auscultation, use of accessory muscles, heart rate, respiratory rate), PEF or FEV_1, oxygen saturation, and other tests as indicated

FEV_1 or PEF > 50%
- Inhaled beta$_2$-agonist by metered-dose inhaler or nebulizer, up to three doses in first hour
- Oxygen to achieve O_2 saturation $\geq$ 90%
- Oral systemic corticosteroids if no immediate response or if patient recently took oral systemic corticosteroid

FEV_1 or PEF < 50% (Severe Exacerbation)
- Inhaled high-dose beta$_2$-agonist and anticholinergic by nebulization every 20 min or continuously for 1 h
- Oxygen to achieve O_2 saturation > 90%
- Oral systemic corticosteroid

Impending or Actual Respiratory Arrest
- Intubation and mechanical ventilation with 100% O_2
- Nebulized beta$_2$-agonist and anticholinergic
- Intravenous corticosteroid

Admit to Hospital Intensive Care (see box below)

Repeat Assessment
Symptoms, physical examination, PEF, O_2 saturation, other tests as needed

Moderate Exacerbation
FEV_1 or PEF 50–80% predicted/personal best
Physical examination: Moderate symptoms
- Inhaled short-acting beta$_2$-agonist every 60 min
- Systemic corticosteroid
- Continue treatment 1–3 h, provided there is improvement

Severe Exacerbation
FEV_1 or PEF < 50% predicted/personal best
Physical examination: Severe symptoms at rest, accessory muscle use, chest retraction
History: High-risk patient
No improvement after initial treatment
- Inhaled short-acting beta$_2$-agonist hourly or continuous + inhaled anticholinergic
- Oxygen
- Systemic corticosteroid

Good Response
- FEV_1 or PEF $\geq$ 70%
- Response sustained 60 min after last treatment
- No distress
- Physical examination: Normal

Incomplete Response
- FEV_1 or PEF $\geq$ 50% but < 70%
- Mild to moderate symptoms

Individualized decision re hospitalization (see text)

Poor Response
- FEV_1 or PEF < 50%
- P_{CO_2} > 42 mmHg
- Physical examination: Symptoms severe, drowsiness, confusion

Discharge Home
- Continue treatment with inhaled beta$_2$-agonists
- Continue course of oral systemic corticosteroid
- Patient education
  – Review medicine use
  – Review/initiate action plan
  – Recommend close medical follow-up

Admit to Hospital Ward
- Inhaled beta$_2$-agonist + inhaled anticholinergic
- Systemic (oral or intravenous) corticosteroid
- Oxygen
- Monitor FEV_1 or PEF, O_2 saturation, pulse

Admit to Hospital Intensive Care
- Inhaled beta$_2$-agonist hourly or continuously + inhaled anticholinergic
- Intravenous corticosteroid
- Oxygen
- Possible intubation and mechanical ventilation

Discharge Home
- Continue treatment with inhaled beta$_2$-agonists
- Continue course of oral systemic corticosteroid
- Patient education
  – Review medicine use　　– Review/initiate action plan
  – Recommend close medical follow-up

ABBREVIATIONS: FEV_1, forced expiratory volume in 1 s; PEF, peak expiratory flow.

Table 16-13

Signs of Increased Risk for Death from Asthma

- Past history of sudden severe asthma attacks
- Prior intubation for asthma, prior admission to an ICU for asthma
- 2 or more hospitalizations within the past 12 months
- 3 or more emergency department visits in the past 12 months
- Use of more than 2 canisters of inhaled beta-agonists per month
- Current chronic use of oral steroids
- Difficulty perceiving severe airflow obstruction
- Low socioeconomic status and urban residence
- Illicit drug use (child, adolescent, or parent)
- Serious mental health problems in the child or parent
- Allergic sensitivity to outdoor molds

ABBREVIATION: ICU, intensive care unit.

Asthma in Adults

Much of the information that has already been presented for childhood asthma also applies to adults. This section of the chapter will highlight differences between adult and childhood asthma in the areas of recognition, diagnosis, and management.

Current estimates are that between 9 and 10 million adults have recognized asthma. As in children, allergies play a major role in the pathogenesis of asthma in adults. Allergies are associated with 70 percent of asthma in adults less than 30 years old and with 50 percent of asthma in adults over age 30. Therefore, an allergic basis of asthma should always be considered in adults.

Many exacerbations of asthma in adults are triggered by infections. Common preventive measures such as good hand washing and wide availability of nasal tissues for use during colds may decrease the spread of viral infections. Other exacerbations are linked to smoking, both in the person with asthma who continues to smoke and through exposure to environmental tobacco smoke. Other industrial and occupational exposures are estimated to be related to between 5 and 10 percent of adult asthma cases. Many irritants found in the workplace may affect the susceptible adult. Common agents associated with occupational asthma include metal salts, wood dusts, and animal and insect materials. More information about occupational asthma is provided in Chap. 18.

Although not always considered causes of asthma, several concomitant conditions may worsen asthma. These include sinusitis, gastroesophageal reflux, pregnancy, hyperthyroidism, and emotional stress.

Diagnosis

DIFFERENTIAL DIAGNOSIS

As in children, the diagnosis of asthma is based on documented recurrent episodes of airway obstruction that are reversible with bronchodilator medications. Pulmonary function testing can be needed to confirm the diagnosis. As in the child, the diagnosis of intermittent asthma requires proof of prolonged symptom-free periods. New asthma is usually diagnosed before the age of 40, although previously unrecognized asthma can be newly identified at any age.

In adults, wheezing, coughing, and chest tightness have a more extensive differential diagnosis than in children. Tumors, cardiac disease, gastric reflux, and lung damage from smoking should all be considered in the adult who presents with a chronic cough or wheezing.

Furthermore, diagnosing asthma in older adults may be complicated by the presence or presumed presence of COPD. Also called chronic bronchitis and/or emphysema, COPD is almost always a sequel to many (>20) years of smoking. After 5 to 10 years of smoking, no changes may be seen on pulmonary function testing, but by 20 years of smoking the FEV_1 and FVC are usually decreased, and after 30 years of smoking clinical symptoms are the rule. Like asthma, COPD may also present with wheezing and at least partially reversible airway obstruction and bronchial hyperresponsiveness. A family history of COPD, α-antitrypsin deficiency, or long-term smoking helps to direct the evaluation toward COPD. Evaluating for an underlying nonreversible component of airway obstruction may require treatment of the acute wheezing episode with 2 weeks of oral or inhaled corticosteroids to alleviate acute reversible obstruction, leaving only the underlying nonreversible obstruction. New-onset wheezing in a smoker of 20 to 30 years should be considered as possible COPD with acute exacerbations until proven otherwise.

Episodes of recurrent pulmonary emboli may also mimic asthma. These can be difficult to distinguish without pulmonary function testing, especially challenge testing, which should be normal with pulmonary emboli. Pulmonary imaging and assessment of ventilation/perfusion differences should be completed any time recurrent pulmonary emboli are considered. The sudden worsening of stable asthma in an adult with a fracture or cancer, or in a pregnant woman at or near term or in the postpartum period should trigger a consideration of pulmonary emboli.

An uncommon cause of asthma in adults is allergic bronchopulmonary aspergillosis (ABPA). Originally thought to be limited to England, ABPA has been found in the midwestern United States. The prevalence is unknown, but asthma associated with pulmonary infiltrates should trigger consideration of ABPA. ABPA can be diagnosed with serologic testing for IgG antibodies to *Aspergillus*. Consultation with an allergist or pulmonary specialist with experience in diagnosis of this uncommon condition may be helpful.

Coexisting asthma and nasal polyposis is a warning sign for sensitivity to aspirin and other nonsteroidal anti-inflammatory drugs (NSAIDs). Most people with aspirin sensitivity will also complain of chronic or recurrent sinusitis. The treatment is avoidance of aspirin and NSAIDs. In special cases, aspirin desensitization can be accomplished, although this procedure carries a significant risk of anaphylaxis.

HISTORY

It is important to understand the exact nature of the person's symptoms and exacerbations. Clinicians should inquire into episodes of wheezing, coughing (especially a recurrent nocturnal cough), shortness of breath, exercise intolerance, nighttime restlessness, and chest tightness, because patients may fail to connect some symptoms with asthma. Therefore, it is helpful to have a list of symptoms to review.

A history of seasonal variations, aspirin sensitivity, chronic rhinitis or sinusitis, or allergies increases suspicion of asthma and especially allergic asthma. A family history of asthma also increases the likelihood of asthma in the patient. The pattern of symptoms assessed should include any indications of worsening with work attendance, especially early in the workweek, improvement during vacations, problems when visiting homes with pets, or improvement when traveling.

PHYSICAL EXAMINATION

The physical examination in a patient with asthma may be entirely normal or may reveal signs of concomitant allergy-related conditions such as rhinitis, sinusitis, conjunctivitis (edema of the eye, often without erythema), nasal polyps, bad breath, and signs of postnasal drip. Otitis media in an adult should raise particular suspicion of the presence of allergic disease. Clubbing of the fingers should immediately suggest other diagnoses, such as cardiac disease, pulmonary neoplasia, or COPD. Signs of nicotine stains on fingers suggest chronic cigarette use and may suggest COPD rather than asthma.

Between exacerbations, the chest examination may be normal or may show signs of chronic hyperinflation (hyperresonance and increased anterior-posterior diameter). During an exacerbation or with persistent asthma, wheezing may be present. Severe symptoms can be associated with accessory muscle use, diminished wheezing and breath sounds, anxiety, patient refusal to lie down, dyspnea, tachypnea, and tachycardia. Cyanosis is a sign of impending respiratory failure from whatever cause.

TESTING

Adults should have pulmonary function testing to confirm the diagnosis of asthma. Optimally, testing is done before and after inhalation of a short-acting beta-agonist. Challenge testing should be considered in those with normal FEV_1 and without a contraindication (e.g., known or suspected coronary artery disease). Any suspicion of another etiology should be evaluated either concomitantly or prior to challenge testing.

Pulmonary function testing can help distinguish chronic bronchitis and COPD from asthma. In asthma the airflow obstruction should be reversible, and restriction patterns should be nonexistent or minimal. In COPD the obstruction is usually not or only minimally reversible (less than 12 percent improvement), and mixed restrictive and obstructive patterns are common.

Other appropriate tests for adults with asthma or suspected asthma are based on the patient's age, symptoms, and co-morbid conditions. Common tests that are ordered include a chest x-ray to rule out infiltrates, masses, or congestive heart failure and allergy testing.

Evaluation for allergies is appropriate in patients with a family history of asthma and allergy, seasonal variations in symptoms, or other indications of allergic disease. "New" allergies can occur at any age, but in adults they are usually preceded by a change in allergen exposure, such as a new pet in the house. If specific suspect antigens can be identified, allergen-specific RAST tests may be ordered. When allergen specificity is unclear or many allergens seem to be candidates for symptoms, a screening battery of tests may be appropriate. As in children, these batteries can be tailored to specific regions of the country. Skin prick testing may be appropriate in adults with persistent and poorly controlled asthma or adults who are unable to comply with drug therapy, and in whom immunotherapy is being considered.

Management

The goals of asthma management are the same for adults and children. They include preventing chronic or troublesome symptoms, maintaining normal or near-normal lung function, maintaining normal activity levels, preventing the need for emergent or hospital care, and limiting the side effects of the treatment regimen.

As with all chronic diseases, management is based on the foundation of informed and involved patients. Understanding the role of inflammation and the impact of allergens, irritants, and exercise on the tissues in the pulmonary tree may make it easier for patients and families to comply with allergy or irritant avoidance and a regimen of chronic drug treatment.

PHARMACOLOGIC THERAPY

The drugs used in managing adult asthma are the same as those used in children. In adults, concern about the effects of corticosteroids on linear growth is less important, but it is replaced with increased concern about the development of steroid-induced osteoporosis, cataracts, and glaucoma. As in children, the total dose of corticosteroids in adults should be kept at the lowest level needed to control symptoms. Adding leukotriene inhibitors and long-acting bronchodilators should be tried whenever the doses of inhaled corticosteroids reach the high end of the recommended dosage range. Regimens that combine corticosteroids and long-acting beta-agonists may be useful in adults with moderate or severe asthma. Cromoglycates have limited use in adults with asthma. The simplest dosing schedule possible, one that avoids dosing during work hours, is preferable.

Initial therapy should be based on the assessed asthma severity. Like children, adults need routine visits scheduled at regular 3- to 6-month intervals to assess asthma control and monitor exacerbations and drug use. Treatment can be stepped up or down at these regular visits. Exacerbations may be treated at home, at the workplace, in the clinician's office, in the ED, or in the hospital. Patients should always return for reevaluation within 2 weeks of any exacerbation requiring an office or ED visit or hospitalization.

IMMUNOTHERAPY

The value of immunotherapy (allergy shots) in controlling symptoms in adults with asthma has been shown in several trials.[29] Immunotherapy treatment for longer than 2 years without substantial improvement is inappropriate. Many primary care physicians work with an allergist to co-manage these patients and may administer allergy injections in the primary care office after evaluation and an initial trial of immunotherapy in the allergist's office. Co-management is particularly important in rural and inner city areas, where access to an allergist is difficult.

CHRONIC DISEASE CARE

At each visit, someone in the physician's office must evaluate (by direct observation) the patient's inhaler technique. Recent studies suggest that over 50 percent of poor control is due to poor inhaler technique, resulting in little disposition of medications in the large and small airways.[30] Each visit should also include specific questions about weekly and monthly estimates of the number of canisters of short-acting bronchodilators used. Use of more then one canister per month or the need for urgent care or ED visits strongly suggests inadequate control.

Evaluation of the patient's and family's satisfaction with the level of control and ability to do usual and desired activity as well as asthma care in general should be included in each visit. Reassessing the goals of asthma care can refocus attention on important aspects of care.

Education is the foundation of a partnership. Adults often learn differently from children, but repetition emphasizes messages for all learners. Careful listening can also teach the physician a lot about the effect of disease on the patient and explain many of the reasons for inadequate asthma control.

References

1. Silverman M: Asthma and wheezing in young children. *N Engl J Med* 332(3):181–182, 1995.
2. Drazen JF, Israel E, Boushey HA, et al: Comparison of regularly scheduled with as-needed use of albuterol in mild asthma. *N Engl J Med* 335: 841–847, 1996.
3. Mannino DM, Homa DM, Pertowski CA, et al: Surveillance for asthma—United States, 1960–1995. *MMWR CDC Surveill Summ* 47(1):1–27, 1998.
4. Yawn BP, Wollan PC, Kurland MJ, et al: A longitudinal study of asthma prevalence in a community population of school age children. *J Pediatr*, in press.
5. Joseph CL, Foxman B, Leickly FE, et al: Prevalence of possible undiagnosed asthma and associated morbidity among urban schoolchildren. *J Pediatr* 129(5):735–742, 1996.
6. Maier WC, Arrighi HM, Morray B, et al: The impact of asthma and asthma-like illness in Seattle school children. *J Clin Epidemiol* 51(7):557–568, 1998.
7. Siersted HC, Boldsen J, Hansen HS, et al: Population based study of risk factors for underdiagnosis of asthma in adolescence: Odense schoolchild study. *Br Med J* 316(7132):651–655; discussion 655–656, 1998.
8. Brown CM, Anderson HA, Etzel RA: The state's challenge. *Public Health Rep* 112:198–205, 1997.
9. Crespo CJ: Update on national data on asthma. Unpublished data. Presented at the National Asthma Education and Prevention Program meeting, Leesburg, VA, March 27–28, 1998.

10. McFadden ER: Diseases of the respiratory system, in Braunwald E, Fauci AS: *Harrison's Principles of Internal Medicine*, 15th ed. New York, McGraw-Hill; 2001: pp 1456–1463.

11. Newacheck PW, Halfon N: Prevalence, impact, and trends in childhood disability due to asthma. *Arch Pediatr Adolesc Med* 154:287–293, 2000.

12. Rand CS, Butz AM, Kolodner K, et al: Emergency department visits by urban African American children with asthma. *J Allergy Clin Immunol* 105(1 pt 1):83–90, 2000.

13. Martinez FD, Wright AL, Taussig LM, et al: Asthma and wheezing in the first six years of life. *N Engl J Med* 332:133–138, 1995.

14. Nelson DA, Johnson CC, Divine GW, et al: Ethnic differences in the prevalence of asthma in middle class children. *Ann Allergy Asthma Immunol* 78:21–26, 1997.

15. *Actions against Asthma.* Washington, DC, U.S. Department of Health and Human Services; 2000.

16. Annenberg Center for Health Sciences at Eisenhower: Atopic factors in upper respiratory disease: diagnosing and managing nasal symptoms. (Monograph.)

17. Vollmer WM, Osborne ML, Buist AS: 20-year trends in the prevalence of asthma and chronic airflow obstruction in an HMO. *Am J Respir Crit Care Med* 157(4 pt 1):1079–1084, 1998.

18. US Department of Health and Human Services: *Guidelines for the Diagnosis and Management of Asthma. Expert Panel Report 2.* NIH Publication No. 97-4051, 1997.

19. Busse WW, Lemanske RF Jr: Asthma. *N Engl J Med* 344:350–362, 2001.

20. Evidence Report. Management of Chronic Asthma. Rockville, MD, Technology Evaluation Center, Agency for Health Care Research and Quality, August 2001.

21. Nash DR: Allergic rhinitis. *Pediatr Ann* 799–808, 1998.

22. Powell CV, Primhak RA: Asthma treatment, perceived respiratory disability, and morbidity. *Arch Dis Child* 72:209–213, 1995.

23. The Childhood Asthma Management Program Research Group: Long-term effects of budesonide or nedocromil in children with asthma. *N Engl J Med* 343(15):1054–1063, 2000.

24. Silverstein MD, Yunginger JW, Reed CE, et al: Attained adult height after childhood asthma: effect of glucocorticoid therapy. *J Allergy Clin Immunol* 99:466–474, 1997.

25. Agertoft L, Pedersen S: Effect of long-term treatment with inhaled budesonide on adult height in children with asthma. *N Engl J Med* 343:1064–1069, 2000.

26. Van Bever HP, Desager KN, Lijssens N, et al: Does treatment of asthmatic children with inhaled corticosteroids affect their adult height? *Pediatr Pulmonol* 27:369–375, 1999.

27. Asthma and wheezing in young children (editorial). *N Engl J Med* 332:181–182, 1995.

28. *Asthma Management and Prevention. A Practical Guide for Public Health Officials and Health Care Professionals.* NIH Publication No. 96-3659A, 1995.

29. Abramson MJ, Puy RM, Weiner JM: Is allergen immunotherapy effective in asthma? A meta-analysis of randomized controlled trials. *Am J Respir Crit Care Med* 151:969–974, 1995.

30. Vanden Burgt JA, Busse WW, Martin RJ, et al: Efficacy and safety overview of a new inhaled corticosteroid, QVAR (hydrofluoroalkane-beclomethasone extrafine inhalation aerosol), in asthma. *J Allergy Clin Immunol* 106:1210–1226, 2000.

Melissa H. Hunter
Dana E. King

COPD: Management of Acute Exacerbations and Chronic Stable Disease

Despite public education regarding cigarette smoking, chronic obstructive pulmonary disease (COPD) continues to pose a major medical problem. Approximately 20 percent of the adult American population is afflicted with COPD.[1] COPD is the fourth leading cause of death in the United States.[2] Acute bronchitis and acute exacerbations of COPD account for over 16 million physician visits annually and are among the most common illnesses encountered by the primary care clinician.[3,4]

Although there is no precise agreement on the definition of COPD, the American Thoracic Society defines it as a disease process featuring progressive chronic airflow obstruction due to chronic bronchitis, emphysema, or both. The airflow obstruction may be partially reversible, with a small subset of patients exhibiting bronchial hyperresponsiveness.[5]

Chronic bronchitis is defined clinically as excessive cough and production of sputum on most days for at least 3 months during at least 2 consecutive years.[6] Chronic bronchitis affects both small and large airways, with hypertrophy and hyperplasia of glandular structures and goblet cell metaplasia in the large airways.[7] Peribronchiolar fibrosis and airway narrowing can be a prominent feature in the small airways. It has been suggested that the definition of COPD should emphasize the central pathogenic role of an inflammatory process that progresses to obstruction by causing distortion and fibrosis of terminal airways, loss of alveolar attachments tethering small airways, mucus hypersecretion, and smooth muscle contraction.[8,9]

Emphysema is characterized by chronic dyspnea due to destruction of lung tissue and enlargement of air spaces. These changes result in a loss of lung elastic recoil.

Asthma, which also features airflow obstruction, airway inflammation, and increased airway responsiveness to various stimuli, may be distinguished from COPD by the reversibility of the pulmonary function deficits.[10]

For patients with stable COPD, the aims of outpatient management should be to improve the patients' quality of life by preventing acute exacerbations, relieving symptoms, and slowing the progressive deterioration of lung function. The clinical course of COPD is characterized by chronic disability with intermittent acute exacerbations, which occur primarily during winter months. When exacerbations of COPD occur, they are typically manifested by increased sputum production, sputum purulence, and dyspnea.[11] While infectious etiologies account for most exacerbations, exposure to allergens, pollutants, or inhaled irritants may play a role.[12]

Epidemiology

COPD is one of the most serious and disabling conditions of middle-aged and elderly people, causing over 110,000 deaths annually. In the United States, over 16 million people have COPD. Their burden of suffering is reflected in their more than 16 million office visits, 500,000 hospitalizations, and $18 billion in direct health care costs.[13] Cigarette smoking is implicated in 90 percent of cases.

COPD exacts a large toll on its sufferers. Two-thirds of patients have serious chronic dyspnea and nearly 25 percent have profound total body pain, and many patients with these disorders are disabled from work.[14,15] Chronic lung disease also has a major impact on families, including caring for the disabled persons and facing end-of-life decisions. Caregivers face considerable burdens caring for COPD patients at home because of patients' functional limitations, anxieties regarding air hunger, and frequency of exacerbations, often requiring medical attention. The indirect costs in dollars are so large as to be inestimable.

Pathophysiology

COPD is a subset of a group of obstructive lung diseases that also includes cystic fibrosis, bronchiectasis, and asthma. It is characterized as degeneration and destruction of the lung and supporting tissue, resulting in emphysema, chronic bronchitis, or both. Emphysema begins with small airway disease and progresses to alveolar destruction, with a predominance of small airway narrowing and hyperplasia of the mucus glands. Chronic bronchitis is characterized by ongoing inflammation in the bronchial tree.

The pathophysiology of COPD is not completely understood. Both degeneration of alveolar tissue and chronic inflammation of the cells lining the bronchial tree play important roles. Smoking and occasionally other inhaled irritants precipitate an ongoing inflammatory response, resulting in airway narrowing and hyperactivity. This results in airflow obstruction during both inspiration and expiration, mainly as a result of airway edema, excess mucus production, and poor ciliary function.[14]

The mechanisms of airflow obstruction are different in emphysema and chronic bronchitis. In patients with emphysema, the alveolar and tissue destruction leads to loss of elastic recoil. This loss of recoil inhibits the ability of the tiniest airways to remain open during inspiration and expiration, leading to collapse of the smallest bronchioles.[16] Increasing pressure with forced expiration causes airways to collapse more, making the airflow obstruction worse with greater effort by the patient. In chronic bronchitis, hypertrophy of glandular structures and mucus-producing cells causes mild to moderate obstruction of airways. Even greater airflow obstruction occurs as a result of the inflammatory response and the accompanying fibrosis and narrowing of small airways.[17] With disease progression, patients have increasing symptoms of airflow obstruction, including difficulty in clearing secretions, chronic productive cough, wheezing, and dyspnea. Patients quickly become colonized with bacteria, which leads to further inflammation, recurrent infection, and formation of diverticulae in the bronchial tree.

Exacerbations of COPD can be caused by many factors, but most often they are the result of bacterial or viral infection. Other causes include environmental irritants, heart failure, and discontinuation of medications.[8] Bacterial infection is present in 70 to 75 percent of exacerbations, with up to 60 percent of infections being due to *Streptococcus pneumoniae, Haemophilus influenzae*, and *Moraxella catarrhalis*.[9] Organisms such as *Chlamydia pneumoniae* have been implicated in about 10 percent of exacerbations (Table 17-1).[20] In the remaining 25 to 30 percent of cases, viruses are the most common culprit.[21] More serious exacerbations requiring mechanical ventilation have been associated with *Pseudomonas* species and are most common in patients with severe disease and a history of frequent exacerbations.

Risk Factors for COPD

Causes of COPD include smoking, genetic factors (including α_1-antitrypsin deficiency), occupational exposures, air pollution, passive smoking, and possibly hyperresponsive airways. Up to 90 percent of COPD is caused by smoking. Although precise distinctions between chronic bronchitis and emphysema are difficult to detect clinically, it is commonly believed that chronic bronchitis is responsible for as much as 85 percent of COPD.

Table 17-1

Most Common Infectious Causes of COPD Exacerbations

Mild/moderate exacerbations	*Streptococcus pneumoniae*
	Haemophilus influenzae
	Moraxella catarrhalis
	Chlamydia pneumoniae
	Mycoplasma pneumoniae
	Viral
Severe exacerbations	*Pseudomonas* spp.
	Other gram-negative enteric bacilli

SOURCE: Adapted from Soler et al,[19] Fein and Fein,[20] and Sethi.[21]

Little is known about the natural history of COPD since initiation of the modern era of treatment; however, the severity of a patient's symptoms is strongly influenced by the rate of decline in forced expiratory volume in 1 s (FEV_1). One major factor influencing this rate of decline is cigarette smoking. Rate of decline exhibits a very strong relationship with smoking and with the amount smoked.[22] Age, correlated with number of years of cigarette smoking, is also a risk factor for more rapid decline of lung function.

Exposures other than cigarette smoke also have been associated with an accelerated rate of decline of FEV_1.[23–25] These include occupational exposures, exposure to passive smoke, alcohol ingestion, and exposure to high amounts of air pollution. Not all of the determinants of the rate of decline in FEV_1 are external; genetic factors may also play a role. It is felt, however, that individuals who have airflow limitation have presumably had an accelerated rate of decline in FEV_1 in the past, and are likely to experience accelerated rates of decline in FEV_1 in the future.[22] This observation has been called the "horse racing effect" and suggests that genetic features possibly leading to accelerated rates of decline in FEV_1 are probably present throughout the individual's lifetime.[26]

The only genetic factor that influences COPD that is well established at present is deficiency of α_1-protease inhibitor.[27] The lack of this serum protein, a trait that is inherited in an autosomal recessive fashion, can be associated with accelerated rates of development of emphysema in nonsmokers and markedly accelerated rates in smokers. Description of this condition has led to the concept that proteolytic activity by a substance known as neutrophil elastase, in excess of antiprotease protective mechanisms, can lead to alveolar wall destruction characteristic of emphysema. Further studies looking at ways to modify the activity of neutrophil elastase are ongoing.

Additionally, it is hypothesized that oxidants from cigarette smoking may contribute to the development of COPD. However, the role of antioxidants in the management of COPD

remains unclear.[28] Research targeting other molecular and cellular mediators is currently in progress.

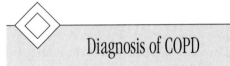

Diagnosis of COPD

Diagnostic testing for COPD centers on chest imaging and spirometry, although in actual practice the diagnosis is based appropriately on clinical factors such as symptoms of dyspnea, sputum production, and a history of smoking. When objective measures are employed to establish the diagnosis of COPD, the FEV_1 has been used most often because it is easiest to quantify.[13]

Chest radiography is useful for diagnosis in COPD, but radiographic changes often are not evident until the disease has progressed to advanced stages. When changes are present, however, chest radiography can often offer objective evidence for COPD. In severe cases of emphysema, chest radiographs demonstrate flattening of the diaphragm, irregularity in the lucency of the lung fields, enlargement of the retrosternal space, and blunting of the costophrenic angle.[14] Observational studies show that in exacerbations of COPD, chest radiographs are useful because they detect a high rate of abnormalities.[29–31]

Spirometry can be useful for measuring FEV_1 and forced vital capacity (FVC), which can give an estimate of the level of airflow obstruction. The peak expiratory flow rate (PEFR), a test easily performed in a physician's office, also can be useful as a screening test and diagnostic clue when full spirometry is not readily available. The diagnosis of COPD should be considered when the PEFR falls below 350 L/min in adults.[14] Symptoms of COPD usually begin when FEV_1 falls below 80 percent of predicted values for weight and age. Patients can become dyspneic on exertion when levels fall to 50 percent of predicted values, and dyspneic at rest with further drops.

FEV_1 also can be used to stage the severity of COPD. The two main systems for staging COPD are based on FEV_1 (Table 17-2).[32] There is disagreement between the two organizations (the American Thoracic Society and the British Thoracic Society) that created the system. One reason for this disagreement may be that FEV_1 values do not correlate with symptoms or Po_2 levels in patients with COPD as well as they do in patients with asthma.[32] However, FEV_1 is the objective measure that correlates best with mortality and frequency of exacerbations.[32] Spirometric assessment is of limited usefulness during acute exacerbations of COPD and is best performed when the patient is stable.

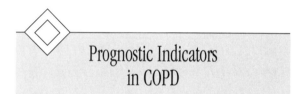

Prognostic Indicators in COPD

Over the past four decades, numerous attempts have been made to determine what factors influence the survival of patients with COPD. Most of these studies have examined the survival of stable outpatients; only limited data regarding the survival of patients with acute exacerbations of COPD requiring hospitalization exist. Data from the last decade show that 60-year-old smokers with chronic bronchitis have a 10-year mortality of 60 percent, four times that of age-matched nonsmoking asthmatics.[33]

Table 17-2

Staging Systems for COPD Using FEV_1 (Percent Predicted)

SYSTEM	MILD	MODERATE	SEVERE
ATS	≥50%	35–49%	<35%
BTS	60–79%	40–59%	<40%

ABBREVIATIONS: FEV_1, forced expiratory volume in 1 s; ATS, American Thoracic Society; BTS, British Thoracic Society.
SOURCE: Information from Bach et al,[32] with permission.

Several studies examined factors influencing the survival of outpatients with COPD, with the strongest predictors of mortality being the patient's age and baseline postbronchodilator FEV_1 (Table 17-3).[34–36] Younger patients with COPD generally have lower mortality rates unless there is an accompanying α_1-antitrypsin deficiency, a rare genetic abnormality that causes panlobular emphysema in adults and is responsible for approximately 1 percent of COPD cases. It should be suspected when COPD develops in patients under the age of 45 without a history of chronic bronchitis or tobacco use or when multiple family members develop obstructive disease at an early age. Reversible changes after bronchodilator administration are a sign of less advanced disease and improved survival.

Decreases in FEV_1 on serial testing are associated with increased mortality rates, i.e., patients with a faster decline in FEV_1 have a higher rate of death. The major risk factor associated with an accelerated rate of decline in FEV_1 is continued cigarette smoking. Smoking cessation in patients with early COPD improves lung function initially and slows the annual loss of FEV_1.[22,25,37] Other factors that predict improved survival chances include higher oxygen partial pressure (Po_2) levels, a history of atopy, and higher diffusion and exercise capacity.[34,38–40] Performance status and oral steroid usage have also been linked to survival,[41] while coexistent cardiopulmonary disease and number of previous exacerbations have been identified as risk factors for hospitalization or returning to the physician following institution of antibiotic therapy.[42] Other factors found to decrease survival rates include malnutrition/weight loss, dyspnea, hypoxemia ($Pa_{O_2} < 55$ mmHg), presence of right-sided heart failure, resting tachycardia, and increased P_{CO_2} (> 45 mmHg).[34,43,44]

Recommendations for clinical monitoring of patients with COPD include serial FEV_1 measurement, pulse oximetry, and the time required to walk a predetermined distance, although decline in FEV_1 has the most predictive value.[45]

Table 17-3

Factors Influencing Survival in Chronic Bronchitis

RISK FACTOR	EFFECT ON SURVIVAL
Age	Decreased mortality in younger patients
Postbronchodilator FEV_1	Increased mortality with decreased FEV_1; decreased mortality if reversible component of obstruction present
Rate of FEV_1 decline	Decreased mortality with slower decline
Cigarette smoking	Increased mortality with continued use/greater consumption
History of atopy	Decreased mortality
Higher diffusion capacity	Decreased mortality
P_{O_2} level	Decreased mortality with increased levels; $P_{O_2} < 55$ mmHg increases mortality
Hypercapnia ($P_{CO_2} > 45$ mmHg)	Increased mortality
Right heart failure	Increased mortality
Malnutrition	Increased mortality
Resting tachycardia	Increased mortality

ABBREVIATIONS: FEV_1, forced expiratory volume in 1 s; P_{O_2}, partial oxygen pressure; P_{CO_2}, carbon dioxide partial pressure.
SOURCE: Information from Hughes et al,[36] with permission.

Once FEV_1 falls below 1 L, 5-year survival is approximately 50 percent.[40] FEV_1 less than 750 mL or less than 50 percent predicted on spirometric testing is associated with worsening disease and poorer prognosis.

For those patients with acute exacerbations, outcomes are similarly heterogeneous. In studies looking at outcomes from acute exacerbations of COPD in both emergency room and outpatient settings, relapse is more likely for patients with lower pretreatment and posttreatment FEV_1, those who receive more bronchodilator treatments or corticosteroids during their visit, and those who have higher rates of previous relapse.[32] While nearly 50 percent of exacerbations are not reported to physicians, those exacerbations that require hospitalization are associated with inpatient mortality rates of 3 to 4 percent.[46] For hospitalized patients with severe underlying lung disease with acute exacerbations, acute respiratory failure may develop, requiring mechanical ventilation in 20 to 60 percent of cases. Mortality rates are substantially higher for those patients requiring admission to an intensive care unit (ICU), ranging from 11 to 24 percent while in hospital and 43 to 46 percent at 1 year after hospitalization.[47–51] Additional factors associated with in-hospital mortality include age $\geq$ 65 years, length of hospital stay before ICU admission, and severity of respiratory and nonrespiratory organ system dysfunction.[50] Additionally, 50 percent of those hospitalized for acute exacerbations of COPD are expected to be readmitted at least once in the following 6 months.[47,52]

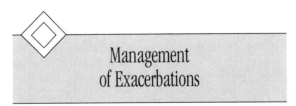

Management of Exacerbations

One challenging problem facing clinicians is providing the most effective treatment for patients with exacerbations of COPD. Since there is no curative therapy available, it is important to focus on relief of symptoms and restoration of functional capacity. COPD patients are often at a poorer baseline functional status than other hospitalized patients, with few respiratory reserves. Any infection that worsens a patient's condition can lead to a decline in pulmonary function in a relatively short period of time.

The American Thoracic Society has recommended strategies for management of acute exacerbations of chronic bronchitis and emphysema (AECB).[5] These strategies include the use of oxygen (when hypoxia is present), use of beta$_2$-agonists, addition or increase of anticholinergics, administration of intravenous (IV) steroids, use of antibiotics when indicated, and consideration of IV methylxanthines such as aminophylline. (See Table 17-4 for details regarding pharmacologic agents.) Hospitalization may be necessary to provide antibiotics, appropriate supportive care, and monitoring of oxygen status. Supplemental oxygen, via either external devices or mechanical ventilation to maintain oxygen delivery to vital tissues, may also be indicated.

Assuring Oxygenation

Initial therapy should focus on maintaining oxygen saturation ≥90 percent. Oxygen status can be monitored clinically by serial measurement of arterial blood gases or pulse oximetry. Oxygen supplementation usually is supplied by a nasal cannula at 1/2 to 4 L/min, depending on the patient's need. When the patient cannot maintain oxygen saturation >90 percent via a nasal cannula, a face mask may be required. With more severe exacerbations, intubation and/or positive-pressure methods are often necessary for adequate oxygenation. Such interventions are more likely to be needed when hypercapnia is present, when exacerbations are frequent, and when altered mental status is evident.[20]

Bronchodilator Therapy

Inhaled beta$_2$-agonists (see Table 17-4) should be administered as soon as possible during the exacerbation. Providing albuterol or a similar agent by nebulizer with saline and oxygen enhances delivery of medication to airways.[53] Metered-dose inhalers (MDIs) provide effective delivery of beta-agonists if patients are able to use them. Salmeterol (Serevent), a long-acting beta-agonist, has been shown in clinical trials to offer relief of symptoms in COPD patients, but it should be used only for chronic stable outpatients and not for relief of acute exacerbations.[54] The twice-daily dosing of salmeterol is an added benefit for long-term compliance and may be convenient for many patients. Oral beta-agonists are generally not used because of the greater chance of side effects than with inhaled forms.

Anticholinergic Agents

While many patients will already be using anticholinergic therapy when they present to the clinician with an acute exacerbation of chronic bronchitis, its use should be optimized during an exacerbation. Anticholinergic drugs (e.g., ipratropium) are extremely effective in COPD patients and provide the same or greater bronchodilation than beta-agonists.[20] They have few adverse effects in inhaled form because of their minimal systemic absorption and may be added to beta-agonist therapy when delivered by nebulizer or MDI. A common error of inexperienced clinicians is to underdose ipratropium; because of its safety profile and lack of systemic absorption, it can be used at recommended doses (see Table 17-4) with only minimal concern about toxicity or side effects.

There are no known or significant drug interactions. The only known contraindication is soy or peanut allergy, since patients with food allergies have a higher rate of developing allergic-type reactions to ipratropium. At least three clinical studies that used ipratropium bromide for treatment of COPD reported no adverse effects of ipratropium when it was used alone.[55–57] The recommended maximum dose is 12 puffs per 24 h or nebulizer therapy four times a day, but it is sometimes used more frequently in severe exacerbations (every 4 h).

Table 17-4

Pharmacologic Therapy for Chronic Obstructive Lung Disease (COPD)

Class of Drug	Drug	Dosage Range	Side Effects and Warnings*	Comments	Cost†
Beta₂-agonists	**Short-Acting Agents**				
	—Albuterol MDI	1–2 puffs q4–6h up to max 6–8 puffs q2h	Caution in patients with cardiovascular disease, hyperthyroidism, seizure disorder	Used for maintenance therapy and acute exacerbations	$20 per MDI
	—Albuterol nebulized	0.25–0.5 mL 5% solution q4–6h			$30 per 25 3-mL doses
	Long-Acting Agents				
	—Salmeterol MDI	2 puffs q12h		Not to be used for acute treatment	$67 per MDI
Anticholinergic agents	—Ipratropium MDI	2–4 puffs q6h to max 6–8 puffs q4h	Caution in patients with BPH or angle-closure glaucoma	No significant drug interactions known	$39 per MDI
	—Ipratropium nebulized	Up to 500 µg divided TID-QID for acute severe episodes			$45 per 25 2.5-mL doses
Corticosteroids	Methylprednisolone	1–2 mg/kg IV q6–12 h	Caution in patients with CHF, diabetes mellitus, TB, impaired hepatic function, immunocompromised states Side effects include psychosis, GI upset/PUD, immuno-suppression	Osteoporosis and steroid withdrawal with long-term use	$13–38
	Prednisone	60 mg/day tapering for total of 2 weeks			$4 per 2-week course
Methylxanthines	Aminophylline	0.3–0.7 mg/kg/h IV	Caution in patients with arrhythmias, CHF, seizure disorders, impaired hepatic or renal function Side effects include GI upset, agitation, tremor	Narrow therapeutic index Increased levels with cimetidine, ciprofloxacin, erythromycin	$100 per 20 mL of 25 mg/mL
	Theophylline	300–600 mg QD		Smoking decreases serum levels	$12–24 per month
Antidepressants	Bupropion	150 mg PO BID for 7–12 weeks	Caution in patients with eating and seizure disorders Side effects include GI upset, insomnia	Exact mechanism of action unknown Advise patients to attempt quitting 7–14 days after initiation of therapy	$92 per month
Nicotine replacements	Nicotine patch	Apply QD × 6–12 weeks 7 mg/14 mg/21 mg titrated in decreasing doses	Caution in patients with arrhythmias, CHF, PUD Side effects include local pruritus, insomnia	No significant interactions with drugs For use in patients smoking > 10 cigarettes per day	$49 for 2-week supply
	Nicotine gum	2–4 mg prn			$29–32 for 48 pieces of gum

ABBREVIATIONS: MDI, metered-dose inhaler; BPH, benign prostatic hypertrophy; IV, intravenous; CHF, congestive heart failure; TB, tuberculosis; GI, gastrointestinal; PUD, peptic ulcer disease.

*For more detailed information, consult the package insert provided by the manufacturer of each drug.

†Estimated cost to the pharmacist (rounded to the nearest dollar) based on average wholesale prices in *Red Book*. Montvale, NJ, Medical Economics Data, 1999. Cost to the patient will be higher, depending on prescription filling fee.

Adding ipratropium to beta-agonist therapy is beneficial for patients. The combination has been shown to improve FEV_1 and shorten the duration of stays in the emergency department.[56,58] Combination products (e.g., Combivent) may help simplify medication regimens and aid compliance, especially in outpatient and long-term therapy.

Antibiotic Therapy

Antibiotic therapy has been demonstrated to be beneficial in the treatment of exacerbations of COPD and should be initiated at the beginning of treatment for exacerbations even if no clear evidence for infection is present (see Table 17-5).[20] A meta-analysis including nine clinical trials of antibiotic use for patients with chronic bronchitis exacerbations demonstrated the benefit of antibiotic therapy.[59] Therapy for moderate exacerbations of chronic bronchitis

should be directed against *S. pneumoniae*, *H. influenzae*, and *M. catarrhalis*. *Chlamydia* and *Mycoplasma* occur less often. Augmented penicillins such as Augmentin, doxycycline, double-strength trimethoprim-sulfamethoxazole, or a newer macrolide are preferred treatment for initial outpatient management.[20] Patients over age 65 or with more frequent exacerbations (≥ four episodes/year) should be treated with an augmented penicillin or fluoroquinolone because of increased concerns about bacterial resistance. Inpatients should receive intravenous ampicillin/sulbactam, a third-degree cephalosporin, a newer macrolide, or a fluoroquinolone, similar to treatment for pneumonia, as guided by local bacterial resistance patterns.[60,61] In more severe cases, infection with gram-negative bacteria (especially *Klebsiella* and *Pseudomonas* spp.) is more likely. Consequently, in these cases treatment should include a third-generation cephalosporin or augmented penicillin, plus a fluoroquinolone or aminoglycoside for synergy.

Table 17-5

Commonly Used Antibiotics for Exacerbations of COPD

Mild/moderate exacerbations	Amoxicillin/clavulanate 500 mg/125 mg PO TID
	Doxycycline 100 mg PO BID
	Trimethoprim-sulfamethoxazole DS (double-strength) PO BID
	Macrolides: Clarithromycin 500 mg PO BID
	Azithromycin 500 mg initially, then 250 mg QD
	Quinolones: Levofloxacin 500 mg PO QD
	Gatifloxacin 400 mg PO QD
	Moxifloxacin 400 mg PO QD
Moderate/severe exacerbations*	Cephalosporins: Ceftriaxone 1–2 g IV QD
	Cefotaxime 1 g IV q8–12h
	Ceftazidime 1–2 g IV q8–12h
	Anti-pseudomonal penicillins:
	Piperacillin tazobactam 3.375 g IV q6h
	Ticarcillin/clavulanate 3.1 g IV q4–6h
	Quinolones: Levofloxacin 500 mg IV QD
	Gatifloxacin 400 mg IV QD
	Aminoglycoside: Tobramycin 3–5 mg/kg/day q8–12h

*Drugs often used in combination for synergy.
SOURCE: Information from Hodgkin,[34] Anthonisen et al,[35] Kanner,[37] and Bates et al,[38] with permission.

Antibiotic resistance poses an increasing problem, especially for infections due to *S. pneumoniae*, beta-lactamase-producing *H. influenzae*, and *M. catarrhalis*, forcing clinicians to use broader-spectrum antibiotics for empiric therapy.[49] For patients requiring mechanical ventilation, respiratory samples for culture are useful in guiding antibiotic therapy.

Corticosteroid Therapy

A short course of systemic steroids may provide important benefits in patients with COPD exacerbations. A recent clinical study at Veterans Administration hospitals involving 271 patients demonstrated moderate improvement in clinical outcomes, including shorter hospital stays and increases in FEV_1.[62] There were no significant differences in patients treated with steroids for 2 weeks versus 8 weeks, justifying shorter therapy to reduce adverse effects. Six other clinical trials have been done using corticosteroids in patients with exacerbations of COPD. The results have shown that a short course of therapy reduces the rate of relapse and improves spirometry.[32]

Methylprednisolone is commonly used intravenously at an initial dose of 1 to 2 mg/kg q6–12h. Once the patient has improved and is tolerating oral intake, methylprednisolone can be discontinued and changed to oral prednisone at a starting dose of 60 mg/day for 2 weeks. Many clinicians prescribe a tapering dose of prednisone at the end of 2 weeks to avoid adverse effects of sudden withdrawal or rebound symptoms.

Currently, there are no criteria available for deciding which patients benefit most from steroid treatment; thus all patients should receive systemic steroids for serious exacerbations of COPD unless important contraindications exist.

Adverse effects that can be seen with steroid administration include hyperglycemia, secondary infection, and behavioral changes.[63]

Methylxanthines

The use of methylxanthines (aminophylline, theophylline) is of questionable benefit in patients with COPD exacerbations. Although of some help in improving diaphragmatic function in COPD patients, methylxanthines may be potentially toxic and may exhibit serious drug interactions.[64] The results of three randomized studies that have been done to evaluate whether methylxanthines improve lung function or outcomes have been equivocal.[65–67] Nevertheless, with close monitoring and attention to potential adverse effects, these medications are sometimes used in the treatment of patients who are not responding to other bronchodilators.

Doses of aminophylline for use in COPD range from 10 to 15 mg/kg/day to achieve therapeutic levels of 8 to 12 µg/mL to improve diaphragm function. Increased serum levels can be expected with concurrent use of cimetidine, ciprofloxacin, or erythromycin.[68] Smoking promotes methylxanthine metabolism and therefore decreases serum levels of theophylline.[14]

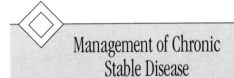

Management of Chronic Stable Disease

Nonpharmacologic Management

One of the first aspects of the management of COPD patients is encouragement of a healthy lifestyle and patient education about the disease. To maximize therapeutic options, initiation of regular exercise and nutritional management should occur, and smoking (if present) should be stopped. Weight loss should be encouraged in those obese patients labeled as "blue bloaters." Thin patients should be considered for nutritional supplementation. Comprehensive pulmonary rehabilitation should also be considered in the management of any patient with COPD. Use of home health care services is also a key to the successful management of chronic bronchitis in outpatient settings. Hospice care may be appropriate for select cases.

Smoking cessation is the single most important factor in the treatment of COPD. There are a number of interventions available to aid patients with smoking cessation. These include behavioral modification and pharmacologic agents such as nicotine replacement, as well as newer therapies including antidepressants like bupropion. A combination of pharmacologic and behavioral approaches appears to yield optimal quit rates. Receiving even minimal counseling from a health care provider improves the effectiveness of nicotine patches.[69]

Pharmacologic Management

Pharmacologic interventions used in the long-term treatment of stable COPD include the same medications previously discussed in the management of acute exacerbations of chronic bronchitis (see Fig. 17-1). Review of the clinical evidence shows that pharmacologic treatment with anticholinergics, beta$_2$-agonists, and oral steroids provides the greatest benefits.

Anticholinergics such as ipratropium seem to provide some short-term improvement in airway obstruction. Unfortunately, they appear to have no significant effect on rate of decline in FEV$_1$.[70]

Both short- and long-acting beta$_2$-agonists achieve short-term benefits by causing bronchodilation, symptom relief, and improvement in quality of life in COPD patients.[71] Salmeterol's longer duration of action and twice-daily dosing schedule offer advantages in convenience, leading to increased compliance by patients using beta-agonists on a long-term basis. Combining beta$_2$-agonists with anticholinergic agents has been found to provide additional bronchodilation compared to either medication used alone.[72]

Short-term oral steroid treatment (2 to 4 weeks) provides improvement of 20 percent or more in baseline FEV$_1$ in COPD;[73] however, no current evidence is available regarding the long-term effects of steroids on lung function. Controversy exists over the effectiveness of inhaled steroids in patients with COPD; recent studies from the Lung Health Study show no slowing of the rate of decline in FEV$_1$. However, inhaled steroids seem to improve airway reactivity, improve respiratory symptoms, and decrease patients' use of health care services for respiratory problems.[74] Benefits of long-term oral steroid use should be weighed against potential long-term effects, including decreased bone mineral density, hyperglycemia, hypertension, and weight gain.

Antibiotics are generally reserved for episodes of AECB, as discussed earlier. Theophylline may improve FEV$_1$ in the short term, but its benefits should be weighed against its potential side effects and its possible toxicity.

There also may be a role for theophylline in chronic stable disease for patients who cannot operate metered-dose inhalers and/or cannot use other medications because of adverse drug interactions.

Management of Hypoxemia

Apart from smoking cessation, supplemental oxygen is the only therapy shown to reduce mortality in COPD.[75] Patients who are hypoxemic with a P$_{O_2}$ ≤ 55 mmHg or an oxygen saturation of 88 percent or less while sleeping should receive supplemental oxygen. Delivery of home oxygen may be provided through either oxygen therapy via nasal cannula or positive-pressure mask ventilation (i.e., CPAP). Continuous long-term oxygen therapy (LTOT) should also be considered in those patients with stable chronic pulmonary disease with P$_{O_2}$ < 55 mmHg on room air, at rest and awake, as well as for patients with accompanying polycythemia, pulmonary hypertension, right-sided heart failure, and/or hypercapnia (P$_{CO_2}$ > 45 mmHg).

Figure 17-1

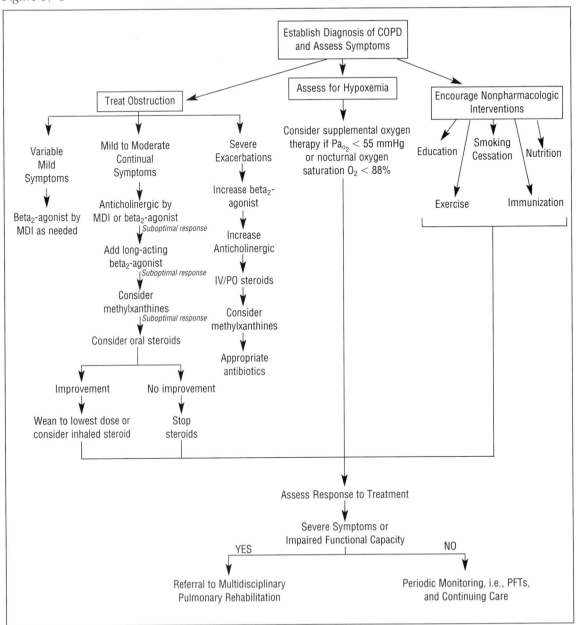

Algorithm for the Management of Chronic Obstructive Pulmonary Disease
ABBREVIATIONS: MDI, metered-dose inhaler; IV, intravenous; PO, by mouth; PFTs, pulmonary function tests.
SOURCE: Adapted from American Thoracic Society,[5] with permission.

CPAP is generally reserved for those patients with chronic hypercapnia. Studies by Clini et al.[76] have shown significant decreases in hospital admissions and length of stay for acute exacerbations of COPD in those patients treated with CPAP and LTOT. Presence of home health care services and nursing care is essential in considering initiation of LTOT and/or CPAP.

Pulmonary Rehabilitation

Pulmonary rehabilitation and exercise are beneficial as adjunctive therapies for those patients whose symptoms are not adequately addressed with pharmacologic therapy, and are most useful for patients with limited activities and decreased quality of life. Rehabilitation exercises that improve the strength of the respiratory musculature have been shown to improve exercise tolerance.[77] The goals of pulmonary rehabilitation are to enhance standard medical therapy and maximize patients' functional capacity. In addition to medical therapy, rehabilitation programs should also include patient and family education; smoking cessation; physical, nutritional, and occupational therapy; and, in selected cases, LTOT and/or CPAP.

Surgical Options

Recent emphasis on surgical interventions for COPD has included lung transplantation and lung volume–reduction procedures. Although transplant surgery began in the 1960s, only with recent advances in immune suppression and improved understanding of timing of interventions and selection of appropriate recipients has transplantation become a realistic option. Lung volume–reduction surgery aims to reduce hyperinflation of one or both lungs by surgical and/or laser resection. Cooper[78] has reported a 1-year 45 percent increase in FEV_1, 25 percent decrease in total lung capacity, and improvement of exercise performance. Preliminary findings in other studies have shown improvement in dyspnea, quality of life, and lung function.[79] Perioperative mortality ranges up to 10 percent, and the cost-effectiveness of this approach should be considered before widespread use of this procedure occurs.[80]

Miscellaneous Concerns

Chronic diseases are frequently accompanied by a host of psychological responses that may interfere with social and family functioning, and clinicians always should consider the possibility that a mood disorder may be present in a patient with COPD. Depression and anxiety are the most commonly reported emotional consequences of COPD, with prevalence of depression reported to range from 50 to 70 percent.[81]

Long-term management and monitoring should include periodic spirometry and measurement of arterial blood gases to assess the need for supplemental LTOT or CPAP once $P_{O_2} < 55$ mmHg or $P_{CO_2} > 50$ mmHg. Sedatives and hypnotics should be avoided in patients who require oxygen because of the possibility of depression of respiratory drive. Influenza immunization is recommended annually and reduces morbidity and mortality of influenza in the elderly by 50 percent.[82] Beneficial effects of pneumococcal vaccination have not been established; however, current recommendations are that patients with COPD should be given immunization at least once. Those who fall into a high-risk category, such as asplenic patients, should be revaccinated every 5 to 10 years.[83] Orcel et al showed a 40 percent reduction in the incidence of acute exacerbations of chronic bronchitis after oral immunization with lyophilized fractions of the eight most common pathogens isolated in respiratory tract infections, but at this time this approach remains experimental.[84]

References

1. Woolcock AJ: Epidemiology of chronic airways disease. *Chest* 96(suppl 3):302S–306S, 1989.
2. U.S. Bureau of the Census: *Statistical Abstract of the United States: 1994*, 114th ed. Washington, DC, U.S. Bureau of the Census; 1994: p. 95.
3. Garibaldi RA: Epidemiology of community acquired respiratory tract infections in adults: incidence, etiology, and impact. *Am J Med* 78(suppl 68):32–37, 1985.
4. Verheij TJM, Kaptein AA, Mulder JD: Acute bronchitis: etiology, symptoms and treatment. *J Fam Pract* 6:66–69, 1989.
5. American Thoracic Society: Standards for the diagnosis and care of patients with chronic obstructive pulmonary disease. *Am J Respir Crit Care Med* 152:S77–S102, 1995.
6. Medical Research Council: Definition and classification of chronic bronchitis for clinical and epidemiological purposes. *Lancet* 1:775–779, 1965.
7. Reid LM: Pathology of chronic bronchitis. *Lancet* 266:275, 1954.
8. Siafakas NM: ERS consensus statement: optimal assessment and management of chronic obstructive pulmonary disease. *Eur Respir Rev* 6:270–275, 1996.
9. Saetta M: Airway pathology of COPD compared with asthma. *Eur Respir Rev* 45:211–215, 1997.
10. Celli BR, Snider GL, Heffner J, et al: Standards for the diagnosis and care of patients with chronic obstructive pulmonary disease. *Am J Respir Crit Care Med* 152:S77–S120, 1995.
11. Anthonisen NR, Manfreda J, Warren CPW, et al: Antibiotic therapy in exacerbations of chronic obstructive lung disease. *Ann Intern Med* 106:196–204, 1987.
12. Gump DW, Phillips CA, Forsyth BR, et al: Role of infection in chronic bronchitis. *Am Rev Respir Dis* 113:465–473, 1976.
13. Snow V, Lascher S, Mottur-Pilson C, for the Joint Expert Panel on Chronic Obstructive Pulmonary Disease of the American College of Chest Physicians and the American College of Physicians–American Society of Internal Medicine: Evidence base for management of acute exacerbations of chronic obstructive pulmonary disease. *Ann Intern Med* 134:595–599, 2001.
14. Goroll AH: Management of chronic obstructive pulmonary disease, in Goroll AH, Mulley AG (eds): *Primary Care Medicine: Office Evaluation and Management of the Adult Patient*, 4th ed. Philadelphia, Lippincott Williams & Wilkins; 2000, pp 293–304.
15. Lynn J, Ely EW, Zhong Z, et al: Living and dying with chronic obstructive pulmonary disease. *J Am Geriatr Soc* 48:S91–S100, 2000.
16. Rennard SI: COPD: overview and definitions, epidemiology, and factors influencing its development. *Chest* 113:235S–241S, 1998.
17. Matsuba K, Wright JL, Wiggs BR, et al: The changes in airways structure associated with reduced forced expiratory volume in one second. *Eur Respir J* 2:834–839, 1989.
18. Voelkel NF, Tuder R: COPD exacerbation. *Chest* 117: S376–S379, 2000.
19. Soler N, Torres A, Ewing S, et al: Bronchial microbial patterns in severe exacerbations of chronic obstructive pulmonary disease (COPD) requiring mechanical ventilation. *Am J Respir Crit Care Med* 157:498–505, 1998.
20. Fein A, Fein AM: Management of acute exacerbations in chronic obstructive pulmonary disease. *Curr Opin Pulm Med* 6(2):122–126, 2000.
21. Sethi S: Infectious etiology of acute exacerbations of chronic bronchitis. *Chest* 117:S380–S385, 2000.
22. Fletcher C, Peto R, Tinker C, et al: *The Natural History of Chronic Bronchitis and Emphysema*. New York, Oxford University Press; 1976: pp 1–272.
23. Becklake M: Occupational exposures: evidence for a causal association with chronic obstructive pulmonary disease. *Am Rev Respir Dis* 134:649–652, 1989.
24. Kauffmann F, Drouet D, Lelouch J: Occupational exposure and 12-year spirometric changes among Paris area workers. *Br J Ind Med* 39:221–232, 1982.
25. Krzyanowski M, Jedrychowski W: Occupational exposure and incidence of chronic respiratory symptoms among residents of Cracow followed for 13 years. *Int Arch Occup Environ Health* 62:311–317, 1990.
26. Burrows B, Knudson RJ, Camilli AE, et al: The "horse-racing effect" and predicting decline in forced expiratory volume in 1 second from screening spirometry. *Am Rev Respir Dis* 135:788–793, 1987.
27. Lucey EC, Stone PJ, Snider GL: Consequences of proteolytic injury, in Crystal RG, Barnes PJ, West JB, et al (eds): *The Lung: Scientific Foundations*, vol 2. Philadelphia, Lippincott-Raven; 1997: pp 2237–2250.

28. British Thoracic Research Committee: Oral *N*-acetylcysteine and exacerbation rates in patients with chronic bronchitis and severe airways obstruction. *Thorax* 40:823–835, 1985.

29. Emerman CL, Cydulka RK: Evaluation of high-yield criteria for chest radiography in acute exacerbation of chronic obstructive pulmonary disease. *Ann Emerg Med* 22:680–684, 1993.

30. Sherman S, Skoney JA, Ravikrishnan KP: Routine chest radiographs in exacerbations of chronic pulmonary disease. *Arch Intern Med* 149:2493–2496, 1989.

31. Tsai TW, Gallagher EJ, Lombardi G, et al: Guidelines for selective ordering of admission chest radiography in adult obstructive pulmonary disease. *Ann Emerg Med* 22:1854–1858, 1993.

32. Bach PB, Brown C, Gelfand SE, McCrory DC: Management of acute exacerbations of chronic obstructive pulmonary disease: a summary and appraisal of published evidence. *Ann Intern Med* 134:600–620, 2001.

33. Burrows B, Bloom JW, Traver GA, Cline MG: The course and prognosis of different forms of chronic airway obstruction in a sample from the general population. *N Engl J Med* 317:1309–1314, 1987.

34. Hodgkin JE: Prognosis in chronic obstructive lung disease. *Clin Chest Med* 2:555–569, 1990.

35. Anthonisen NR, Wright EC, Hodgkin JE: Prognosis in chronic obstructive pulmonary disease. *Am Rev Respir Dis* 133:14–20, 1986.

36. Hughes JR, Goldstein MG, Hurt RD, et al: Recent advances in the pharmacotherapy of smoking. *JAMA* 281:72–76, 1999.

37. Kanner RE: Early intervention in chronic obstructive pulmonary disease: a review of the Lung Health Study results. *Med Clin North Am* 80:523–543, 1996.

38. Bates DV, Knott JMS, Christie RV: Respiratory function in emphysema in relation to prognosis. *Q J Med* 25:137–157, 1956.

39. Boushy SF, Coates EO Jr: Prognostic value of pulmonary function tests in emphysema: with special reference to arterial blood studies. *Am Rev Respir Dis* 90:553–563, 1964.

40. Traver GA, Cline MG, Burrows B: Predictors of mortality in chronic obstructive pulmonary disease. *Am Rev Respir Dis* 119:895–902, 1979.

41. Strom K: Survival of patients with chronic obstructive pulmonary disease. *Am Rev Respir Dis* 147:585–591, 1986.

42. Ball P, Harris JM, Lowson D, et al: Acute infective exacerbations of chronic bronchitis. *Q J Med* 88:61–68, 1995.

43. Burrows B, Earle RH: Prediction of survival in patients with chronic airway obstruction. *Am Rev Respir Dis* 99:865–871, 1969.

44. France AJ, Prescott RJ, Biernacki W, et al: Does right ventricular function predict survival in patients with chronic obstructive lung disease? *Thorax* 43:621–626, 1988.

45. Celli BR: The importance of spirometry in COPD and asthma: effect on approach to management. *Chest* 117:15S–19S, 2000.

46. Mushlin AI, Black ER, Connolly CA, et al: The necessary length of hospital stay for chronic pulmonary disease. *JAMA* 266:80–83, 1991.

47. Connors AF Jr, Dawson NV, Thomas C, et al: Outcomes following acute exacerbation of severe chronic obstructive lung disease. The SUPPORT investigators (Study to Understand Prognoses and Preferences for Outcomes and Risks of Treatments). *Am J Respir Crit Care Med* 154:959–967, 1996.

48. Burk RH, George RB: Acute respiratory failure in chronic obstructive pulmonary disease: immediate and long-term prognosis. *Arch Intern Med* 132:865–868, 1973.

49. Portier F, Defouilloy C, Muir JF: Determinants of immediate survival among chronic respiratory insufficiency patients admitted to an intensive care unit for acute respiratory failure: a prospective multicenter study. The French Task Group for Acute Respiratory Failure in Chronic Respiratory Insufficiency. *Chest* 101:204–210, 1992.

50. Seneff MG, Wagner DP, Wagner RP, et al: Hospital and 1-year survival of patients admitted to intensive care units with acute exacerbation of chronic obstructive pulmonary disease. *JAMA* 274:1852–1857, 1995.

51. Connors AF Jr, McCaffree DR, Gray BA: Effect of inspiratory flow rate on gas exchange during mechanical ventilation. *Am Rev Respir Dis* 124:537–543, 1981.

52. Weinberger M, Oddone EZ, Henderson WG: Does increased access to primary care reduce hospital readmissions? Veterans Affairs Cooperative Study Group on Primary Care and Hospital Readmission. *N Engl J Med* 334:1441–1447, 1996.

53. Madison JM, Irwin RS: Chronic obstructive pulmonary disease. *Lancet* 352:467–473, 1998.

54. Kerstjens HAM: Stable chronic obstructive pulmonary disease. *Br Med J* 319:495–500, 1999.

55. Backman R, Hellstrom PE: Fenoterol and ipratropium bromide for treatment of patients with chronic bronchitis. *Curr Ther Res* 38:135–140, 1985.

56. Shrestha M, O'Brien T, Haddox R, et al: Decreased duration of emergency department treatment of chronic obstructive pulmonary disease exacerbations with the addition of ipratropium bromide to beta-agonist therapy. *Ann Emerg Med* 20:1206–1209, 1991.

57. Patrick DM, Dales RE, Stark RM, et al: Severe exacerbations of COPD and asthma: incremental benefit of adding ipratropium to usual therapy. *Chest* 98:295–297, 1990.

58. Cydulka RK, Emerman CL: Effects of combined treatment with glycopyrrolate and albuterol in acute exacerbation of chronic obstructive pulmonary disease. *Ann Emerg Med* 25:470–473, 1995.

59. Saint S, Bent S, Vittinghoff E, Grady D: Antibiotics in chronic obstructive pulmonary disease exacerbations. A meta-analysis. *JAMA* 273:957–960, 1995.

60. Fiel S: Guidelines and critical pathways for severe hospital-acquired pneumonia. *Chest* 119(2):412S–418S, 2001.

61. King DE, Malone R, Lilley SH: New classification and update on the quinolone antibiotics. *Am Fam Physician* 61:2741–2748, 2000.

62. Niewoehner DE, Erbland ML, Deupree RH, et al: Effect of systemic glucocorticoids on exacerbations of chronic obstructive pulmonary disease. Department of Veterans Affairs Cooperative Study Group. *N Engl J Med* 340:1941–1947, 1999.

63. Keatings VM, Jatakanon A, Worsdell YM, Barnes PJ: Effects of inhaled and oral glucocorticoids on inflammatory indices in asthma and COPD. *Am J Respir Crit Care Med* 155:542–548, 1997.

64. Heath JM, Mongia R: Chronic bronchitis: primary care management. *Am Fam Physician* 57:2365–2372, 2376–2378, 1998.

65. Wrenn K, Slovis CM, Murphy F, et al: Aminophylline therapy for acute bronchospastic disease in the emergency room. *Ann Intern Med* 115:241–247, 1991.

66. Rice KL, Leatherman JW, Duane PG, et al: Aminophylline for acute exacerbations of chronic pulmonary disease: a controlled trial. *Ann Intern Med* 107:305–309, 1987.

67. Seidenfeld JJ, Jones WN, Moss RE, et al: Intravenous aminophylline in the treatment of acute bronchospastic exacerbations of chronic obstructive pulmonary disease. *Ann Emerg Med* 13:248–252, 1984.

68. Cada DJ (ed): Respiratory agents, in *Facts and Comparisons*. St. Louis, Facts and Comparisons, 2001: pp 654–659.

69. Daughton D, Susman J, Sitorius M, et al: Transdermal nicotine therapy and primary care: importance of counseling, demographic, and participant selection factors on 1-year quit rates: the Nebraska Primary Practice Smoking Cessation Trial Group. *Arch Fam Med* 7:4225–4430, 1998.

70. Braun SR, McKenzie WN, Copeland W, et al: A comparison of the effect of ipratropium bromide and albuterol in the treatment of chronic obstructive airway disease. *Arch Intern Med* 149:544–547, 1989.

71. Boyd G, Morice AH, Pounsford JC, et al: An evaluation of salmeterol in the treatment of chronic obstructive pulmonary disease (COPD). *Eur Respir J* 10:815–821, 1997.

72. Combivent Inhalation Aerosol Study Group: In chronic obstructive pulmonary disease, a combination of ipratropium and albuterol is more effective than either agent alone: an 85-day multicenter trial. *Chest* 5:1411–1419, 1994.

73. Callahan CM, Dittus RS, Katz BP: Oral corticosteroid therapy for patients with stable chronic obstructive pulmonary disease: a meta-analysis. *Ann Intern Med* 114:216–223, 1991.

74. Lung Health Study Research Group: Effect of inhaled triamcinolone on the decline in pulmonary function in chronic obstructive pulmonary disease. *N Engl J Med* 343:1902–1909, 2000.

75. Nocturnal Oxygen Therapy Trial Group: Continuous or nocturnal oxygen therapy in hypoxemic chronic obstructive lung disease. *Ann Intern Med* 93:391–398, 1990.

76. Clini E, Vitacca M, Faglio K, et al: Long-term home care programmes may reduce hospital admissions in COPD with chronic hypercapnia. *Eur Respir J* 9:1605–1610, 1996.

77. Cousar JI, Martinez FJ, Celli BR: Pulmonary rehabilitation that includes arm exercise reduces metabolic ventilatory requirements for simple arm elevation. *Chest* 103:37–41, 1998.

78. Cooper JD: The history of surgical procedures for emphysema. *Am Thorac Surg* 63:312–319, 1997.

79. Trulock EP: Lung transplantation. *Am J Respir Crit Care Med* 155:789–818, 1997.

80. Cooper JD, Trulock EP, Triantafillou AN, et al: Bilateral pneumonectomy (volume reduction) for chronic obstructive pulmonary disease. *J Thorac Cardiovasc Surg* 109:106–119, 1995.

81. Schlosser M: Psychological assessment of COPD inpatients. *Eur Respir J* 2(suppl 8):444s, 1989.

82. Nichol KL, Margolis KL, Wuorenma J, et al: The efficacy and cost effectiveness of vaccination against influenza among elderly persons living in the community. *N Engl J Med* 331:778–784, 1994.

83. Butler JC, Breinan RF, Campbell JF, et al: Pneumonococcal polysaccharide vaccine efficacy: an evaluation of current recommendations. *JAMA* 270:1826–1831, 1993.

84. Orcel B, Delclaux B, Baud M, et al: Oral immunization with bacterial extracts for protection against acute bronchitis in elderly institutionalized patients with chronic bronchitis. *Eur Respir J* 7:446–452, 1994.

William M. Simpson, Jr.

Chapter
18

Common Occupational
Respiratory Diseases

The respiratory tract is a common site of injury or illness that is associated with exposure to toxic substances in the workplace. The airways are exposed to at least 14,000 L of workplace air during the typical 40-h workweek. If work is physically heavy and the respiratory rate increases, this volume can increase up to 12 times.[1] At higher levels of ventilation, breathing shifts from nasal to a combination of oral and nasal, decreasing the filtering action of the nasal passages and increasing the exposure of the lower airways to inhaled materials.

Clinicians should consider an occupational cause for lung disease symptoms when a working or retired adult presents for evaluation of respiratory problems. Recognition of an occupational cause is made difficult in some cases by a short latent period, so that symptoms are produced after the workday is over, and in others by a long (sometimes decades) latent period between exposure and disease manifestations.

Since the respiratory tract has limited ways to respond to injury, one type of respiratory disease can be caused by many different occupational exposures. In addition, one respiratory exposure type may cause several different types of pulmonary disease.

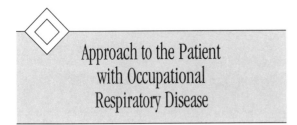

Approach to the Patient with Occupational Respiratory Disease

Most occupational respiratory diseases can be diagnosed with a combination of history, physical examination, imaging studies, and pulmonary function testing. Usually, the most effective course is to determine what type of respiratory condition is causing the patient's symptoms and then use the occupational history to identify the most likely cause or causes.

History

A detailed history of the patient's chief complaint and environmental and occupational exposures is essential to making the appropriate diagnosis. A job title alone rarely gives necessary information about exposures in the workplace. The question "What do you do?" must be followed by "How do you do it?" to obtain a meaningful picture of the types of risk to which the patient is exposed. Because of the latent period between some exposures and disease manifestations, previous employment exposures must also be identified and quantified, at least in general terms. Home and hobby exposures also must be considered, along with other personal habits, since they may all contribute to respiratory exposure and potentially to respiratory illness.

Higher-risk workplaces are those that have visible smoke, dust, or mist and those in which there is painting, spraying, or drying of coated surfaces. Heavier exposures occur when very small particles are generated; when work processes involve friction, grinding, heat, or blasting; and when work is done in enclosed spaces.[2]

By law, the employer must make a Material Safety Data Sheet (MSDS) for chemicals used in the workplace available on request. Previous measurements of air quality also may be available from the employer or may be requested. Consultation with an industrial hygienist or occupational medicine physician can be helpful if further detailed investigations of the work site seem indicated.

Physical Examination

The physical examination is rarely specific for a particular occupational lung disease. However, a complete physical examination is necessary to ensure that no disease manifestations are missed—even if they point to a nonoccupational cause of illness. More often, both occupation-related and non-occupation-related illnesses exist in the same patient.

Imaging Studies

A chest x-ray should be a part of the evaluation when occupational lung disease is suspected. When dust exposure is suspected, the x-ray should be interpreted by a "B reader," a physician certified by the National Institute for Occupational Safety and Health. Computed tomography (CT) scanning may be indicated when pleural or mediastinal disease is suspected. High-resolution CT is useful in assessing the presence and severity of diffuse lung processes such as emphysema or interstitial lung diseases, which are common to many occupational respiratory illnesses.

Pulmonary Function Testing

Office spirometry and peak expiratory flow measurements are useful for the initial evaluation of patients with suspected occupational lung diseases. More details on the use of pulmonary function tests are provided in Chap. 3.

Forced vital capacity (FVC), forced expiratory volume in 1 s (FEV_1), and the FEV_1/FVC ratio are the best parameters for defining the presence and severity of airway obstruction and the most reliable assessment of overall respiratory impairment. Peak expiratory flow measurements are useful in determining airway obstruction, especially when used serially to measure lung function during different parts of the workday and different days of the week. Changes in the peak flow that correspond to certain activities or exposures can help pinpoint where the problem lies.

More sophisticated testing may be indicated to better define restrictive diseases, problems of gas exchange, nonspecific hyperresponsiveness of airways (methacholine challenge), or responses to specific allergens. Pulmonary exer-

cise testing can be performed to determine the presence and severity of respiratory impairment, especially when the patient's symptoms appear more severe than is predicted on the basis of routine pulmonary function testing.

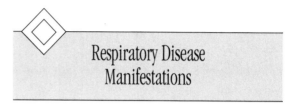

Respiratory Disease Manifestations

Major occupational respiratory disease types are discussed here, with attention to etiologies and key points in the history, physical findings, and diagnostic testing. In all cases, prevention is preferable to treatment. Since general principles of prevention can be applied at all levels of respiratory tract exposure, they will be discussed first. Treatment for occupational forms of respiratory disease is generally identical to that for nonoccupational forms of lung disease, so this aspect of care will not be discussed unless there are aspects of treatment that are specific to occupationally related disease.

Prevention of Occupational Respiratory Disease

Limitation of exposure to potential irritants, allergens, sensitizers, dusts, and carcinogens is the basis for prevention of occupational respiratory disease. Methods for limiting exposure include replacing known toxins with nontoxic or less toxic components, engineering controls (enclosing dusty parts of a process or those that cause exposure to toxins of all types, wetting down dusts, adequate ventilation systems, etc.), use of personal protective equipment, and worker education about appropriate procedures to limit exposures and proper methods for dealing with leaks and spills. All of these interventions are outside the normal activity of the clinician, but any clinician who sees a patient with a possible work-related respiratory illness should consider contacting the patient's employer to ensure that these preventive measures have been optimally applied. If preventive interventions have been undertaken and respiratory illnesses still occur, further evaluation of the work site by an industrial hygienist or occupational medicine specialist may be indicated.

Rhinitis and Laryngitis

Table 18-1 lists common causes of occupational rhinitis and laryngitis. Nasal hairs and nasal turbinates filter large particles (>10 μm) and water-soluble gases. The initial mucosal response when exposed to these agents is vascular dilatation and increased permeability, leading to congestion and rhinorrhea. Nasal mucosal irritants usually produce burning or stinging,

Table 18-1

Common Causes of Occupational Rhinitis and Laryngitis

Allergic sensitizers
   Acid anhydrides
   Animal danders (proteins)
   Dust from baking flour
   Dusts from animal feeds and grains
   Latex on cornstarch granules (on latex gloves)
   Pollens and mold spores
   Psyllium
Irritants
   Acidic or alkaline cleaning solutions or
      powders
   Ammonia
   Environmental tobacco smoke
   Hypochlorous acid (bleach)
   Metalworking fluids
   Ozone
   Sulfur dioxide
   Volatile organic compounds (in sprays,
      paints, pesticides, solvents, and many
      other compounds)

whereas allergens produce sneezing and itching.[3] Occupational rhinitis is distinguished from perennial or seasonal rhinitis by its improvement when the patient is away from work. Allergic occupational rhinitis often precedes occupational asthma. Previous allergic disease and a family history of allergic disease increase the risk of developing allergic occupational rhinitis.

The larynx, as a result of its small cross-sectional area, is the site of deposition of irritating particulate matter and inflammatory mediator drainage from the nasal passages. The resulting edema and inflammation of the vocal cords produce laryngitis.[4] Some irritants, such as chlorine gas from mixing bleach and detergents or mono- or dichloramine from mixing detergents with ammonia, produce vocal cord dysfunction that results in a narrowing of the vocal cord aperture during inspiration, producing an asthma-like wheeze.

Tracheitis, Bronchitis, Bronchiolitis

Table 18-2 lists common causes of occupational bronchitis and bronchiolitis.

Soluble gases are absorbed by the upper respiratory tract, whereas less soluble gases may penetrate to the alveolar level. Particle deposition in the airways is determined by the size of the particle: Particles > 10 μm lodge in the nose and pharynx, those < 5 μm pass through to the alveoli, and those of intermediate size lodge in the intervening portions of the respiratory tract. Therefore, the solubility of gases and the size of the particles produced or used in industrial processes can predict the likely site of pathology.[5]

Asthma

Occupational asthma is defined as airway hyperreactivity and/or airflow obstruction in response to an agent contacted in the work environment. Many agents found in the workplace have been implicated as a cause of asthma (Table 18-3).

Table 18-2

Common Causes of Occupational Bronchitis and Bronchiolitis

Bronchitis
Cement dust
Rock and mineral dusts
Smoke from welding or cutting with an
acetylene torch
Sulfur dioxide
Bronchiolitis
Acetaldehyde
Ammonia
Chlorine gas
Hydrogen fluoride
Hydrogen sulfide
Nitrogen dioxide (from freshly stored hay in
silos), nitric acid, nitrous acid, and
nitric oxide
Phosgene

Table 18-3

Common Causes of Occupational Asthma

Asthma with latency
Acid anhydrides (used in adhesives, circuit
boards, and polymers)
Aldehydes
Acrylates (used in paints and adhesives)
Animal danders (proteins)
Cobalt (in carbide-tipped tools)
Dusts from flours and grains
Dusts from wood (in furniture making and
cabinetry)
Ethylenediamine and other amines
Formaldehyde and glutaraldehyde
Isocyanates (in polyurethane paints, roofing
foam)
Latex
Asthma without latency
Bleach
Chlorine gas
Contaminants in metalworking fluids
Strong acids

Workers may develop sensitivity to an agent despite years of previously uneventful exposure to that agent. Both immunologic and nonimmunologic mechanisms can play roles. The list of potential causes for occupational asthma continues to grow, suggesting that the absence of previous reports of an association should not rule out the possibility of an occupationally related cause.[6]

In general, triggers for occupational asthma can be divided into two groups: high-molecular-weight compounds (HMWC) and low-molecular-weight compounds (LMWC). HMWC are proteins, polysaccharides, and peptides that produce an allergic response mediated by IgE and sometimes IgG antibodies. Patients usually have a history of atopy, and positive skin test reactions are usually present. Inhalation challenges with HMWC induce an immediate asthmatic response or a biphasic reaction (immediate and late), and on rare occasions an isolated late response.

Alternatively, LMWC act as haptens that combine with a carrier protein to form an allergen, usually in nonatopic individuals. Inhalation challenge with a LMWC induces a late-phase response in about half of subjects and a biphasic response in the other half. An isolated immediate response is rare.

A little more than 1 worker in 100 in the United States disability system reports occupational asthma. This is probably an underestimate, since workers affected by occupational asthma typically leave the industry or job. Occupational asthma has now become the most prevalent occupational lung disease, surpassing asbestosis and silicosis.

Characteristically, occupational asthma affects only a portion of those exposed. Individual susceptibility is related to host factors: atopy, smoking, and, in some cases, nonspecific bronchial hyperreactivity (NSBH)—although most authorities consider NSBH to be the result of exposure to the agent itself. A latent period of months or years between first exposure and asthma symptoms is frequently reported.

Asthma symptoms can occur at work within a few minutes of exposure or, often, after a delay of several hours. Some workers report worst symptoms in the evening or at night, hours after leaving the work site. Frequently symptoms worsen as the workweek progresses and may improve on the weekends or during vacations (at least early in the illness). At later stages, recovery may occur only days or weeks after exposure ceases. NSBH may be manifest as further symptoms on exposure to cold air or exercise.

The natural history of this disorder is variable. As noted, symptoms frequently force the worker to leave the particular job type or site. Of those workers who remain on the job with continuing exposure, all eventually require treatment for their asthma and some deteriorate despite medical therapy. Complete avoidance of exposure to the sensitizing agent should be recommended once the diagnosis of occupational asthma is confirmed, since life-threatening attacks can occur.

To establish a diagnosis of occupational asthma, the diagnosis of asthma must first be made, followed by confirmation that the asthma is related to occupational exposure. A new persistent cough should trigger consideration of asthma as a diagnosis, although other etiologies are certainly possible. Any new-onset asthma in an adult should trigger a search for a possible occupational cause.

In addition to HMWC and LMWC as causes of sensitization and occupational asthma, some agents may produce asthma without sensitization. Airway irritation (by dust, fumes, smoke, and cold) and airway inflammation (from acids, ammonia, or chlorine) as well as anticholinesterase effects produced by organophosphate pesticides can produce occupational asthma. Endotoxins found in cotton dust are felt to be the inciting agents in byssinosis (or cotton worker's lung), another form of occupational asthma.

Once the diagnosis of occupational asthma is made, reduction or elimination of exposure to the offending agent is the primary intervention. With irritant-induced asthma, engineering interventions and personal protective equipment may lower exposures to levels that do not induce bronchospasm. With sensitizer-induced asthma, the worker should be removed from any exposure to the sensitizing agent because exposure to even minute quantities may precipitate bronchospasm.

Chronic Obstructive Pulmonary Disease

Chronic obstructive pulmonary disease is most commonly caused by cigarette smoking, but occupational dusts can cause or contribute to chronic airflow limitation or emphysema.[7] Cadmium, used in electronics and metal plating, can cause emphysema. Coal dust causes emphysema with nodular fibrosis with long-term exposure (see discussion of coal worker's pneumoconiosis later in this chapter). Cotton dust, crystalline silica (used in sandblasting and found in sandy soil), and toluene diisocyanate (used in the manufacturing of paints, plastics, and circuit boards) can cause chronic airflow limitation. No specific treatment is available for any of these conditions. Limitation of exposure is the most reasonable preventive strategy.

Interstitial Lung Disease

Most inhaled dust is either trapped by the upper airways or cleared by the large airway ciliated epithelium. Fine dust can overwhelm these defenses and produce alveolar and interstitial inflammation, leading to interstitial disease.

FIBROTIC DISEASES
Asbestosis, silicosis, and coal worker's pneumoconiosis are the most common pneumoconioses in the United States, causing approximately 4000 deaths per year.

ASBESTOSIS Asbestosis refers to a diffuse interstitial fibrosis caused by inhalation of asbestos fibers. While there are several forms of asbestos, all three of the main commercial types (chrysotile or white asbestos, amosite or brown asbestos, and crocidolite or blue asbestos) have been associated with the major asbestos-related conditions.[8] Major occupational exposures occur with asbestos mining and milling, manufacture or installation of insulation in ships and buildings, manufacture of brake linings and clutch facings, asbestos cement and textile manufacture, and manufacture of asbestos-containing products for acoustical and fireproofing purposes.

The initiation and progression of asbestosis are related to the type and size of the fibers, the duration and intensity of exposure, history of cigarette smoking, and individual susceptibility. Once asbestosis has begun, it may progress despite removal from continued exposure. The latency period between exposure and clinically apparent disease is 10 to 20 years.

Symptoms of asbestosis are indistinguishable from those of any other progressive interstitial fibrosing disorder and include progressive dyspnea and a nonproductive cough. The most characteristic physical finding is "Velcro"-quality bibasilar crackles that do not clear with cough and are heard over the posterolateral chest in mid to late inspiration.

The most useful radiographic finding in asbestosis is the presence of bilateral pleural thickening. Pericardial and diaphragmatic calcification are almost pathognomonic signs of asbestos exposure.

The substitution of other fibrous materials for asbestos and the institution of strict environmental controls where asbestos is still used have led to a dramatic reduction in occupational exposure to asbestos in the last two decades.

There is no known treatment for asbestosis. Further exposure to asbestos should be eliminated, since the risk of further parenchymal scarring appears to increase with cumulative exposure. Any other factors that contribute to respiratory disease, particularly cigarette smoking, should be eliminated, if possible.

COAL WORKER'S PNEUMOCONIOSIS   Coal worker's pneumoconiosis (CWP) is a parenchymal lung disease caused by inhalation of coal dust. Miners who work at the coal face in underground operations and drillers in surface mines are at greatest risk of developing the disease.[8] Because a heavy coal dust burden is necessary for induction of the disease, it is rarely seen in those who have less than 20 years of underground exposure.

The coal macule is the primary lesion of CWP. It develops when the inhaled dust burden overwhelms the ability of the cilia and alveolar macrophages to remove it. Prolonged retention of coal dust causes lung fibroblasts to secrete a layer of reticulin around the dust collection, which may gradually enlarge and weaken the bronchiole wall, leading to focal centrilobular emphysema.

CWP is often asymptomatic. Cough and sputum production are often the result of chronic bronchitis from dust inhalation rather than of CWP. The chest radiograph shows small rounded opacities in the lung parenchyma that are indistinguishable from those seen in silicosis.

Treatment of CWP is limited to elimination of further coal dust exposure and symptomatic and supportive therapy.

SILICOSIS   Silicosis refers to a parenchymal lung disease resulting from inhalation of silicon dioxide, or silica, in crystalline form. Workers with potential exposure include miners, sandblasters, stone carvers, and ceramic workers.[9]

Exposure to silica can produce an acute illness, a subacute illness, or a chronic illness. Acute illness usually occurs after intense exposure to fine dust over a several-month period, while subacute illness follows 2 to 5 years of moderate exposure. The chronic pattern usually occurs following 10 or more years of exposure to dust with less than 30 percent quartz.

Acute silicosis occurs rarely but is usually fatal. The chest x-ray in acute silicosis shows consolidation without silicotic nodules and alveolar spaces filled with fluid similar to that seen in pulmonary alveolar proteinosis.

In contrast, chronic silicosis has few specific signs or symptoms. The diagnosis of chronic silicosis is made by chest x-ray showing small round opacities (<10 mm in diameter) in both lungs, primarily in the upper lobes. Hilar lymph nodes may calcify in an "eggshell" pattern; this is pathognomonic of silicosis but occurs in only a small proportion of cases. For reasons that are not well understood, fungal diseases and mycobacterial disease, both typical and atypical, are seen more commonly in patients with silicosis.

No treatment for silicosis is known, so interventions are directed to prevention of further exposure and surveillance for tuberculosis.

OTHER PNEUMOCONIOSES In addition to the exposures discussed previously, other mineral dusts can cause fibrotic interstitial disease. These include diatomaceous earth (used in gardening) and kaolin (which causes silicosis-like disease in kaolin millers and miners), graphite (which causes a disease similar to CWP in graphite miners and those who work in the purification process), mica (used in the production of paints, wallpaper, lubricants, cements, and other building products), and talc (which can cause a disease with features of both silicosis and asbestosis in talc miners). Fibers of aluminum oxide, a metal dust produced in the processing of bauxite ore, can also cause pneumoconiosis.

GRANULOMATOUS DISEASES

CHRONIC BERYLLIUM DISEASE Chronic beryllium disease (CBD) is a granulomatous inflammatory disease with histologic findings identical to those in sarcoidosis.[10] Beryllium is a lightweight metal with a wide range of applications in the aerospace, electronics, and power production industries. Exposure of workers occurs in smelting, casting, grinding, and machining the metal. CBD occurs after sensitization to the metal through a cell-mediated (type IV) mechanism. Latency from initial exposure to active disease ranges from months to years.

CBD usually affects the lungs, but skin, liver, spleen, salivary gland, kidney, and bone involvement may occur. Respiratory symptoms of CBD are usually insidious in onset and limited to dyspnea on exertion, cough, and fatigue. Physical findings may be absent in early disease and are usually limited to dry rales even in advanced cases. Chest x-rays reveal only ill-defined nodularities and hilar adenopathy. Because of the similarity between sarcoidosis and CBD, demonstration of beryllium sensitization is necessary to confirm the diagnosis. A lymphocyte proliferation test is available to confirm beryllium sensitization in lymphocytes from peripheral blood or bronchoalveolar lavage specimens.

Since CBD is a hypersensitivity syndrome, workers with CBD should be removed from further contact with beryllium. Steroids are the only available therapy. Serial pulmonary function testing and chest x-rays should be used to follow the response to therapy and guide steroid dose and duration of use decisions.

HYPERSENSITIVITY PNEUMONITIS Hypersensitivity pneumonitis, also known as extrinsic allergic alveolitis, is an immunologically mediated inflammatory disease of lung parenchyma induced by inhalation of organic dusts[11] (Table 18-4). Granulomatous changes occur early in the process, along with lymphocytic alveolitis. Termination of exposure to the antigen usually results in improvement or complete resolution of symptoms. Continued exposure leads to progressive interstitial fibrosis. Since only a small portion of exposed persons develop hypersensitivity pneumonitis, the mechanism of the disease may be a genetically determined failure to down-regulate normal host defense responses. Interestingly, environmental factors may also be involved, since several small studies have shown that hypersensitivity pneumonitis occurs more frequently in nonsmokers than in smokers.

Table 18-4

Occupational Exposures Causing Hypersensitivity Pneumonitis

ANTIGENS	EXPOSURE
Amoebae	
Naegleria gruberi	Contaminated water ("humidifier lung")
Acanthamoeba castellani	
Animal proteins	
Avian proteins	Bird droppings, feathers
Rodent proteins	Urine, sera, pelts
Wheat weevil	Infested flour
Chemicals	
Toluene diisocyanate	Paints, coatings, polyurethane foam
Trimellitic anhydride	Epoxy resins, paints
Bacteria	
Bacillus subtilus	Detergents
Thermoactinomycetes	Moldy grain
Faenia rectivirgula	Moldy hay ("farmer's lung")
Thermoactinomycetes sacchari	Moldy sugar cane fiber ("bagassosis")
Thermoactinomycetes candidus	Water reservoirs ("humidifier lung")
Fungi	
Penicillium casei	Moldy cheese
Penicillium frequentans	Moldy cork dust ("suberosis")
Aspergillus clavatus	Moldy malt
Cryptostroma corticale	Moldy maple bark
Aureobasidium pullulans, Graphium spp	Moldy redwood dust ("sequoiosis")

Hypersensitivity pneumonitis should be suspected in patients with episodic respiratory symptoms and evidence of fleeting infiltrates on x-ray or restrictive disease on pulmonary function testing. Symptoms of hypersensitivity pneumonitis usually occur within 6 h of heavy exposure to the offending antigen. Chills, fever, malaise, myalgia, cough, headache, and dyspnea are usually present. Physical findings are often only an ill-appearing patient with bibasilar inspiratory crackles on chest examination. Chest x-ray may be completely normal or show a diffuse reticulonodular pattern.

Recurrent low-level exposures may produce chronic interstitial lung disease with fibrosis. Progressive respiratory impairment with dyspnea, cough, fatigue, and weight loss may develop without noted acute episodes. Physical findings of cyanosis, clubbing, and inspiratory crackles indicate the insidious development of significant respiratory dysfunction.

Avoidance of contact with the offending agent is key to management of hypersensitivity pneumonitis. Steroids can be useful in patients with severe or progressive symptoms. Generally prednisone can be given at a dose of 1 mg/kg/day, with serial chest x-rays and pulmonary function testing to evaluate response.

Inhalation Fevers

Inhalation fever refers to several syndromes characterized by debilitating flulike symptoms after exposure to a variety of organic dusts or chemical and metal fumes (Table 18-5). In contrast to hypersensitivity pneumonitis and occupational asthma, which require susceptibility or sensitization, inhalation fevers have high attack rates; most people with high-level exposure develop symptoms.[12] Release of cytokines from alveolar macrophages and airway epithelial cells induces leukocytosis, with associated fever beginning within 6 h after exposure and usually lasting 12 h or less. Nonsteroidal anti-inflammatory agents and avoidance of future exposure are indicated for this self-limited syndrome.

Pleural Disorders

Asbestos is the primary cause of occupationally induced pleural diseases, which include benign pleural effusions, pleural plaques, and malignant mesotheliomas. Talc and mica also can cause benign pleural disease, and zeolite can cause mesothelioma.[13]

BENIGN PLEURAL EFFUSIONS

Up to 3 percent of workers exposed to asbestos develop benign pleural effusions. Those with heavy exposure have more effusions and develop them after shorter latent periods, but the minimum time until effusions develop is usually 5 years. Most workers with effusions are asymptomatic. Physical examination of those with large effusions reveals dullness to percussion and decreased breath sounds. Bilateral involvement occurs in about 10 percent of asbestos effusions. Chest x-rays may also show pleural thickening along with the effusion(s). Thoracentesis reveals a sterile exudate, sometimes with increased eosinophils. Other causes of pleural effusion, especially tuberculosis and malignancy, must be excluded by regular follow-up and repeat thoracentesis if pleural fluid persists. In most cases the effusion clears spontaneously within a year without obvious residual pleural disease, but recurrences are relatively common.

PLEURAL PLAQUES

Pleural plaques are the most common radiographic findings caused by chronic asbestos exposure. Plaques usually occur over the central portions of the hemidiaphragm and along the inferior posterolateral aspects of the lower ribs. Bilateral plaques are almost always caused by asbestos exposure.

Table 18-5
Common Occupational Causes of Inhalation Fever

AGENT	SYNDROME
Metals	
Zinc	Metal fume fever
Teflon pyrolysis products	
Polytetrafluoroethylene	Polymer fume fever
Bioaerosols	
Contaminated water	Humidifier fever
Moldy silage, compost, wood chips	Organic dust toxic syndrome
Sewage sludge	Sludge fever
Cotton, jute, hemp, flax dust	Mill fever
Grain dust	Grain fever

A worker with a history of asbestos exposure and pleural plaques on chest x-ray should be evaluated for asbestosis. If no evidence of parenchymal disease is found, periodic reevaluation is indicated to recognize future development of the disease. Diffuse pleural thickening can also be related to past asbestos exposure.

Because of the risk of bronchogenic carcinoma in individuals exposed to asbestos, cigarette smoking should be especially discouraged in this group. Neither diffuse pleural thickening nor pleural plaques is believed to undergo malignant transformation to mesothelioma

MESOTHELIOMA

Up to 80 percent of mesotheliomas occur in asbestos-exposed individuals. Exposure histories indicate that relatively light exposures are associated with mesothelioma and that latent periods of 25 to 40 years are usual. Exposure to zeolite and thoracic irradiation are other risk factors for mesothelioma.

Symptoms of mesothelioma are usually non-pleuritic chest pain and dyspnea. Pain may be referred to the upper abdomen or shoulder if there is diaphragmatic involvement. Fatigue and diminished appetite with weight loss are often reported.

The histologic tumor type influences clinical findings. Epithelial and mixed mesotheliomas are associated with large pleural effusions, whereas mesenchymal tumors rarely have an associated effusion. Epithelial tumors are more likely to have local invasion; mesenchymal tumors have a greater incidence of extrapulmonary metastases.

Chest x-ray often reveals an effusion without a meniscus or, in advanced cases, tumor encasing the lung with a contracted hemithorax. Cytology of pleural fluid is often suggestive of malignant mesothelioma, but thoracotomy or thoracoscopy with multiple biopsies is often required to confirm the diagnosis.

Treatment is palliative. Death from respiratory failure or chronic wasting syndrome usually occurs within months of diagnosis.

Lung Cancer

Occupational exposures to potential carcinogens are preventable. The percentage of lung cancers attributable to occupational factors is estimated to be between 3 and 17 percent.[14] At least 12 substances found in the workplace are classified as human carcinogens, and another small group of chemicals are considered suspected carcinogens (Table 18-6). In addition, workers in several industries (foundries, welding, printing, rubber manufacturing) have been shown to be at

Table 18-6

Known and Suspected Occupational Lung Carcinogens

Known carcinogens
Asbestos
Arsenic and arsenic compounds
Bis(chloromethyl) ether and chloromethyl methyl ether (used in the manufacture of ion-exchange resins, pesticides, water repellants, flame repellants)
Cadmium and cadmium compounds
Chromium and certain chromium compounds (used in alloys and metal plating)
Environmental tobacco smoke
Ionizing radiation
Mustard gas
Nickel
Polyaromatic hydrocarbons
Radon
Silica (crystalline)
Suspected carcinogens
Acrylonitrile
Beryllium
Formaldehyde
Man-made vitreous fibers
Vinyl chloride monomer

slightly increased risk of lung cancer without identification of a specific carcinogenic agent. Evaluation of any patient with lung cancer should include a careful occupational and environmental history.

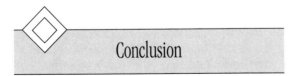

Conclusion

The respiratory tract is exposed to many potential toxins in the workplace. The primary care physician's role is to obtain an occupational and environmental history that will uncover these exposures and allow for optimal evaluation and proper treatment. Early recognition of occupational respiratory disease limits long-term adverse health effects and may prevent further cases in the same or similar workplaces.

References

1. Beckett WS: Occupational respiratory diseases. *N Engl J Med* 342(6):406, 2000.
2. Blanc P, Balmes JR: History and physical examination, in Harber P, Schenker M, Balmes J (eds): *Occupational and Environmental Respiratory Disease.* St Louis, Mosby; 1996.
3. Naclerio R, Solomon W: Rhinitis and inhalant allergens. *JAMA* 278:1842, 1997.
4. Bascom R, Shusterman D: Occupational and environmental exposures and the upper respiratory tract, in Naclerio RM, Durham SR, Mygind N (eds): *Rhinitis: Mechanisms and Management*, vol. 123 of *Lung Biology in Health and Disease.* New York, Marcel Dekker; 1999.
5. Balmes JR: Occupational respiratory diseases. *Prim Care* 27(4):1, 2000.
6. Venables KM, Chan-Yeung M: Occupational asthma. *Lancet* 349:1465, 1997.
7. Kennedy S: Agents causing chronic airflow obstruction, in Harber P, Schenker M, Balmes J (eds): *Occupational and Environmental Respiratory Disease.* St Louis, Mosby; 1996.
8. Occupational lung diseases, in Beers MH, Berkow R (eds): *The Merck Manual of Diagnosis and Therapy*, 17th ed. Whitehouse Station, NJ, Merck Research Laboratories; 1999: p 622.
9. Ibid, p 620.
10. Balmes JR: Beryllium and hard metal-related diseases, in Rosenstock L, Cullen M (eds): *Clinical Occupational and Environmental Medicine.* Philadelphia, WB Saunders; 1994.
11. Rose CS: Hypersensitivity pneumonitis, in Murry JF, Nadel JA (eds): *Textbook of Respiratory Medicine*, 3rd ed. Philadelphia, WB Saunders; 2000.
12. Rose CS, Blanc PB: Inhalation fever, in Rom WN (ed): *Environmental and Occupational Medicine*, 3rd ed. Baltimore, Lippincott-Raven; 1998.
13. Rom WN: Asbestos-related diseases, in Rom WN (ed): *Environmental and Occupational Medicine*, 3rd ed. Baltimore, Lippincott-Raven; 1998.
14. Steenland K, Loomis D, Shy C, Simonsen N: Review of occupational lung carcinogens. *Am J Ind Med* 29:474, 1996.

Richard K. Zimmerman
Inis Jane Bardella

Chapter

19

Immunization for Respiratory Diseases

Vaccination reduces morbidity and mortality and is cost-effective for the prevention of viral and bacterial respiratory infections. Yet vaccination rates remain below national target levels for both children and adults.

In 1997, among children aged 19 to 35 months, 93 percent had received three or more doses of *Haemophilus influenzae* B (Hib) vaccine, and 81 percent had received four doses of diphtheria and tetanus toxoids and pertussis vaccine (DTP) or pediatric diphtheria and tetanus toxoids (DT). Only 78 percent had completed four doses of DTP, three doses of polio virus vaccine, three doses of Hib, and one dose of measles-containing vaccine.[1]

Each year an estimated 20,000 adults die from influenza and thousands more die unnecessarily from pneumococcal infection. A study of the cost-effectiveness of vaccinating noninstitutionalized elderly adults against influenza found that vaccination resulted in reduced hospitalization due to acute and chronic respiratory disease and congestive heart failure, with a direct savings of $117 per person vaccinated per year.[2] For persons 65 years of age and older, cost-effectiveness analyses show that pneumococcal vaccination saves $8.27 per person and adds 1.21 quality-adjusted days of life per person.[3] Nevertheless, both influenza and pneumococcal vaccine are underutilized.

In addition, the current explosion of antibiotic-resistant organisms presents a new role for immunizations. Penicillin resistance to *Streptococcus pneumoniae* is rising, with only 76 percent of isolates being fully susceptible.[4] Immunization may be our most effective defense against serious respiratory illness.

This chapter discusses pediatric and adult vaccines and vaccination recommendations for viral and bacterial infections that are transmitted through respiratory secretions, present with respiratory symptoms, or both.

Table 19-1 summarizes the vaccine recommendations for various medical conditions.

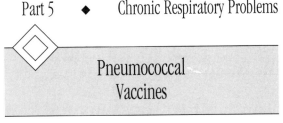

Pneumococcal Vaccines

23-Valent Polysaccharide Vaccine

BURDEN OF PNEUMOCOCCAL DISEASE

Pneumococcal disease causes an estimated 3000 cases of meningitis, 50,000 cases of bacteremia, and 500,000 cases of pneumonia annually in the United States.[5,6] *S. pneumoniae* causes 25 to 35 percent of the cases of community-acquired pneumonia that require hospitalization.[5] Most cases (60 to 87 percent) of pneumococcal bacteremia in adults are associated with patients over 65.[5] Despite appropriate therapy, the overall case-fatality rate for pneumococcal bacteremia is 15 to 20 percent among adults; this climbs to approximately 30 to 40 percent for elderly patients.[5] African Americans have about twice the rate of invasive pneumococcal disease as do whites, depending on the age group considered.

Recent data from a population-based case-control study of nonelderly adults show that cigarette smoking and passive smoking among nonsmokers are independent predictors of invasive pneumococcal disease.[7] Analyses show that there is a dose-response relationship between cigarette use and invasive disease. Surprisingly, the adjusted population-attributable risk was 51 percent for cigarette smoking, 17 percent for passive smoking, and 14 percent for chronic illness.[7] This study also found that African Americans, males, persons with lower education levels, and persons with a preschool-aged child in day care are at higher risk for invasive pneumococcal disease.

Table 19-1

Vaccine Recommendations for Adults with Various Medical Conditions

SPECIFIC ILLNESS	VACCINES TO ADMINISTER	SPECIFICS OF ADMINISTRATION
Alcoholism	Pneumococcal, influenza	Recommended
Aspirin therapy, long-term	Influenza	Recommended for children and teenagers (6 months to 18 years old)
Asplenia (splenic dysfunction or anatomic asplenia), including sickle cell disease and splenectomy	Hib	Consider even for adults; for elective splenectomy, give at least 2 weeks before surgery, if possible
	Meningococcal, pneumococcal[a]	Recommended; for elective splenectomy, give at least 2 weeks before surgery, if possible
Cardiac disease that alters or potentially alters hemodynamics	Influenza, pneumococcal	Recommended
Cerebrospinal fluid leak	Pneumococcal	Recommended
Cirrhosis (alcoholic)	Influenza, pneumococcal, hepatitis A	Recommended
Complement deficiency (terminal component deficiencies)	Meningococcal	Recommended
Diabetes mellitus	Influenza, pneumococcal	Recommended
Factor deficiency (hemophilia) necessitating receipt of a clotting factor concentrate	Hepatitis A	Consider[b]
	Hepatitis B	Recommended[b]
Hemoglobinopathies	Influenza	Recommended
Immunocompromised severely (e.g., leukemia, lymphoma, generalized malignancy, or therapy with chemotherapy, radiation, or large amounts of corticosteroids);[c] vaccinate ≥ 2 weeks before chemotherapy or immunosuppressive therapy	Hepatitis B	Recommended when indicated by risk factor; use 40-μg dose[d]
	Hib	Recommended even if adult (consider if HIV-infected)
	Immunoglobulin	If exposed to measles disease[e]
	Influenza, pneumococcal	Recommended
	VZIG	Post-exposure prophylaxis[f]
Liver disease (chronic)	Hepatitis A	Recommended
Metabolic disease (chronic) that increases the likelihood that influenza infection will be more severe	Influenza	Recommended
Pregnant women	Influenza	Recommended for pregnant women who have a medical condition that increases risk for complications from influenza

Table 19-1

Vaccine Recommendations for Adults with Various Medical Conditions (Continued)

Specific Illness	Vaccines to Administer	Specifics of Administration
Pregnant women	Influenza	Recommended for pregnant women in the second or third trimester during the influenza season
Pulmonary disease (chronic), including asthma and chronic obstructive pulmonary disease	Influenza	Recommended
	Pneumococcal	Recommended except for asthma
Renal disease (chronic)	Influenza, pneumococcal[a]	Recommended
Renal disease requiring dialysis or likely to lead to dialysis or transplantation	Hepatitis B	Recommended; use 40-μg dose[d]
Varicella exposure in susceptible, immunocompetent adult	VZIG	Consider postexposure prophylaxis[f]
Varicella exposure in pregnancy	VZIG	Postexposure prophylaxis;[f] unknown if will protect fetus

[a]Pneumococcal revaccination should be considered 5 or more years after immunization if asplenia, chronic renal failure, or organ transplant have occurred.

[b]Use fine needle (≤23 gauge) and firm pressure at injection site for ≥ 2 min (see Greco et al[74] for details).

[c]Vaccination ideally should occur ≥ 2 weeks before chemotherapy or immunosuppressive therapy. If vaccination occurs either during immunosuppressive therapy or within 2 weeks before the start of such therapy, revaccinate ≥ 3 months after therapy ends. Other sources should be consulted for vaccination recommendations in transplant patients.

[d]Immunocompromised persons should received 40-μg doses of hepatitis B vaccine (special formulation of Recombivax HB or Engerix-B). If Engerix-B is used, a four-dose schedule is indicated. Check titers every 12 months and reimmunize if needed.

[e]Live-virus vaccines are contraindicated in severely immunocompromised persons. Severely immunocompromised persons should receive IG if exposed to measles, even if they have been immunized with MMR. See Centers for Disease Control and Prevention[41] for details.

[f]Before administering VZIG, determine (1) if the patient was exposed *and* (2) if the patient is susceptible (no history of varicella and negative antibody test, if performed). Exposure includes household contact, greater than 1 h of indoor contact, prolonged direct/face-to-face contact, or sharing the same hospital room. Susceptibility is rare; only 5 to 15 percent of adults do not have immunity to varicella. Antibody testing may be helpful in determining the susceptibility of immunocompetent persons without a history of varicella (see Centers for Disease Control and Prevention[109] for details). VZIG is expensive, and supplies are limited.

ABBREVIATIONS: Hib, *Haemophilus influenzae* type B conjugated vaccine; HIV, human immunodeficiency virus; VZIG, varicella zoster immune globulin; IG, immune globulin; MMR, measles, mumps, and rubella vaccine.

HIGH-RISK MEDICAL CONDITIONS

Asplenia, chronic renal disease, alcoholism, and, to a lesser degree, cirrhosis are predisposing factors for pneumonia and *S. pneumoniae* infection;[8–11] pulmonary disease, heart disease, and diabetes mellitus are three of the most common predisposing factors.[8,9,12] It should be noted that asthma alone is not an indication for pneumococcal vaccination.

Immunosuppression increases the risk of pneumonia and *S. pneumoniae* infection.[8,9,12]

High-dose or long-term steroids, cancer, and human immunodeficiency virus (HIV) infection all compromise the immune system, resulting in immunosuppression.

VACCINE EFFICACY

In a meta-analysis of randomized controlled trials of older pneumococcal polysaccharide vaccines, the vaccines were found to be 66 percent effective against definitive pneumococcal pneumonia and 83 percent effective against definitive pneumococcal pneumonia for vaccine types.[13] For the 23-valent polysaccharide vaccine (PPV23) in current use, the efficacy in case-control studies generally ranged from 56 to 81 percent.[5]

IMMUNIZATION RECOMMENDATIONS

PPV23 is recommended for all persons 65 years of age and older, and for persons greater than 2 years of age with asplenia (functional or surgical), chronic renal disease, alcoholism, cirrhosis, pulmonary disease (excluding mild to moderate asthma), heart disease, diabetes mellitus, and any form of immunosuppression. Table 19-2 provides PPV23 vaccination recommendations for children.

The Advisory Committee on Immunization Practices (ACIP) recommends that persons 65 years of age and older who were initially vaccinated before age 65 should receive one revaccination, provided that at least 5 years has elapsed since the initial vaccination.[5] This revaccination recommendation was based on data indicating that efficacy decreased with increasing time since vaccination. Several studies have suggested that revaccination after intervals of at least 4 years was safe (although local reactions increased at intervals of ≤2 years). Asplenic and other immunocompromised persons should receive a second dose of PPV23 5 or more years after the first.[5]

A prime opportunity for vaccination, especially in those ≥ 65 years of age, is at hospital discharge. In one study, 61 to 62 percent of persons aged 65 years or older who were hospitalized with pneumonia had been discharged from a hospital within the previous 4 years.[14]

ADVERSE REACTIONS AND CONTRAINDICATIONS

Since these 1997 ACIP recommendations were published, one article found that 11 percent of revaccinees, compared to 3 percent of placebo recipients, had a 10.2-cm (4-in) or greater self-limited, local reaction. These reactions occurred at vaccination intervals longer than 4 years.[15] Revaccination continues to be recommended, but physicians should be aware that local reactions may occur.

7-Valent Conjugate Vaccine

BURDEN OF PNEUMOCOCCAL DISEASE IN CHILDREN

S. pneumoniae causes approximately 100,000 to 135,000 cases of pneumonia requiring hospitalization and 7 million cases of otitis media in children annually in the United States.[4] Among children under the age of 5, *S. pneumoniae* causes about 17,000 cases of invasive disease, including 200 deaths.[16] Invasive disease consists of bacteremia, meningitis, or infection in a normally sterile site, excluding the middle ear. The 1998 incidence rates for invasive infection were 165 per 100,000 for infants, 203 per 100,000 for children aged 12 to 23 months, 37 per 100,000 for children aged 2 to 4 years, and 4 per 100,000 for children aged 5 to 17.[4] *S. pneumoniae* is the most common bacterial cause of community-acquired pneumonia, sinusitis, and acute otitis media in young children.[16]

Since the introduction of *Haemophilus influenzae* B (Hib) vaccines and the resulting decrease in the prevalence of infections due to *H. influenzae, S. pneumoniae* is now the leading cause of bacterial meningitis in the United States.[17] However, penicillin resistance is rising, and only 76 percent of isolates are fully susceptible.[4] Some isolates are resistant to multiple antibiotics,[18,19] which underscores the importance of immunization against this organism.

HIGH-RISK MEDICAL CONDITIONS

African Americans have rates of invasive pneumococcal disease about two to three times

Table 19-2

Schedule for 23-valent Pneumococcal Polysaccharide Vaccine (PPV23) in Children with High-Risk Conditions Who Have Already Been Given Pneumococcal Conjugate Vaccine

HEALTH CONDITION	SCHEDULE FOR PPV23 FOR HIGH-RISK CHILDREN ≥ 2 YEARS OF AGE	REVACCINATE WITH PPV23?
Healthy	None	No
Sickle cell disease, anatomic or functional asplenia, HIV-infected, immunocompromising conditions	1 dose PPV23 given ≥ 2 months after PCV7	Yes*
Chronic illness	1 dose PPV23 given ≥ 2 months after PCV7	No

*If patient is aged > 10 years, single revaccination ≥ 5 years after previous dose. If patient is aged < 10 years, consider revaccination 3 to 5 years after previous dose. Regardless of when administered, a second dose of PPV23 should not be given earlier than 3 years following the previous PPV23 dose.

SOURCE: Recommendations for revaccination adapted from Centers for Disease Control and Prevention,[5] Table 2, with permission.

higher than Caucasians. Alaskan Natives and Native Americans have rates about three to seven times higher than Caucasians.[16] Children with sickle cell disease or HIV infection also have high rates of disease (e.g., 9000 per 100,000 in HIV-infected children).[7,20]

VACCINE EFFICACY

The older PPV23 vaccine is effective in older children and adults but is not effective in children less than 2 years of age, who are at highest risk for infection. This is because PPV23 elicits a T-independent immune response that does not lead to an amnestic response upon challenge, nor does it reduce nasopharyngeal colonization of *S. pneumoniae.*

A 7-valent pneumococcal conjugate vaccine (PCV7) was licensed in 2000 in the United States. The carrier protein is CRM-197, which has been used in one Hib vaccine. PCV7 elicits a T-dependent immune response that leads to an amnestic response on challenge, is effective in infants, and reduces nasopharyngeal colonization of *S. pneumoniae.* The seven serotypes (4, 6B, 9V, 14, 18C, 19F, and 23F) included in the vaccine account

for about 80 percent of invasive infections in children less than 6 years of age, but only 50 percent of infections in those aged 6 and older.[21]

A randomized, double-blind controlled trial was conducted in Kaiser Permanente of Northern California pediatric patients. The vaccine's efficacy against invasive disease was 97 percent for serotypes included in the vaccine among children who were fully vaccinated. Overall, the efficacy was 89 percent regardless of serotype.[22] The efficacy was 6.4 percent against otitis media and 20 percent against ventilatory tube placement.[22] The vaccine also reduced use of antibiotics and was efficacious against pneumonia with x-ray consolidation. Published analyses show that the vaccination of healthy infants would prevent more than 12,000 cases of meningitis and bacteremia, 53,000 cases of pneumonia, and 1 million episodes of otitis media.[23]

IMMUNIZATION RECOMMENDATIONS

Table 19-3 summarizes the PVC7 immunization schedule. Figure 19-1 summarizes the overall childhood immunization schedule.

The ACIP recommends a full series of pneumococcal conjugate vaccine for infants and catch-up vaccination of children aged ≤ 23 months. Children 24 to 59 months of age should receive immunization if they are at high risk for invasive disease as a result of sickle cell disease, asplenia, HIV infection, chronic illness (e.g., bronchopulmonary dysplasia), or immunocompromising conditions. Penicillin prophylaxis should continue for children with sickle cell disease after vaccination with PCV7. The ACIP recommends that PCV7 should be considered for all children 24 to 59 months of age, with priority given to children aged 24 to 35 months; children who are of Alaska Native, American Indian, and African American descent; and children who attend group child care.

PCV7 is not licensed for use in adults, and no efficacy data are available for adults or children older than 5 years. The serotypes that cause infection change with age, and only 50 percent of the serotypes that cause infection in older children and adults are covered by PCV7, in comparison to 80 to 90 percent for PPV23. Although the ACIP recommends the use of PCV7 in older children who have high-risk conditions, it should not replace the polysaccharide vaccine in older children or adults. Table 19-2 details the use of PVC7 and PPV23 in children with high-risk conditions.

The American Academy of Family Physicians (AAFP) recommends PCV7 for children less than 24 months and for children less than 60 months with high-risk conditions (e.g., sickle cell disease, HIV, functional or anatomic asplenia, immunocompromising conditions, and chronic illness). The AAFP recommends vaccination for children who are African American, Alaskan Native, or American Indian. The AAFP regards the vaccination of children aged 24 to 59 months who attend child care settings and children who have had frequent or complicated acute otitis media in the previous year as an option.

ADVERSE REACTIONS AND CONTRAINDICATIONS

No serious adverse reactions have been associated with PCV7. When given with diphtheria toxoid, tetanus toxoid, and acellular pertussis vaccine (DTaP) but at another site, a fever of 38°C or higher occurred in 15 to 24 percent of those vaccinated with PCV7 compared to 9 to 17 percent of those receiving a control vaccine (experimental meningococcal conjugate vaccine). Among PCV7 vaccinees, 10 to 14 percent develop redness at the injection site and 15 to

Table 19-3

Recommended Schedule for Pneumococcal Conjugate Vaccine (PCV7), Including Catch-up Vaccination

AGE AT FIRST DOSE	PRIMARY SERIES	ADDITIONAL DOSE
2–6 months	3 doses, 2 months apart*	1 dose at 12–<16 months
7–11 months	2 doses, 2 months apart*	1 dose at 12–<16 months
12–23 months	2 doses, 2 months apart*	NA
24–59 months		
• Healthy children	1 dose	NA
• Children with SCD, asplenia, HIV infection, chronic illness, or immunocompromising condition†	2 doses, 2 months apart*	NA

*Minimum interval is 4 weeks.
†Recommendations do not include children who have undergone bone marrow transplant.
ABBREVIATIONS: NA, not applicable; SCD, sickle cell disease; HIV, human immunodeficiency virus.
SOURCE: Modified from Centers for Disease Control and Prevention,[16] with permission.

Recommended Childhood Immunization Schedule
United States, 2002

range of recommended ages | catch-up vaccination | preadolescent assessment

Vaccine ▼ / Age ▶	Birth	1 mo	2 mos	4 mos	6 mos	12 mos	15 mos	18 mos	24 mos	4-6 yrs	11-12 yrs	13-18 yrs
Hepatitis B[1]	Hep B #1 only if mother HBsAg (-)	Hep B #2			Hep B #3						Hep B series	
Diphtheria, Tetanus, Pertussis[2]			DTaP	DTaP	DTaP		DTaP	DTaP		DTaP	Td	
Haemophilus Influenzae Type b[3]			Hib	Hib	Hib	Hib						
Inactivated Polio[4]			IPV	IPV		IPV				IPV		
Measles, Mumps, Rubella[5]						MMR #1				MMR #2	MMR #2	
Varicella[6]						Varicella				Varicella	Varicella	
Pneumococcal[7]			PCV	PCV	PCV	PCV	PCV		PCV	PCV / PPV		
------ Vaccines below this line are for selected populations ------												
Hepatitis A[8]										Hepatitis A series		
Influenza[9]						Influenza (yearly)						

This schedule indicates the recommended ages for routine administration of currently licensed childhood vaccines, as of December 1, 2001, for children through age 18 years. Any dose not given at the recommended age should be given at any subsequent visit when indicated and feasible. ▒ Indicates age groups that warrant special effort to administer those vaccines not previously given. Additional vaccines may be licensed and recommended during the year. Licensed combination vaccines may be used whenever any components of the combination are indicated and the vaccine's other components are not contraindicated. Providers should consult the manufacturers' package inserts for detailed recommendations.

1. Hepatitis B vaccine (Hep B). All infants should receive the first dose of hepatitis B vaccine soon after birth and before hospital discharge; the first dose may also be given by age 2 months if the infant's mother is HBsAg-negative. Only monovalent hepatitis B vaccine can be used for the birth dose. Monovalent or combination vaccine containing Hep B may be used to complete the series; four doses of vaccine may be administered if combination vaccine is used. The second dose should be given at least 4 weeks after the first dose, except for Hib-containing vaccine which cannot be administered before age 6 weeks. The third dose should be given at least 16 weeks after the first dose and at least 8 weeks after the second dose. The last dose in the vaccination series (third or fourth dose) should not be administered before age 6 months.

Infants born to HBsAg-positive mothers should receive hepatitis B vaccine and 0.5 mL hepatitis B immune globulin (HBIG) within 12 hours of birth at separate sites. The second dose is recommended at age 1-2 months and the vaccination series should be completed (third or fourth dose) at age 6 months.

Infants born to mothers whose HBsAg status is unknown should receive the first dose of the hepatitis B vaccine series within 12 hours of birth. Maternal blood should be drawn at the time of delivery to determine the mother's HBsAg status; if the HBsAg test is positive, the infant should receive HBIG as soon as possible (no later than age 1 week).

2. Diphtheria and tetanus toxoids and acellular pertussis vaccine (DTaP). The fourth dose of DTaP may be administered as early as age 12 months, provided 6 months have elapsed since the third dose and the child is unlikely to return at age 15-18 months. **Tetanus and diphtheria toxoids (Td)** is recommended at age 11-12 years if at least 5 years have elapsed since the last dose of tetanus and diphtheria toxoid-containing vaccine. Subsequent routine Td boosters are recommended every 10 years.

3. *Haemophilus influenzae* type b (Hib) conjugate vaccine. Three Hib conjugate vaccines are licensed for infant use. If PRP-OMP (PedvaxHIB® or ComVax® [Merck]) is administered at ages 2 and 4 months, a dose at age 6 months is not required. DTaP/Hib combination products should not be used for primary immunization in infants at ages 2, 4 or 6 months, but can be used as boosters following any Hib vaccine.

4. Inactivated polio vaccine (IPV). An all-IPV schedule is recommended for routine childhood polio vaccination in the United States. All children should receive four doses of IPV at ages 2 months, 4 months, 6-18 months, and 4-6 years.

5. Measles, mumps, and rubella vaccine (MMR). The second dose of MMR is recommended routinely at age 4-6 years but may be administered during any visit, provided at least 4 weeks have elapsed since the first dose and that both doses are administered beginning at or after age 12 months. Those who have not previously received the second dose should complete the schedule by the 11-12 year old visit.

6. Varicella vaccine. Varicella vaccine is recommended at any visit at or after age 12 months for susceptible children, i.e. those who lack a reliable history of chickenpox. Susceptible persons age ≥13 years should receive two doses, given at least 4 weeks apart.

7. Pneumococcal vaccine. The heptavalent **pneumococcal conjugate vaccine (PCV)** is recommended for all children age 2-23 months. It is also recommended for certain children age 24-59 months. **Pneumococcal polysaccharide vaccine (PPV)** is recommended in addition to PCV for certain high-risk groups. See *MMWR* 2000;49(RR-9);1-35.

8. Hepatitis A vaccine. Hepatitis A vaccine is recommended for use in selected states and regions, and for certain high-risk groups; consult your local public health authority. See *MMWR* 1999;48(RR-12);1-37.

9. Influenza vaccine. Influenza vaccine is recommended annually for children age ≥ 6 months with certain risk factors (including but not limited to asthma, cardiac disease, sickle cell disease, HIV, diabetes; see *MMWR* 2001;50(RR-4);1-44), and can be administered to all others wishing to obtain immunity. Children age ≤ 12 years should receive vaccine in a dosage appropriate for their age (0.25 mL if age 6-35 months or 0.5 mL if age ≥ 3 years). Children age ≤ 8 years who are receiving influenza vaccine for the first time should receive two doses separated by at least 4 weeks.

For additional information about vaccines, vaccine supply, and contraindications for immunization, please visit the National Immunization Program Website at **www.cdc.gov/nip** or call the National Immunization Hotline at 800-232-2522 (English) or 800-232-0233 (Spanish).

Approved by the Advisory Committee on Immunization Practices (www.cdc.gov/nip/acip), the American Academy of Pediatrics (www.aap.org), and the American Academy of Family Physicians (www.aafp.org).

23 percent develop tenderness at the injection site.[22] Fever greater than 39°C was uncommon, occurring in 1 to 2.5 percent of vaccinees.

The only contraindication to PCV7 is hypersensitivity (e.g., anaphylaxis) to a previous dose or any component of the vaccine. Simultaneous administration on the same day of PCV7 and PPV23 is not recommended, since the safety has not been evaluated.

Future Considerations

A recent report of the 1998 Active Bacterial Core Surveillance data revealed that pneumococcal resistance to penicillin (24 percent) and multidrug resistance (14 percent) continue to increase across the United States, with the greatest penicillin resistance in children less than 5 years of age (32 percent) and adults 65 years old or greater (24 percent).[24] Serotypes in PPV23 accounted for 88 percent of penicillin-resistant strains, and serotypes in PCV7 account for 78 percent of penicillin-resistant strains.[24] While eliminating inappropriate use of antibiotics is crucial for decreasing antibiotic resistance, prevention of pneumococcal infection through vaccination is an equally important weapon to combat antibiotic-resistant pneumococcal disease.

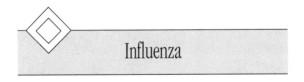

Influenza

Burden of Disease

Influenza is extremely contagious, being easily transmitted, usually by the airborne route, from person to person in semiclosed or crowded environments. Such environments include nursing homes, where influenza attack rates can approach 60 percent,[25,26] with case-fatality rates

up to 30 percent.[27] In each of 10 recent influenza epidemics in the United States, estimated deaths related to this disease totaled more than 20,000.[28] Furthermore, during some epidemics of influenza type A, there have been approximately 172,000 hospitalizations attributable solely to influenza and pneumonia.[29] The cost of a severe influenza epidemic has been estimated at $12 billion.[30]

The elderly, partly because they have a higher incidence of chronic medical conditions, have the highest age-specific case-fatality rate from influenza. More than 90 percent of deaths due to influenza occur in persons 65 years of age or older.[28] Those 65 years old or older also account for a high proportion of individuals hospitalized for influenza-like illness (35 to 46 percent in recent years), although they account for only 9 to 10 percent of patients making an office visit for such a complaint.[31,32]

High-Risk Medical Conditions

As with pneumococcal disease, chronic renal disease, alcoholism, cirrhosis, pulmonary disease, heart disease, and diabetes mellitus are predisposing factors for pneumonia and influenza.[8–12] In contrast to pneumococcal vaccine, influenza vaccine is indicated in individuals with asthma.[33] Pregnant women are at increased risk for complications from influenza during the third trimester, possibly because lung capacity decreases during pregnancy; consequently, pregnant women who will be late in their pregnancy during influenza season should be immunized.[34]

Immunosuppression increases the risk of pneumonia and influenza.[8,9,12] High-dose or long-term steroids, cancer, and HIV infection all compromise the immune system, resulting in immunosuppression. Influenza vaccination is recommended for all of these individuals.

Many individuals with influenza contract their illness from medical personnel. Transmission of influenza from hospital staff to patients was documented in one outbreak of influenza among hospital patients.[35] Another study found that vaccination of staff in long-term care facilities reduced mortality in patients, even though more than 60 percent of patients had also received vaccination.[36] A British randomized controlled trial showed a reduction in patient mortality rates of 9 percent in long-term care institutions in which health care workers were offered vaccination compared to institutions in which vaccination of employees was not offered.[37]

Vaccine Efficacy

When there is a good match between vaccine and circulating viruses, influenza vaccine has been shown to prevent illness in approximately 70 to 90 percent of healthy persons less than 65 years of age. When the match between vaccine and circulating virus is poor, efficacy is less.

A study in Minnesota of working adults aged 18 to 64 years of age found that influenza vaccination reduces episodes of upper respiratory illness (URI) by 25 percent (105 versus 140 episodes per 100 subjects), with a number needed to treat (NNT) of 2.9 to prevent one URI. Vaccination also reduces sick leave from work due to upper respiratory infections by 43 percent (70 versus 122 days per 100 subjects), and reduces visits to physicians' offices for upper respiratory infections by 44 percent (31 versus 55 visits per 100 subjects, NNT of 4.2 to prevent one physician visit).[38]

Depending on the year, one study found that influenza vaccination resulted in a 27 to 39 percent reduction in hospitalizations due to acute and chronic respiratory conditions and a 37 percent reduction in hospitalizations due to congestive heart failure.[2] Although influenza vaccine may be only 30 to 40 percent effective in preventing influenza illness among elderly persons residing in nursing homes, it can be 50 to 60 percent effective in preventing hospitalization and pneumonia and over 80 percent effective in pre-

venting death. Vaccination is 27 to 54 percent effective in reducing mortality from all causes.[2,39]

Immunity from influenza vaccine wanes following vaccination and may not persist beyond a year. It may take up to 2 weeks after vaccination for protection to develop.

Immunization Recommendations

After considering the burden of influenza disease, the low rates of vaccination among persons 50 to 64 years of age who are at high risk for complications, and the cost-effectiveness of vaccination, in 1999 the AAFP lowered the age for annual, routine influenza vaccination to age 50. In the fall of 2000, the ACIP also dropped the recommended age for immunization to 50 years. Beginning each September, when vaccine for the upcoming influenza season becomes available, all persons 50 years of age and older who are seen by health care providers should be offered influenza vaccine so that vaccination opportunities are not missed. In addition, persons 6 months of age or older may receive influenza vaccine if they desire it or have a high-risk condition. Persons of any age with asplenia (functional or surgical), chronic renal disease, alcoholism, cirrhosis, pulmonary disease, asthma, heart disease, diabetes mellitus, hemoglobinopathies, and any form of immunosuppression also should receive influenza vaccine annually (Table 19-1).[33,40,41]

It is recommended that women who will be in the second or third trimester of pregnancy during the influenza season receive influenza vaccination.[33] Pregnant women who have high-risk medical conditions that increase the risk of complications of influenza should be vaccinated before the influenza season regardless of gestational age.

Many residents of institutions for the developmentally disabled have chronic medical conditions such as congenital heart disease that place them at risk for complications from influenza.

Therefore, all residents of these institutions should receive influenza vaccine annually.

Achieving a high rate of vaccination among nursing home residents can reduce the spread of infection in a facility and prevent disease through herd immunity. Therefore, institution protocols for infection control should include standing orders for vaccination of all residents of chronic-care facilities as a group, with consent for annual influenza vaccination of each resident being obtained at the time of admission to the facility. Residents admitted during the winter but after the annual vaccination program should be vaccinated on admission.

It is recommended that persons who provide health care or home care services to chronically ill patients receive influenza vaccine yearly. Annual vaccination against influenza is also indicated for household contacts of persons at high risk for complications of influenza.

Adverse Reactions and Contraindications

Since inactivated influenza vaccines do not contain live virus, they cannot cause influenza. However, influenza vaccine can cause local reactions such as soreness at the injection site. In persons previously exposed to influenza disease or vaccination, placebo-controlled studies show similar rates of systemic reactions such as fever when split virus vaccine is compared to placebo. However, in young children not previously exposed to influenza vaccine, fever, malaise, and myalgia can occur after vaccination. The current vaccines are considerably purer than vaccines produced prior to 1968, and thus cause far fewer adverse events.

The main contraindication to influenza vaccine is anaphylaxis from eggs or other vaccine components. Persons who can eat eggs without experiencing a reaction generally can be vaccinated. A protocol is available for influenza vaccine administration to persons who have a true allergy to egg protein yet need influenza vaccine

because of high-risk conditions.[42] Allergy to duck dander or duck meat is not a contraindication. Influenza vaccine contains small amounts of thimerosal, a mercurial antibacterial agent that acts as a preservative. Severe allergy to this component is rare. Influenza vaccination should be delayed in persons who have an acute, febrile illness. A person who has a contraindication to influenza vaccine may be a candidate for antiviral prophylaxis.

In 1976 the federal government sponsored the National Influenza Immunization Program to give A/New Jersey influenza vaccine to nearly all adults and children in the United States. Included in this program was a nationwide surveillance system to look for possible adverse reactions. The surveillance program identified 7 cases of Guillain-Barré syndrome (GBS) by December 2, 1976, when over 35 million doses had been administered. An active surveillance system discovered more cases, and epidemiologic evidence indicated that some GBS cases were related to vaccination.[43] The attributable risk was approximately 9.5 cases per million vaccinees. This strain of influenza vaccine is no longer in use.

Studies since 1976 are mixed, with some showing no increased risk and one suggesting a slight increase in GBS. If influenza vaccine increases the risk of GBS, the risk is on the order of 1 to 2 cases per million persons vaccinated. There is good evidence that a number of infectious diseases, particularly *Campylobacter jejuni*, *Mycoplasma pneumoniae*, cytomegalovirus, and Epstein-Barr virus, provoke GBS. Even if GBS were a true side effect of vaccination in some years, the risk is substantially less than the risk for severe influenza. The decision about whether or not to vaccinate persons with a history of GBS may be based on two factors: their risk for severe complications if they contract influenza and whether or not GBS was documented to occur following influenza vaccination. It is prudent to not vaccinate persons who are at low risk for complications of influenza disease and have a documented history of GBS following previous influenza vaccination.[33] Even with the known risks, many experts still would vaccinate a person with GBS who is at high risk for complications from influenza.[33]

Future Considerations

Because of the high rate of hospitalizations in young infants from influenza disease and its complications, experts are beginning to consider whether infants should be vaccinated routinely. The vaccine is safe and effective in infants 6 months of age and older. However, issues related to feasibility have been raised. First, vaccine supply needs to be adequate. Second, since two doses of influenza vaccine are needed when children less than 9 years old are vaccinated for the first time, this adds two doses to the already crowded Recommended Childhood Immunization Schedule. Third, many young children would not normally have a visit for well child care that coincided with the influenza vaccination season, so it is unclear how they would be vaccinated. These feasibility issues need to be addressed before a recommendation can be considered further. A live, attenuated, influenza vaccine that is administered by the nasal route may be licensed in the United States within a few years, which would facilitate childhood vaccination.

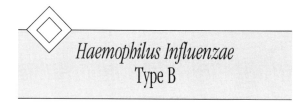

Haemophilus Influenzae Type B

Burden of Disease

Haemophilus influenzae type B is a bacterium that can cause serious disease, primarily in young children. The bacteria are spread by res-

piratory droplets and nasal or oral discharges, and usually infect by way of the nasopharyngeal route.[44]

Before effective vaccines became available, about 1 in 200 children under the age of 5 developed invasive Hib disease.[45] Hib was the most common cause of bacterial meningitis in children;[45] even with prompt and appropriate treatment, this has a 2 to 5 percent mortality rate. The incidence of neurologic sequelae in survivors of bacterial meningitis is 15 to 30 percent,[45,46] with hearing loss being the most common long-term sequela.[47] Other neurologic sequelae include mental retardation, seizures, vision loss, and motor and speech delays.[45,48,49]

Hib is the most common cause of epiglottitis in unimmunized populations.[50,51] The mortality of Hib epiglottitis is 5 to 10 percent, with deaths occurring due to airway obstruction.[52] Hib also causes other invasive diseases, including pneumonia, septic arthritis, cellulitis, pericarditis, osteomyelitis, empyema, and sepsis.[44,53]

High-Risk Medical Conditions

Persons at increased risk for invasive Hib disease should be vaccinated even if they are older than 59 months. Risk factors for invasive disease include anatomic asplenia (e.g., congenital absence or splenectomy), functional asplenia (e.g., sickle cell disease), immunodeficiency (particularly IgG_2 subclass deficiency), immunosuppression from cancer chemotherapy, and infection with HIV. When feasible, vaccination should precede splenectomy and chemotherapy by at least 2 weeks.

As less than 5 percent of cases are linked to contact with a known infection, Hib is not highly contagious. However, the secondary attack rate after household exposure to a known infection is 500 to 600 times higher than the incidence in the general population.[49,54] Because of the concerns about secondary cases, the following guidelines have been published for the care of those exposed to Hib disease. Any child exposed to Hib who then becomes ill should be promptly evaluated for possible Hib disease. Immunization records for all exposed children should be reviewed, and needed doses of vaccine should be administered promptly. If there is a household contact (defined as someone living with the index case or spending at least 4 h a day for 5 of the 7 days preceding the hospitalization of the index case)[47] who is under 4 years of age and is not fully immunized against Hib, then all of the household contacts should receive rifampin prophylaxis. Rifampin also is recommended for all household contacts if the household includes fully immunized but immunocompromised children, or children who are age-appropriately immunized but younger than 12 months of age.[47] Rifampin use is not recommended in pregnant women.

Rifampin is administered once daily for 4 days, in a dose of 20 mg/kg (600 mg maximum dose), or 10 mg/kg in infants less than 1 month of age.[49] Index cases not treated with cephalosporins should also receive rifampin prophylaxis, as ampicillin and chloramphenicol do not eradicate carriage of Hib.[47]

Prophylaxis of contacts in the preschool or day care setting is more controversial. There is some consensus that if there are exposed, incompletely immunized children under the age of 2 years in a day care setting where contact is at least 25 h per week, then prophylaxis is indicated.[47,49] Also, if there have been two or more cases in a 60-day period in a child care facility where there are incompletely immunized children, then prophylaxis is indicated.[47] For the purposes of these guidelines, children are considered fully immunized if they received at least one dose of conjugate vaccine at 15 months of age or older; two doses of conjugate vaccine between 12 and 14 months of age; or a two- or three-dose primary series (depending on the preparation) during the first year of life, with a booster on or after the first birthday.[47]

Vaccine Efficacy

The first Hib vaccine available for use in the United States was approved in 1985 for children at least 18 months of age. However, two-thirds of all cases of invasive Hib occur in children less than 18 months of age, whose immune systems are too immature to respond well to the polysaccharide antigen in this first preparation.[45] Thus, the vaccine's usefulness was limited by its low efficacy in some populations and its lack of immunogenicity in infants.[45]

Since that time, four conjugate Hib vaccines have been licensed in the United States. PRP-D (ProHIBit) contains Hib purified polyribosyribitol phosphate (PRP) conjugated with diphtheria toxoid. Although it appeared efficacious in infants in Finnish trials,[55,56] results in the United States were disappointing.[57] As a result, PRP-D is approved only as a booster for children 12 months of age and older.[53] The other three conjugate vaccines are approved for use in infants and have an efficacy estimated at 93 to 100 percent for a completed series.[58–60] PRP-OMP (PedvaxHIB) contains Hib PRP conjugated with the outer membrane protein of *Neisseria meningitidis* group b (however, it is not intended for use against *N. meningitidis*).[59] HbOC (HibTITER) contains a subunit of Hib polysaccharide conjugated with a mutant (CRM-197) diphtheria toxin. PRP-T (OmniHib/ActHIB) contains PRP conjugated with tetanus toxoid. All of the conjugate vaccines except for PRP-OMP use protein antigens found in diphtheria and tetanus vaccines (DT/DTP/DTaP). There is evidence that suggests a better immune response to these conjugate vaccines if the recipient receives DT/DTP/DTaP vaccine before or simultaneous with Hib vaccination.[45] Children who are not candidates for DT/DTP/DTaP vaccination may benefit from preferential use of PRP-OMP for Hib immunization.

Introduction of conjugated Hib vaccines in 1989, for use in children 15 months of age or older, and subsequent approval in 1990 of the use of conjugated vaccines in infants has had a tremendous impact on the incidence of invasive Hib disease in the United States. Between 1987 and 1997, the incidence of invasive *H. influenzae* disease in children under 5 declined 97 percent.[61]

TriHIBit is a combination of DTaP and Hib that is licensed for the fourth dose of the series. Data suggest that some acellular DTaP-Hib combination vaccines can lead to reduced responses to the Hib component when given in infancy. Hence, acellular DTaP-Hib combination vaccines should not be used in infancy until the Food and Drug Administration has approved their use.

Cases of invasive Hib disease have occurred in fully immunized children, but they are rare. Immunologic evaluation of these children should be considered, as a small but significant percentage of them are found to have an immunoglobulin deficiency.[47]

Immunization Recommendations

HbOC and PRP-T are given as a four-dose series at 2, 4, 6, and 12 to 15 months of age. PRP-OMP is given as a three-dose series at 2, 4, and 12 to 15 months of age if PRP-OMP is the only Hib vaccine given. If a child starts the series late, then a modified schedule may be indicated. The minimal interval between doses in the primary series is 1 month. The booster dose—that is, the dose recommended at 12 to 15 months of age—should be spaced at least 2 months from the previous dose. PRP-D is approved as a booster for children 12 months of age and older.[53] Table 19-4 summarizes the Hib immunization schedules for on-time and late immunization.

Conjugate Hib vaccines, including COMVAX, should not be used in children less than 6 weeks of age because earlier doses may induce immune tolerance, preventing adequate antibody response to further doses of Hib vaccine.

Children who develop invasive Hib disease at less than 24 months of age should be considered unimmunized and should be vaccinated starting in the convalescent phase. Generally, administration of Hib vaccine after 59 months of age is not necessary, since a majority of children should be immune as a result of asymptomatic infection.

VACCINE INTERCHANGEABILITY

Recent studies have shown that Hib conjugate vaccines (Hib) are generally interchangeable.[62–64] In fact, antibody titers are often higher if Hib vaccines from different manufacturers are used. When both PRP-OMP and another Hib vaccine (e.g., HbOC or PRP-T) are given in the first year of life, then the number of doses is determined by the HbOC or PRP-T product (i.e., three doses are recommended for the infant series, with a fourth dose recommended at 12 to 15 months of age).

Adverse Reactions and Contraindications

Adverse reactions to conjugate Hib vaccines are usually mild. Fever has been noted infrequently (1 to 4.6 percent of recipients).[65] Swelling, erythema, or tenderness at the injection site have been reported in 5 to 30 percent of recipients and usually resolve within 12 to 24 h.[66] The Institute of Medicine (IOM) reviewed adverse reactions to many childhood vaccines and did not find any serious adverse event linked to conjugate Hib vaccines.[67]

The permanent contraindication to administering Hib vaccines is anaphylaxis to a previous dose of Hib or to a vaccine component. Thimerosal is a preservative in some Hib vaccines. HbOC and PRP-T contain diphtheria or tetanus toxoid; therefore, children who have severe reactions to DTP/DTaP or DT vaccines may benefit from preferential use of PRP-OMP, which does not contain thimerosal. Severe acute illness usually warrants postponement of vaccination until the patient has recovered from the

Table 19-4

Detailed Vaccination Schedule for *Haemophilus influenzae* Type B Conjugate Vaccines

Vaccine	AGE AT FIRST DOSE (MONTHS)	PRIMARY SERIES	BOOSTER
HbOC or	2–6	3 doses, 2 months apart	12–15 months
PRP-T	7–11	2 doses, 2 months apart	12–18 months
	12–14	1 dose	2 months later
	15–59	1 dose	—
PRP-OMP	2–6	2 doses, 2 months apart	12–15 months
	7–11	2 doses, 2 months apart	12–18 months
	12–14	1 dose	2 months later
	15–59	1 dose	—
PRP-D (Connaught)	15–59	1 dose	—

ABBREVIATIONS: Hib, *Haemophilus influenzae* type B; HbOC, Hib vaccine conjugated with a pediatric dose of diphtheria toxoid; PRP-T, Hib vaccine conjugated with tetanus toxoid; PRP-OMP, Hib vaccine conjugated with *Neisseria meningitidis* group B; PRP-D, Hib vaccine conjugated with a pediatric dose of diphtheria toxoid.
SOURCE: Modified from Epidemiology & Prevention of Vaccine-Preventable Diseases. 4th ed. Centers for Disease Control and Prevention, Atlanta, GA, September 1997:110 (public domain), with permission.

acute phase of illness. Hib vaccines contain neomycin, but allergy to this agent is a delayed-type (cell-mediated) immune response and is not a contraindication to vaccination.[68]

Future Considerations

One study has suggested that large amounts of tetanus toxoid carrier protein given simultaneously with PRP-T could result in a reduced response to Hib.[68] This might occur when new conjugate vaccines against other diseases are developed. Research is also ongoing to develop combination vaccines that incorporate Hib.

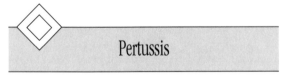

Pertussis

Burden of Disease

Almost half (47 percent) of reported cases of pertussis occur in infants, and most reported cases (72 percent) occur in children younger than 5 years of age.[69] The hospitalization rate is 69 percent for reported cases of pertussis in infants younger than 12 months of age.[69] The case-fatality rate is 0.6 percent for infants younger than 12 months of age. Pneumonia occurs in about 15 percent of pertussis cases and is the leading cause of death from pertussis. Seizures occur in 2.2 percent of cases of pertussis, and encephalopathy occurs in 0.7 percent of cases. Encephalopathy, which may be caused by hypoxia or minute cerebral hemorrhages, is fatal in approximately one-third of cases and causes permanent brain damage in another one-third.

Before routine pertussis vaccination of children, peaks in pertussis incidence occurred approximately every 3 to 4 years, and virtually all children were eventually infected. Between 1925 and 1930, 36,013 persons died in the United States as a result of complications from pertussis. More than 1 million cases of pertussis were reported in the United States from 1940 through 1945.[70] After pertussis vaccination became widespread in the mid-1940s, the incidence of pertussis dropped by more than 95 percent, although an epidemic of 6586 cases occurred in 1993.

Vaccine Efficacy

In studies conducted in the United States, DTP vaccination was found to be between 70 and 90 percent effective in preventing pertussis disease.[70,71] In studies conducted in Europe, DTaP vaccines demonstrated efficacies between 59 and 89 percent, and DTP vaccines had efficacy rates ranging from 36 to 98 percent.[72–75] However, it is difficult to compare the results of various studies because of differences in (1) study type, (2) degree of blinding, (3) case definition of pertussis, (4) criteria for confirmation of pertussis infection, (5) ethnicity of the study population, (6) number of children studied, (7) timing of the vaccine schedule, and (8) manufacturer of whole-cell vaccine used for comparison. Some of the DTaP and DTP vaccines studied in Europe are not available in the United States.

The protection afforded by pertussis vaccination wanes with time. For whole-cell (DTP) vaccines, protection against pertussis disease is lost by 12 years after the last dose.

Immunization Recommendations

DTaP at 2, 4, 6, and 12 to 18 months of age with a booster at 4 to 6 years of age is recommended for all children because of the reduced risk of adverse reactions when compared with DTP. Completing the recommended series is important for optimal efficacy. Based on a case definition of a cough of at least 14 days with paroxysms, whoop, or vomiting, one study found that the efficacy of whole-cell vaccine is 36 percent after one dose, 49 percent after two doses, and 83 percent after three doses.[76] Although five doses of a DTP or DTaP vaccine are recommended, persons who receive their fourth dose on or after their fourth birthday do not need the fifth dose.

Premature infants should be vaccinated with full doses at the appropriate chronological age. Full doses should be used because fractional doses are not as immunogenic as full doses and do not lessen the risk of adverse reactions.

Although adults and adolescents are the primary source of pertussis infection in young infants,[77] morbidity from pertussis in adolescents and adults is low. Furthermore, the incidence of adverse reactions after administration of whole-cell pertussis vaccine to older children and adults is relatively high—half of such individuals who receive monovalent or combination whole-cell pertussis vaccine develop induration at the injection site.[78,79] Therefore, whole-cell pertussis vaccine alone or in combination with other vaccines is not indicated for use in those older than 7 years. No acellular vaccines have been licensed for use in persons 7 years of age or older, although there is considerable interest in this.

Adverse Reactions and Contraindications

DTaP vaccines have common adverse reaction rates less than half those of DTP vaccines. Furthermore, the rates of adverse reactions are similar for DTaP and DT.[80–83] Administration of a DTaP vaccine has been associated with seizures, persistent crying, and hypotonic-hyporesponsive episodes, but at lower rates than after administration of a DTP vaccine. Table 19-5 compares the frequency of reactions to DTaP and DTP vaccines.

Certain infrequent adverse events occurring after pertussis vaccination are warnings against further doses: (1) temperature of $\geq 40.5°C$ (105°F) within 48 h of a previous dose (not due to another identifiable cause), (2) collapse or shocklike state (hypotonic-hyporesponsive episode) within 48 h of a previous dose, (3) persistent, inconsolable crying lasting 3 h or more, occurring within 48 h of a previous dose, or (4) convulsions within 3 days of a previous dose.

Table 19-5

Percentage of Infants with Mild or Local Reactions by the Third Evening after Pertussis Vaccination at Ages 2, 4, and 6 Months

VACCINE	TEMPERATURE ≥37.8°C	SWELLING > 20 MM	SEVERE FUSSINESS*
Connaught/Biken/CB-2/Tripedia	24.5	3.7	3.7
Lederle/Takeda/LPT-4F₁/ACEL-IMUNE	19.8	3.2	4.6
SmithKline Beecham/SKB-3P/Infanrix	31.6	5.8	5.0
Overall for 13 DTaP vaccines	24.5	4.2	4.7
DTP vaccines overall	60.4	22.4	12.4

*Fussiness was classified as severe when the infant cried persistently and could not be comforted.
ABBREVIATIONS: DTaP, pediatric dose of diphtheria toxoid, tetanus toxoid, and acellular pertussis vaccine; DTP, pediatric dose of diphtheria toxoid, tetanus toxoid, and whole-cell pertussis vaccine.
SOURCE: Adapted from data in Decker et al,[78] with permission.

If the pertussis component is withheld because of a contraindication or warning, then pediatric DT is administered instead. In the case of true anaphylaxis, both diphtheria and pertussis components are permanently contraindicated. In such cases, referral may be made to an allergist to assess whether tetanus toxoid can be given and for possible desensitization to tetanus toxoid.

DTaP vaccination should be postponed for infants with an evolving neurologic disorder, unevaluated seizures, or a neurologic event between doses of pertussis vaccine. Vaccination should be resumed after evaluation and treatment of the condition.

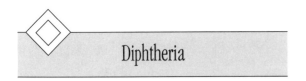

Diphtheria

Burden of Disease

In 1921, 206,000 cases of diphtheria were reported in the United States, with 15,520 deaths.[84] This number fell to 19,000 cases in 1945 (15 cases per 100,000 population) after introduction of the diphtheria vaccine.[84] From 1980 through 1999, 49 cases of diphtheria were reported in the United States (an average of 3 cases per year), mostly in unimmunized or inadequately immunized individuals.

In former states of the Soviet Union, where diphtheria had been well controlled for the previous 30 years, vaccination levels dropped after dissolution of the Soviet Union. This drop in vaccination is held accountable for the diphtheria epidemics in these states in 1994 and 1995.[85,86]

Serologic surveys in the United States show that 40 percent of individuals ≥ 60 years of age lack protective levels of antibody to diphtheria.[87–89] Given the low levels of vaccination and antibody among older persons in the United States, it is possible that an epidemic of diphtheria could spread to the United States from another country.

Vaccine Efficacy

A protective level of diphtheria antitoxin is reached after three toxoid doses in adults or four in infants for 95 percent of vaccinees. The clinical efficacy of diphtheria toxoid is estimated at 97 percent.[84]

Immunization Recommendations

Children with a contraindication to pertussis vaccination should complete the DTaP series with DT vaccine. Persons 7 years of age and older should receive adult tetanus and diphtheria toxoids (Td), which contain about the same quantity of tetanus toxoid as the DTP/DTaP or pediatric DT vaccines but only one-third to one-eleventh as much diphtheria toxoid. Td vaccine should be used for the primary three-dose series in those receiving the first dose at 7 years or older and for routine booster doses every 10 years.[70]

Adults who have not had a primary series of tetanus and diphtheria toxoids or whose vaccination history is uncertain should have three doses of Td. The first two doses of Td vaccine should be given at least 4 weeks apart and the third dose 6 to 12 months after the second dose. According to the ACIP, adults who have completed the primary vaccination series should receive a booster dose of Td vaccine every 10 years.[90] The American Academy of Family Physicians, the American College of Physicians, and the Infectious Diseases Society of America recommend Td boosters every 10 years or a single booster at age 50 years.[91,92] The United States Preventive Services Task Force recommends periodic boosters, allowing intervals of 10 to 30 years.[93]

Adverse Reactions and Contraindications

While a palpable nodule at the injection site can persist for several weeks, fever, injection site abscess, and severe systemic reactions to diphtheria toxoid are rare.[84] Local reactions such as erythema, induration, and tenderness are common and self-limited.[84]

Persons who experience an Arthus-type hypersensitivity reaction or a fever of greater than 39.4°C (103°F) after a previous dose of tetanus toxoid probably have high serum antitoxin titers and should not be given a dose of Td more often than every 10 years.[70]

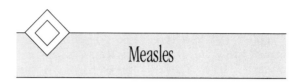

Measles

Burden of Disease

Measles is highly contagious, with an attack rate for unvaccinated household contacts of over 90 percent.[94] Before the introduction of vaccine, measles caused illness in approximately 3 to 4 million persons yearly, with 500 reported deaths annually in the United States. Epidemics occurred every 2 to 3 years, and more than 90 percent of persons contracted measles by age 15. Following the introduction of measles vaccine in 1963, the incidence of measles dropped by more than 98 percent, although a major epidemic in 1989–1991 caused 55,467 reported cases and 136 deaths.[95]

Vaccine Efficacy

The measles vaccine currently used in the United States contains a live, highly attenuated virus. Following measles vaccination, seroconversion rates are 95 percent for children vaccinated at 12 months of age and 98 percent for children vaccinated at 15 months of age.[70] The vaccine induces both humoral and cellular immunity. Antibody persists for at least 17 years and is probably lifelong in almost all vaccinated persons who initially seroconvert. Subclinical reinfection may occur in persons following vaccination, but there is no evidence that persons with subclinical disease transmit wild virus to others. Of the few whose antibody level wanes, most are probably still immune because they have secondary immune responses upon revaccination.

When measles outbreaks occurred among school-aged children in the United States in the 1980s despite high vaccination levels,[96,97] measles vaccination guidelines were reassessed. In 1989, the ACIP recommended a second dose of measles-containing vaccine at age 4 to 6 years (entry to kindergarten or first grade) to provide protection for most of those who did not respond to the initial measles vaccination.[97] Studies have found that failure of seroconversion after the initial dose of measles vaccine occurs at a rate of 2 to 5 percent.[70] In comparison, the rate of secondary vaccine failure, also known as waning immunity, has been found to be less than 0.2 percent.[98]

Immunization Recommendations

Two doses of measles-mumps-rubella (MMR) vaccine are recommended for children. The first dose should be given at age 12 to 15 months, and a second dose at 4 to 6 years of age, although it may be given any time 1 month or longer after the first dose. Children 7 years of age or older who did not previously receive the second dose of MMR can receive the catch-up dose at any visit.

All adults born in 1957 or later should receive one dose of MMR vaccine unless they have documentation of at least one dose of measles-, rubella-, and mumps-containing vaccine on or after their first birthday, or documentation of presumptive immunity. Documentation of immunity includes physician diagnosis of measles and mumps, but not rubella; serologic evidence; or documented vaccinations against measles, mumps, and rubella. In general, serologic screening to determine immunity is not recommended, is costly, and can be a barrier to vaccination.

Live attenuated Edmonston B measles vaccine and killed (inactivated) measles vaccine (KMV) were licensed in the United States in 1963. Persons who received KMV (which was last used in 1967) may contract an atypical form of measles[49] characterized by fever, pneumonia, pleural effu-sions, edema, and an atypical rash (including maculopapules, urticaria, petechiae, and purpura). Hence, persons known to have received KMV or those vaccinated between 1963 and 1967 with a vaccine of unknown type should receive two doses of live measles vaccine.[99] Persons who received measles vaccine not known to be Edmonston B, with either immune globulin or measles immune globulin, should be considered susceptible to measles and should receive at least one dose of measles vaccine.

Adverse Reactions and Contraindications

Although one study raised concerns about decreased immunogenicity when MMR was administered to children who had a viral illness,[100] recent studies show no difference in vaccine efficacy when administered to children with a mild illness.[101–103] HIV-infected persons who are not severely immunosuppressed should receive MMR vaccine when otherwise indicated based on age.[104]

Pregnancy is a contraindication to administration of live-virus vaccines because of the theoretical risk that the live virus could damage the fetus. Furthermore, women should avoid becoming pregnant within 28 days of receiving MMR. On the other hand, inadvertent administration of a live-virus vaccine during pregnancy is not an indication for pregnancy termination because there are no data to link live-virus vaccination with increased risk of fetal malformations.

Contraindications to Immunizations

The permanent contraindication to any vaccine is anaphylaxis to a previous dose or to a vaccine component. However, contact dermatitis from neomycin is a delayed-type (cell-mediated) immune response and is not a contraindication to vaccination.[67]

Four conditions are temporary contraindications to vaccination: severe acute illness, immunosuppression, pregnancy, and recent receipt of blood products. Severe acute illness (e.g., pneumonia requiring antibiotics and bronchodilators) usually warrants postponement of vaccination until the patient has recovered from the acute phase of illness.

Immunosuppression due to an immune deficiency disease or malignancy or therapy with high-dose corticosteroid drugs, alkylating agents, antimetabolites, or radiation is generally a contraindication to administration of a live-virus vaccine. Inactivated vaccines may be given to immunosuppressed persons because they do not contain live organisms that can replicate; however, immunosuppression may decrease the response to vaccination. There are two exceptions to this general principle: (1) HIV-infected persons who are not severely immunosuppressed should receive MMR vaccine when otherwise indicated based on age, and (2) varicella vaccine remains contraindicated in patients with cellular immunodeficiencies, but according to the ACIP it now may be given to those with humoral immunodeficiencies.[104]

Overly cautious health care providers have misinterpreted a number of other conditions as posing contraindications to vaccination,[105–109] including local reactions to vaccine administration, low-to-moderate fevers following previous doses of vaccine, a family history of severe adverse events related to administration of DTP vaccine, mental retardation, seizures, or allergies. Indicated immunization should not be omitted or delayed because of any of these conditions.

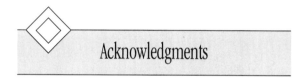

Acknowledgments

The authors acknowledge Ilene T. Burns, M.D., M.P.H., for her work on *Haemophilus influenzae* type B disease and immunization.

References

1. Centers for Disease Control and Prevention, National Immunization Program: *Epidemiology and Prevention of Vaccine-Preventable Diseases*, Atlanta, Centers for Disease Control and Prevention; 1999.
2. Nichol KL, Margolis KL, Wuorenma J, Von Sternberg TL: The efficacy and cost effectiveness of vaccination against influenza among elderly persons living in the community. *N Engl J Med* 331: 778–784, 1994.
3. Sisk JE, Moskowitz AJ, Whang W: Cost-effectiveness of vaccination against pneumococcal bacteremia among elderly people. *JAMA* 278:1333, 1997.
4. Centers for Disease Control and Prevention: *Active Bacterial Core Surveillance (ABCs) Report, Emerging Infections Program Network, Streptococcus pneumoniae, 1998*. Atlanta, Centers for Disease Control and Prevention, Emerging Infections Program Network; 1998.
5. Centers for Disease Control and Prevention: Prevention of pneumococcal disease: recommendations of the Advisory Committee on Immunization Practices (ACIP). *MMWR* 46:1–24, 1997.
6. Jernigan DB, Cetron MS, Breiman RF: Minimizing the impact of the drug-resistant *Streptococcus pneumoniae* (DRSP): a strategy from the DRSP working group. *JAMA* 275:206–209, 1996.
7. Nuorti JP, Butler JC, Farley MM, et al: Cigarette smoking and invasive pneumococcal disease. *N Engl J Med* 342:681–689, 2000.
8. Young CL, MacGregor RR: Alcohol and host defenses: infectious consequences. *Infect Med* 6: 163–175, 1989.
9. Burman LA, Norrby R, Trollfors B: Invasive pneumococcal infections: incidence, predisposing factors, and prognosis. *Rev Infect Dis* 7:133–142, 1985.
10. Musher DM: *Streptococcus pneumoniae*, in Mandell GL (ed): *Principles and Practice of Infectious Diseases*, 5th ed. Philadelphia, Churchill Livingstone; 2000: pp 2128–2147.
11. Riedo FX, Plikaytis BD, Broome CV: Epidemiology and prevention of meningococcal disease. *Pediatr Infect Dis J* 14:643–657, 1995.
12. Barker WH, Mullooly JP: Pneumonia and influenza deaths during epidemics: implications for prevention. *Arch Intern Med* 142:85–89, 1982.

13. Fine MJ, Smith MA, Carson CA, et al: Efficacy of pneumococcal vaccination in adults: a meta-analysis of randomized controlled trials. *Arch Intern Med* 154:2666–2677, 1994.

14. Fedson DS, Harward MP, Reid RA, Kaiser DL: Hospital-based pneumococcal immunization. Epidemiologic rationale from the Shenandoah study. *JAMA* 264:1117–1122, 1990.

15. Jackson LA, Benson P, Sneller VP: Safety of revaccination with pneumococcal polysaccharide vaccine. *JAMA* 281:243–248, 1999.

16. Centers for Disease Control and Prevention: Preventing pneumococcal disease among infants and young children: recommendations of the Advisory Committee on Immunization Practices (ACIP). *MMWR* 49:1–38, 2000.

17. Schuchat A, Robinson K, Wenger JD, et al: Bacterial meningitis in the United States in 1995. *N Engl J Med* 337:970–976, 1997.

18. Breiman RF, Butler JC, Tenover FC, et al: Emergence of drug-resistant pneumococcal infections in the United States. *JAMA* 271:1831–1835, 1994.

19. Kellner JD, Ford-Jones EL: *Streptococcus pneumoniae* carriage in children attending 59 Canadian child care centers. *Arch Pediatr Adolesc Med* 153:495–502, 1999.

20. Levine OS, Farley M, Harrison LH, et al: Risk factors for invasive pneumococcal disease in children: a population-based case-control study in North America. *Pediatrics* 103(3), 1999. *http://www.pediatrics.org/cgi/content/full/103/3/e28*.

21. Butler JC, Brieman RF, Lipman HB, et al: Serotype distribution of *Streptococcus pneumoniae* infections among preschool children in the United States, 1978–1994: implications for development of a conjugate vaccine. *J Infect Dis* 171:885–889, 1995.

22. Black S, Shinefield H, Fireman B, et al: Efficacy, safety and immunogenicity of heptavalent pneumococcal conjugate vaccine in children. *Pediatr Infect Dis J* 19:187–195, 2000.

23. Lieu TA, Ray GT, Black SB, et al: Projected cost-effectiveness of pneumococcal conjugate vaccination of healthy infants and young children. *JAMA* 283:1460–1468, 2000.

24. Whitney CG, Farley MM, Hadler J, et al: Increasing prevalence of multi-drug resistant *Streptococcus pneumoniae* in the United States. *N Engl J Med* 343:1917–1924, 2000.

25. Strassburg MA, Greenland S, Sorvillo FJ, et al: Influenza in the elderly: report of an outbreak and a review of vaccine effectiveness reports. *Vaccine* 4:38–44, 1986.

26. Meiklejohn G, Hall H: Unusual outbreak of influenza A in a Wyoming nursing home. *J Am Geriatr Soc* 35:742–746, 1987.

27. Goodman RA, Orenstein WA, Munro TF, et al: Impact of influenza A in a nursing home. *JAMA* 247:1451–1453, 1982.

28. Centers for Disease Control and Prevention: Prevention and control of influenza: recommendations of the Advisory Committee on Immunization Practices (ACIP). *MMWR* 46(RR-9):1–26, 1997.

29. Barker WH: Excess pneumonia and influenza associated hospitalization during influenza epidemics in the United States, 1970–78. *Am J Public Health* 76:761–765, 1986.

30. Williams WW, Hickson MA, Kane MA, et al: Immunization policies and vaccine coverage among adults. The risk for missed opportunities. *Ann Intern Med* 108:616–625, 1988.

31. Chapman LE, Tipple MA, Folger SG, et al: Influenza—United States, 1988–89. *MMWR* 42:9–22, 1993.

32. Kent JH, Chapman LE, Schmeltz LM, et al: Influenza surveillance—United States, 1991–92. *MMWR* 41:35–43, 1992.

33. Centers for Disease Control and Prevention: Prevention and control of influenza: recommendations of the Advisory Committee on Immunization Practices (ACIP). *MMWR* 49(RR-3):1–38, 2000.

34. Neuzil KM, Reed GW, Mitchel EF, et al: Impact of influenza on acute cardiopulmonary hospitalizations in pregnant women. *Am J Epidemiol* 148:1094–1102, 1998.

35. Centers for Disease Control: Suspected nosocomial influenza cases in an intensive care unit. *MMWR* 37:3–9, 1988.

36. Potter J, Stott DJ, Elder AG, et al: Influenza vaccination of health care workers in long-term care hospitals reduces the mortality of elderly patients. *J Infect Dis* 175:1–6, 1997.

37. Carman WF, Elder AG, Wallace LA, et al: Effects of influenza vaccination of health-care workers on mortality of elderly people in long-term care: a randomized controlled trial. *Lancet* 355:93–97, 2000.

38. Nichols KL, Lind A, Margolis KL, et al: The effectiveness of vaccination against influenza in

healthy, working adults. *N Engl J Med* 333:889–893, 1995.

39. Fedson DS, Wajda A, Nicol JP, et al: Clinical effectiveness of influenza vaccine in Manitoba. *JAMA* 270:1956–1961, 1993.

40. Centers for Disease Control and Prevention: Update on adult immunization: recommendations of the Immunization Practices Advisory Committee (ACIP). *MMWR* 40(RR-12):1–94, 1991.

41. Centers for Disease Control and Prevention: Recommendations of the Advisory Committee on Immunization Practices (ACIP): use of vaccines and immune globulins in persons with altered immunocompetence. *MMWR* 42(RR-4):1–18, 1993.

42. Murphy KR, Strunk RC: Safe administration of influenza vaccine in asthmatic children hypersensitive to egg proteins. *J Pediatr* 106:931–933, 1985.

43. Schonberger LB, Bregman DJ, Sullivan-Bolyai JZ, et al: Guillain-Barre syndrome following vaccination in the National Influenza Immunization Program, United States, 1976–1977. *Am J Epidemiol* 110:105–123, 1979.

44. Benenson AS: *Control of Communicable Diseases in Man*. Washington, DC, American Public Health Association; 1990.

45. Centers for Disease Control and Prevention: Recommendations for use of *Haemophilus* b conjugate vaccines and a combined diphtheria, tetanus, pertussis, and *Haemophilus* b vaccine. Recommendations of the Advisory Committee on Immunization Practices (ACIP). *MMWR* 42(RR-13):1–15, 1993.

46. Dashefsky B: Life-threatening infections. *Pediatr Emerg Care* 7:244–253, 1991.

47. Peter G: *Red Book: Report of the Committee on Infectious Diseases*. Elk Grove Village, IL, American Academy of Pediatrics; 1997.

48. Clements DA: *Haemophilus influenzae* type b, in Krugman S (ed): *Infectious Diseases of Children*. St. Louis, Mosby-Year Book; 1992: pp 127–142.

49. Centers for Disease Control and Prevention, National Immunization Program: *Epidemiology and Prevention of Vaccine-Preventable Diseases*. Atlanta, Centers for Disease Control and Prevention; 1997.

50. Senior BA, Radkowski D, MacArthur C, et al: Changing patterns in pediatric supraglottitis: a multi-institutional review, 1980–1992. *Laryngoscope* 104:1314–1322, 1994.

51. Valdepena HG, Wald ER, Rose E, et al: Epiglottitis and *Haemophilus influenzae* immunization: the Pittsburgh experience—a five-year review. *Pediatrics* 96:424–427, 1995.

52. Ward JI, Zangwill KM: *Haemophilus influenzae*, in Feigin RD (ed): *Textbook of Pediatric Infectious Diseases*. Philadelphia, WB Saunders; 1998: pp 1464–1482.

53. American Academy of Pediatrics Committee on Infectious Diseases: *Haemophilus influenzae* type b conjugate vaccines: recommendations for immunization with recently and previously licensed vaccines. *Pediatrics* 92:480–488, 1993.

54. Barbour ML, Phil D: Conjugate vaccines and the carriage of *Haemophilus influenzae* type b. *Emerging Infect Dis* 2:176–182, 1996.

55. Peltola H, Kayhty H, Virtanen M, Makela PH: Prevention of *Hemophilus influenzae* type b bacteremic infections with the capsular polysaccharide vaccine. *N Engl J Med* 310(24):1561–1566, 1984.

56. Peltola H, Kayhty H, Sivonen A, Makela H: *Haemophilus influenzae* type b capsular polysaccharide vaccine in children: a double-blind field study of 100,000 vaccinees 3 months to 5 years of age in Finland. *Pediatrics* 60(5):730–737, 1977.

57. Osterholm MT, Rambeck JH, White KE, et al: Lack of efficacy of *Haemophilus* b polysaccharide vaccine in Minnesota. *JAMA* 260:1423–1428, 1988.

58. Committee on Infectious Diseases: Report of the Committee on Infectious Diseases (Red Book). Elk Grove Village, IL, American Academy of Pediatrics; 1991.

59. Force RW, Lugo RA, Nahata MC: *Haemophilus influenzae* type B conjugate vaccines. *Ann Pharmacother* 26:1429–1440, 1992.

60. Immunization PAC: Recommendations for use of *Haemophilus* b conjugate vaccines and a combined diphtheria, tetanus, pertussis, and *Haemophilus* b vaccine. Recommendations of the Advisory Committee on Immunization Practices (ACIP). *MMWR* 42(RR-13):1–15, 1993.

61. Centers for Disease Control and Prevention: Progress toward eliminating *Haemophilus influenzae* type b disease among infants and children—United States, 1987–1997. *MMWR* 47:993–998, 1998.

62. Greenberg DP, Lieberman JM, Marcy SM, et al: Enhanced antibody responses in infants given dif-

ferent sequences of heterogeneous *Haemophilus influenzae* type b conjugate vaccines. *Pediatrics* 126:206–211, 1995.

63. Bewley KM, Schwab JG, Ballanco GA, Daum RS: Interchangeability of *Haemophilus influenzae* type b vaccines in the primary series: evaluation of a two-dose mixed regimen. *Pediatrics* 98(5): 898–904, 1996.

64. Anderson EL, Decker MD, Englund JA, et al: Interchangeability of conjugated *Haemophilus influenzae* type b vaccines in infants. *JAMA* 273:849–853, 1995.

65. Pinson JB, Weart CW: New considerations for *Haemophilus influenzae* type b vaccination. *Clin Pharm* 11:332–336, 1992.

66. Centers for Disease Control and Prevention, National Immunization Program: *Epidemiology and Prevention of Vaccine-Preventable Diseases.* Atlanta, Centers for Disease Control and Prevention; 1997.

67. Stratton KR, Howe CJ, Johnston RB Jr: *Adverse Events Associated with Childhood Vaccines: Evidence Bearing on Causality.* Washington, DC, National Academy Press; 1994.

68. Centers for Disease Control and Prevention: General recommendations on immunization: recommendations of the Advisory Committee on Immunization Practices (ACIP). *MMWR* 43(RR-1):1–38, 1994.

69. Dagan R, Eskola J, Leclerc C, Leroy O: Reduced response to multiple vaccines sharing common protein epitopes that are administered simultaneously to infants. *Infect Immun* 66:2093–2098, 1998.

70. Farizo KM, Cochi SL, Zell ER, et al:. Epidemiological features of pertussis in the United States, 1980–1989. *Clin Infect Dis* 14:708–719, 1992.

71. Centers for Disease Control and Prevention: *Epidemiology and Prevention of Vaccine-Preventable Diseases—the Pink Book.* Atlanta, Department of Health and Human Services; 1997.

72. Blennow M, Granstrom M: Long term serologic follow-up after pertussis immunization. *Pediatr Infect Dis J* 9:21–26, 1990.

73. Centers for Disease Control and Prevention: Pertussis vaccination: use of acellular pertussis vaccines among infants and young children. *MMWR* 46:1–25, 1997.

74. Greco D, Salmaso S, Mastrantonio P, et al: A controlled trial of two acellular vaccines and one

75. whole-cell vaccine against pertussis. *N Engl J Med* 334:341–348, 1996.

75. Schmitt HJ, von Konig CH, Neiss A, et al: Efficacy of acellular pertussis vaccine in early childhood after household exposure. *JAMA* 275(1):37–41, 1996.

76. Trollfors B, Taranger J, Lagergard T, et al: A placebo-controlled trial of a pertussis-toxoid vaccine. *N Engl J Med* 338:1045–1050, 1995.

77. Onorato IM, Wassilak SG, Meade B: Efficacy of whole-cell pertussis vaccine in preschool children in the United States. *JAMA* 267:2745–2749, 1992.

78. Nelson JD: The changing epidemiology of pertussis in young infants. The role of adults as reservoirs of infection. *Am J Dis Child* 132:371–373, 1978.

79. Volk VK, Gottshall RY, Anderson HD, et al: Antibody response to booster dose of diphtheria and tetanus toxoids. *Public Health Rep* 78:161–164, 1963.

80. Linnemann CC Jr, Ramundo N, Perlstein PH, et al: Use of pertussis vaccine in an epidemic involving hospital staff. *Lancet* 2:540–543, 1975.

81. Morgan CM, Blumberg DA, Cherry JD, et al: Comparison of acellular and whole-cell pertussis-component DTP vaccines. A multicenter double-blind study in 4- to 6-year-old children. *Am J Dis Child* 144:41–45, 1990.

82. Pichichero ME, Badgett JT, Rodgers GC Jr, et al: Acellular pertussis vaccine: immunogenicity and safety of an acellular pertussis vs. a whole cell pertussis vaccine combined with diphtheria and tetanus toxoids as a booster in 18- to 24-month old children. *Pediatr Infect Dis J* 6:352–363, 1987.

83. Aoyama T, Hagiwara S, Murase Y, et al: Adverse reactions and antibody responses to acellular pertussis vaccine. *J Pediatr* 109:925–930, 1986.

84. Decker MD, Edwards KM, Steinhoff MC, et al: Comparison of 13 acellular pertussis vaccines: adverse reactions. *Pediatrics* 96:557–566, 1995.

85. Centers for Disease Control and Prevention: *Epidemiology and Prevention of Vaccine-Preventable Diseases.* Atlanta, Public Health Foundation; 2000: p 1.

86. Centers for Disease Control and Prevention: Diphtheria outbreak—Russian Federation, 1990–1993. *MMWR* 42:840–847, 1993.

87. Centers for Disease Control and Prevention: Update: diphtheria epidemic—new independent

states of the former Soviet Union, January 1995–March 1996. *MMWR* 45:693, 1996.

88. Weiss BP, Strassburg MA, Feeley JC: Tetanus and diphtheria immunity in an elderly population in Los Angeles County. *Am J Public Health* 73:802–804, 1983.

89. Crossley K, Irvine P, Warren JB, et al: Tetanus and diphtheria immunity in urban Minnesota adults. *JAMA* 242:2298–2300, 1979.

90. Ruben FL, Nagel J, Fireman P: Antitoxin responses in the elderly to tetanus-diphtheria (TD) immunization. *Am J Epidemiol* 108:145–149, 1978.

91. Centers for Disease Control and Prevention: Diphtheria, tetanus, and pertussis: recommendations for vaccine use and other preventive measures: recommendations of the Immunization Practices Advisory Committee (ACIP). *MMWR* 40:1–28, 1991.

92. American Academy of Family Physicians: *Summary of Policy Recommendations for Periodic Health Examination*. AAFP Policy Action, November 1996, pp 2–14.

93. American College of Physicians Task Force on Adult Immunization, Infectious Diseases Society of America: *Guide for Adult Immunization*. Philadelphia, American College of Physicians; 1994.

94. U.S. Preventive Services Task Force: *Guide to Clinical Preventive Services*. Baltimore, Williams & Wilkins; 1996.

95. Markowitz LE, Katz SL: Measles vaccine, in Plotkin SA (ed): *Vaccines*. Philadelphia, WB Saunders; 1994: pp 229–276.

96. LeBaron CW, Birkhead GS, Parsons P, et al: Measles vaccination levels of children enrolled in WIC during the 1991 measles epidemic in New York City. *Am J Public Health* 86:1551–1556, 1996.

97. Markowitz LE, Preblud SR, Orenstein WA, et al: Patterns of transmission in measles outbreaks in the United States, 1985–1986. *N Engl J Med* 320:75–81, 1989.

98. Immunization PAC: Measles prevention. Recommendations of the Immunization Practices Advisory Committee (ACIP). *MMWR* 38(suppl 9): 1–18, 1989.

99. Anders J, Jacobson R, Poland G, et al: Secondary failure rates of measles vaccine: a metaanalysis of published studies. *Pediatr Infect Dis J* 15:62–66, 1996.

100. Centers for Disease Control and Prevention: Measles, mumps, and rubella—vaccine use and strategies for elimination of measles, rubella and congenital rubella syndrome and control of mumps: recommendations of the Advisory Committee on Immunization Practices (ACIP). *MMWR* 47(RR-8):1–57, 1998.

101. Krober MS, Stracener CE, Bass JW: Decreased measles antibody response after measles-mumps-rubella vaccine in infants with colds. *JAMA* 265:2095–2096, 1991.

102. Ratnam S, West R, Gadag V: Measles and rubella antibody response after measles-mumps-rubella vaccination in children with afebrile upper respiratory tract infection. *J Pediatr* 127:432–434, 1995.

103. King GE, Markowitz LE, Heath J, et al: Antibody response to measles-mumps-rubella vaccine of children with mild illness during the time of vaccination. *JAMA* 275:704–707, 1996.

104. Edmonson MB, Davis JP, Hopfensperger DJ, et al: Measles vaccination during the respiratory virus season and risk of vaccine failure. *Pediatrics* 98(5):905–910, 1996.

105. Centers for Disease Control and Prevention: Prevention of varicella: updated recommendations of the Advisory Committee on Immunization Practices (ACIP). *MMWR* 48(RR-6):1–5, 1999.

106. Taylor JA, Darden PM, Slora E, et al: The influence of provider behavior, parental characteristics, and a public policy initiative on the immunization status of children followed by private pediatricians: a study from pediatric research in office settings. *Pediatrics* 99:209–215, 1997.

107. Zimmerman RK, Bradford BJ, Janosky JE, et al: Barriers to measles and pertussis immunization: the knowledge and attitudes of Pennsylvania primary care physicians. *Am J Prev Med* 13:89–97, 1997.

108. Zimmerman RK, Schlesselman JJ, Baird AL, Mieczkowski TA: A national survey to understand why physicians limit childhood immunizations. *Arch Pediatr Adolesc Med* 151:657–664, 1997.

109. Centers for Disease Control and Prevention: Prevention of varicella: recommendations of the Advisory Committee on Immunization Practices (ACIP). *MMWR* 45(RR-11):1–36, 1996.

Robert Mallin

Smoking Cessation

Smoking is the leading cause of preventable death in the United States. More than 400,000 smokers die in the United States every year from smoking-related diseases, accounting for 26 percent of all deaths in men and 17 percent of deaths in women.[1] In addition to those deaths that are directly attributable to smoking, more than 20,000 more people die from asthma, pneumonia, influenza, and other respiratory causes indirectly attributed to smoking.[2] Chronic obstructive pulmonary disease (COPD) alone results in over 60,000 deaths yearly, and between 79 and 85 percent of these deaths are directly attributable to smoking.[3] Smoking is responsible for the majority of the more than 150,000 deaths from lung cancer.[4] Smoking is also a major cause of death due to cardiovascular disease and contributes to several other nonrespiratory malignancies.

Smokers also have more respiratory infections than nonsmokers and respond less favorably to treatment of these infections. Smokers' mortality from pneumonia and influenza is higher than that of nonsmokers.[5] The higher mortality rate and greater morbidity from infections is thought to be related to several factors. Cigarette smoking impairs the immune system and predisposes smokers to infection in a variety of ways (Table 20-1). In addition to immune system damage, there is damage to pulmonary function.

Table 20-1

Impact of Smoking on Immune System

Higher leukocyte count
Higher levels of C5, C9, and C1 inhibitor
Lower levels of IgG, IgM, and IgA
Elevated levels of IgE
Poor response to influenza vaccination
Decreased phagocytosis and intracellular killing
Decreased migration of macrophages
Decreased antibody production

Smoking causes long-term damage to the pulmonary mucociliary system, which impairs the clearance of mucus, contributing to the development of chronic bronchitis.

Patients who quit smoking have fewer respiratory infections than continuing smokers. After 1 month without cigarettes, respiratory symptoms of cough, sputum production, and wheezing improve. Age-adjusted mortality rates for former smokers with respiratory infections approach those of people who never smoked over a period of 10 to 15 years for men and 3 to 5 years for women.[2]

Although there has been a reduction from the over 40 percent prevalence of smoking in 1965, 23.5 percent of adults continue to smoke and the rate of smoking among teenagers and young adults is increasing.[6] Despite the increase in research on smoking, increased awareness of its consequences, and considerable publicity regarding tobacco company litigation, a third of all young adults (ages 18 to 24 years) smoke tobacco. This represents a 32 percent increase in smoking rates between 1991 and 1997.[7]

Some 70 percent of individuals who smoke say that they would like to quit.[8] Without help from their health care provider, however, only 8 percent are able to quit. The advice of a physician improves the quit rate to 10 percent.[9] The addition of nicotine replacement and bupropion in the context of social or behavioral support increases the quit rate to as much as 35 percent.

Treatment for smoking is effective and should be offered at every visit to patients who smoke. Since patients are especially receptive to a smoking cessation message from their physician during an illness episode, the primary care physician treating a respiratory infection in a smoker has a golden opportunity to be heard during that visit. What follows in this chapter is a practical approach to the patient who smokes that will increase the likelihood of the patient's quitting.

Identification and Assessment

Awareness that a patient is a smoker is the most important first step in being able to help the patient break his or her tobacco dependence. Simply providing clinicians with the smoking status of a patient increases the rate of intervention for smoking threefold.[10] One method for identifying smokers is to include the patient's smoking status in the vital signs section of the medical record. A check mark to indicate smoking status will alert the clinician to the patient who smokes.

Assessing the Level of Drug Dependence

More detailed information about nicotine dependence in smokers can be gathered through the administration of other instruments. The Fagerström test for nicotine dependence (Table 20-2) or the CAGE questionnaire for smoking (Table 20-3) will give the clinician further information about the patient's degree of physical dependence on or addiction to nicotine.[11] The Fagerström test allows clinicians to gauge the level of physical dependence on nicotine and can be used to help select the most appropriate dose when nicotine replacement therapy is prescribed. The CAGE questionnaire for smoking is less quantitative than the Fagerström test, but it can serve as a clue to nicotine addiction. As with the CAGE questionnaire for alcohol, two positive responses on the smoking CAGE are highly correlated with nicotine dependence or addiction.

Assessing the Patient's Readiness to Change

Once the diagnosis of nicotine dependence is made, the next step is to assess the patient's readiness to change and quit smoking. The

Table 20-2
Brief Fagerström Test

> ***How soon after waking do you smoke your first cigarette?***
>   < 5 minutes = 3 points
>   5–30 minutes = 2 points
>   31–60 minutes = 1 point
> ***How many cigarettes do you smoke each day?***
>   > 30 cigarettes = 3 points
>   21–30 cigarettes = 2 points
>   11–20 cigarettes = 1 point
> ***Scoring***
>   5–6 = heavy nicotine dependence
>   3–4 = moderate nicotine dependence
>   0–2 = light nicotine dependence

SOURCE: Rustin TA: Nicotine, in Deluca AF, David J, Hersey B, Rottenstein M (eds): *ASAM's Review Course in Addiction Medicine.* Chevy Chase, MD, American Society of Addiction Medicine; 1998, with permission.

Table 20-3
CAGE Questionnaire for Smoking

> 1. Have you ever tried to or felt the need to Cut down on your smoking?
> 2. Do you ever get Annoyed when people tell you to quit smoking?
> 3. Do you ever feel Guilty about smoking?
> 4. Do you ever smoke within a half-hour of waking? (Eye-opener)

SOURCE: Modified from Lairson DR, Harrist R, Martin DW, et al: Screening patients with alcohol problems: severity of patients identified by the CAGE. *J Drug Educ* 22:337–352, 1992, with permission.

Transtheoretical Model developed by Prochaska and DiClemente[12] has been useful in helping to gain an understanding of the processes through which individuals proceed as they make major changes in their life. Prochaska and DiClemente have identified five stages associated with a patient's readiness to change.

Precontemplation represents the first stage, in which the patient does not believe that he or she has a problem with smoking or refuses to consider stopping tobacco use. Intensive counseling or prescribing nicotine replacement at this stage is unlikely to result in success. However, if clinicians bring up the issue of smoking during this stage, it may be useful in moving patients into the next stage at some point in time.

The second stage, called the *contemplation stage*, represents a point at which patients recognize that smoking is a problem and decide that they want to stop. At this point in time, smoking cessation suggestions by the clinician will be met with more interest, and the patient is likely to ask more detailed questions about methods available to help stop smoking. However, this is still a preliminary stage; the patient is not yet ready to take action.

In the next stage, the *preparation* stage, the patient may make specific plans to stop smoking, such as setting a stop date and deciding upon a method to help with smoking cessation.

The *action* stage follows, in which the patient actually stops smoking. Finally comes the *maintenance* stage, in which the individual continues to abstain from smoking. Frequently patients will cycle through the first four stages several times before reaching maintenance and stable abstinence.[12]

Motivational Interviewing

To select the most appropriate intervention for a given patient, it is important for the clinician to ascertain the patient's stage of change. Therapy can then be matched to what will be most effective for the patient given the current stage. For example, offering a patient in the precontemplation stage a prescription for nicotine replacement is unlikely to be successful because the patient is not considering quitting. This amounts to asking the patient to move from precontemplation to action without taking the necessary steps in between. Rather than trying to move the patient along so quickly, it would be more appropriate

to make suggestions that might help move the patient to the next stage, contemplation. So for this patient, instead of talking about the success rates with various nicotine replacement products, the clinician's goal should be to help the patient to think about his or her smoking and consider the possibility that there is a problem that needs attention. Thus the goal is to take the patient to the next stage of change rather than to get the patient to quit on the first visit.

Brief Interventions

Brief interventions have components that should be addressed as the patient moves from one stage of change to the next. These include (1) educating the patient about the effects of smoking, (2) recommending changes in behavior, (3) providing a list of options to achieve behavioral change, (4) discussing the patient's reactions to providers' feedback and recommendations, and (5) following up to monitor and reinforce behavioral change.[13] This process is known as motivational interviewing or enhancement. It uses empathy rather than confrontation as the primary factor in effecting change. It acknowledges that it is the patient and not the physician who is responsible for changing behavior.[14]

The first step in this process is to inquire about smoking status and assess the individual's readiness to quit. If the patient at first does not appear ready to stop smoking, discussion can be postponed to the next visit. On a subsequent visit, a discussion of a list of pros and cons may reveal that the patient now agrees that smoking is a problem and would like to consider quitting. When this occurs, the patient moves into the contemplation stage. Options to consider at this stage include further education about the effects of smoking and encouragement to consider the positive aspects of not smoking, such as reduced cost, improved health, and positive self-image.

Once the patient agrees that the benefits of not smoking outweigh the pleasure derived from smoking and acknowledges wanting to quit, the patient has entered the preparation stage. At this point, options include discussion of the various nicotine replacement systems, the use of bupropion, and the need for social and family support. In addition, a clear plan should be developed, including a quit date, a plan to avoid triggers, and a plan for follow-up care. Tasks for the patient and physician during preparation include setting a quit date, getting support, preparing the environment, and making recommendations for nicotine replacement and the use of bupropion.

Encouraging the patient in the preparation stage to set a definite quit date is important. Often a meaningful date such as a birthday or anniversary provides the patient with increased motivation. Once the date is set, a plan should be constructed. This should include gathering support from family and others who are important in the patient's life. Instruct patients to tell those around them of their decision to quit smoking and the date, and suggest that they ask for support. Use of a support group or a program in the community can be helpful. Preparation of the environment should include removing all cigarettes, ashtrays, and other smoking paraphernalia from the patient's home, car, and office. Requesting that the patient ask others not to smoke in the patient's presence is another important feature of preparation. Counseling patients to avoid alcohol is a good strategy as well, since drinking lowers the chance of success.

The action stage begins on the quit date. In preparation, the patient should have begun bupropion, acquired the nicotine replacement of choice, and removed tobacco and related paraphernalia from the home. During the action phase, behavioral support through self-help or professionally run group meetings, frequent office visits, or telephone calls from support personnel can be effective in enhancing the effectiveness of the cessation attempt.[15]

The purpose of these contacts should be to support abstinence in the recently abstinent smoker. Asking the patient to report any per-

ceived benefits from having stopped, any side effects from medications, and any current or anticipated difficulty in maintaining abstinence is important. These contacts should be made at least weekly in the first month after stopping cigarette use and again when stopping nicotine replacement or bupropion.

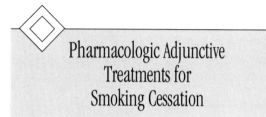

Pharmacologic Adjunctive Treatments for Smoking Cessation

Nicotine Replacement

Nicotine replacement therapy doubles the cessation rate regardless of the delivery system used.[16] Currently there are four delivery systems for nicotine replacement: nicotine gum, patch, nasal spray, and inhaler. There are some data that indicate that in heavily dependent smokers, combining multiple delivery methods, such as the gum and patch, may be more effective than a single method alone.[17] To determine the appropriate dose of the nicotine patch to use, the Fagerström score can be used (Table 20-4).[18]

Adverse reactions to the transdermal nicotine systems are not often a cause for discontinuation

Table 20-4

Nicotine Replacement Dose

Brief Fagerström Score	Nicotine Patch Strength
5–6	21-mg patch
3–4	14-mg patch
0–2	7-mg patch

Source: Rustin TA: Nicotine, in Deluca AF, David J, Hersey B, Rottenstein M (eds): *ASAM's Review Course in Addiction Medicine.* Chevy Chase, MD, American Society of Addiction Medicine; 1998, with permission.

of therapy. Mild skin irritation under the patch may be noticed by 30 to 50 percent of patients and is generally easily dealt with by rotation of the patch sites. Sleep disruption is usually resolved by removing the patch at bedtime. Smoking while using the patch is discouraged. In addition to the discomfort of the higher nicotine levels that occur with concomitant smoking and patch use, combining the two delivery forms raises the chances for relapse to virtually 100 percent. Concerns about sudden cardiac death when smoking with the patch have been allayed by two clinical trials of smokers with heart disease that showed no increase in rates of morbidity or mortality associated with the use of the patch.[19] The appropriate duration of use of nicotine patches is 8 to 12 weeks, with tapering to the next lower dose after an initial 4- to 6-week period.

Nicotine gum is available as nicotine pola-crilex in 2-mg and 4-mg strengths. The gum is most effective at the 4-mg dose, using 10 to 15 pieces a day initially. This initial dose can usually be reduced 50 percent after the first 2 weeks. The most important side effect of using the gum appears to be gastrointestinal upset associated with swallowing large amounts of nicotine when the gum is improperly used. The gum is intended to be "parked" in the buccal area and chewed once or twice every few minutes. If the gum is chewed too quickly, nicotine is ingested with saliva, and nausea or dyspepsia can result.

Nicotine in the form of an inhaler has recently become available. Currently four inhalers a day are considered necessary to result in adequate nicotine levels. This requires frequent dosing, as each inhaler contains five hundred puffs. Side effects include mouth and throat irritation.

Nicotine nasal spray is also available to deliver nicotine. Five sprays per hour up to a maximum of 40 per day is the recommended level. Nasal and throat irritation, rhinorrhea, and nausea are common side effects.

Since all of the nicotine replacement systems appear to be efficacious, decisions regarding which is the most appropriate are usually guided by patient preference. For example, patients who find that they need to be doing something with their hands may prefer the nicotine inhaler rather than the patch.

Bupropion

Bupropion, developed as an antidepressant, is believed to reduce the craving for smoking by its effect on the norepinephrine and dopamine neurotransmitter systems. Bupropion has been shown to enhance quit rates to levels similar to or higher than those that can be achieved with nicotine replacement. Jorenby and colleagues found that bupropion treatment resulted in abstinence rates at 12 months of 30 percent, compared with 16 percent with nicotine therapy alone. Combination therapy of bupropion plus nicotine replacement resulted in even higher quit rates, 36 percent at 12 months.[20]

Bupropion should be begun initially at 150 mg daily for 3 days, then increased to 150 mg twice a day. A quit date should be set to coincide with the end of 2 weeks of bupropion therapy. Bupropion is usually continued at 150 mg twice daily for the next 8 to 12 weeks. A history of seizure disorder, eating disorders, or uncontrolled hypertension is a contraindication to bupropion. The most common side effects include a dry mouth and sleep disturbance.

Other Drugs

Many pharmaceutical agents to alleviate the symptoms of nicotine withdrawal have been tried. Silver acetate tablets have been used for many years as smoking cessation aids. Their use gives cigarettes an unpleasant taste. There is no support in the medical literature for using silver acetate as an effective adjunct for smoking cessation.

Alprazolam and other benzodiazepines have been used to reduce the anxiety associated with nicotine withdrawal. However, these have not proved effective in the improvement of smoking cessation rates.

Clonidine initially appeared to be useful in the treatment of nicotine withdrawal. However, long-term quit rates are not improved when clonidine is used alone.[16]

In summary, of the pharmacologic recommendations for treatment of nicotine dependence, it would appear that combination therapy with nicotine replacement and bupropion is the most effective. A summary of available medications is provided in Table 20-5. Bupropion should be started 2 weeks prior to the quit date, and nicotine replacement should be added on the quit date. The use of the Fagerström test will help in the initial dosing of nicotine, but careful monitoring and creative use of delivery systems may be necessary in some smokers.

Dealing with Relapse

Relapse is an expected event in the treatment of addiction. Most patients will relapse within the first 6 to 12 months of a smoking cessation attempt. This reality should be reflected in the physician's approach to the patient who resumes smoking. Encouragement, followed by an attempt to find out what worked and what did not work in the treatment plan, is a useful approach.

Often patients will not return immediately after a relapse and may smoke for months prior to another visit. At that point, reevaluation of their readiness for change is necessary, and the entire process may need to be restarted right from the precontemplation stage.

Conclusion

Nicotine dependence is a tenacious and difficult addiction to treat successfully. Perseverance on the part of both patient and practitioner is most effective in achieving permanent abstinence. The use of nicotine replacement and bupropion dramatically improves results, and the application of readiness to change strategies as well as motivational interviewing techniques is essential for success.

Table 20-5

Effective Pharmacotherapy for Nicotine Withdrawal

Drug/Delivery	Initial Dose	Maintenance Dose	Duration of Therapy	Approximate Cost/Month
Nicotine				
Gum 4 mg	10–15 pieces/day 21, 14, 7 mg	5–8 pieces/day	8 weeks–5 years	$90
Patch	See Table 20-4	Taper to next lowest dose in 4–6 weeks	8–12 weeks	$115
Inhaler	4 inhalers per day	4/day taper	8–12 weeks	$120
Nasal spray	5 sprays per hour	8–80 sprays per day	8–12 weeks	$100
Bupropion	150 mg QD × 3	150 mg BID	7–12 weeks	$90

References

1. Emmons KM: Smoking cessation and tobacco control: an overview. *Chest* 116:490–492, 1999.
2. Fiore MC, Piasecki TM, Baker LJ, Deeren SM: Cigarette smoking: the leading preventable cause of pulmonary disease, in Bone RC (ed): *Pulmonary and Critical Care Medicine*. St Louis, Mosby-Year Book; 1998.
3. Public Health Service: *Reducing the Health Consequences of Smoking: 25 Years of Progress—A Report of the Surgeon General*. Rockville, MD, U.S. Department of Health and Human Services, Public Health Service, DHHS Publication No (CDC) 89–8411, 1989.
4. Filderman AE, Matthay RA: Bronchogenic carcinoma, in Bone RC (ed): *Pulmonary and Critical Care Medicine*. St Louis, Mosby-Year Book; 1998.
5. Rogot E, Murray JL: Smoking and causes of death among U.S. veterans: 16 years of observation. *Public Health Rep* 95:213–222, 1980.
6. Centers for Disease Control and Prevention: State-specific prevalence of cigarette smoking among adults and children's and adolescent's exposure to environmental tobacco smoke—United States. *MMWR* 46(44):1038–1043, 1997.
7. Rigotti NA, Lee JE, Weschler H: US college students' use of tobacco products. *JAMA* 284:699–705, 2000.
8. Centers for Disease Control and Prevention: Cigarette smoking among adults: United States. *MMWR* 42(12):230–233, 1993.
9. Jorenby DE, Fiore MC: The Agency for Health Care Policy and Research smoking cessation clinical practice guideline. Basics and beyond. *Prim Care* 26:513–528, 1999.
10. Fiore MC, Bailey WC, Cohen SJ: *Smoking Cessation*. Clinical Practice Guideline No. 18. Rockville MD, U.S. Department of Health and Human Services, Public Health Service, Agency for Health Care Policy and Research. AHCPR Publication No. 96-0692, 1996.
11. Rustin TA: Assessing nicotine dependence. *Am Fam Physician* 62:579–584, 591–592, 2000.
12. Prochaska JO, DiClemente CC, Norcross JC: In search of how people change. Applications to addictive behaviors. *Am Psychol* 47:1102–1114, 1992.
13. Barnes HN, Samet JH: Brief interventions with substance-abusing patients. *Med Clin North Am* 81:867–879, 1997.
14. Miller WR, Rollnick S: *Motivational Interviewing*. New York, Guilford Press; 1991.
15. Fiore MC, Novotny TE, Pierce JP, et al: Methods used to quit smoking in the United States: do cessation programs help? *JAMA* 263:2760–2765, 1990.
16. Prochaska AV: New developments in smoking cessation. *Chest* 117:4, 2000.
17. Kornitzer M, Bousten M, Drammaix M, et al: Combined use of nicotine patch and gum in smoking cessation: a placebo-controlled clinical trial. *Prev Med* 24:41–47, 1993.
18. Heartherton TF, Kozlowski LT, Frecker RC, Fagerström KO: The Fagerström test for nicotine dependence: a revision of the Fagerström tolerance questionnaire. *Br J Addict* 86:1119–1127, 1991.
19. Gourlay SG, Forbes A, Martiner T, et al: Prospective study of factors predicting the outcome of transdermal nicotine treatment in smoking cessation. *Br Med J* 304:842–846, 1994.
20. Jorenby DE, Leischow SJ, Nides MA, et al: A controlled trial of sustained-release bupropion, a nicotine patch, or both for smoking cessation. *N Engl J Med* 340:685–691, 1999.

Index

Note: Page numbers followed by f indicate figures; those followed by t indicate tables.